Neurosurgical infectious
disease

# Neurosurgical Infectious Disease
## Surgical and Nonsurgical Management

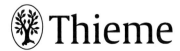

# Neurosurgical Infectious Disease
## Surgical and Nonsurgical Management

**Walter A. Hall, MD, MBA**
Professor of Neurosurgery
Department of Neurological Surgery
SUNY Upstate Medical University
Syracuse, New York

**Peter D. Kim, MD, PhD**
Neurosurgeon
Department of Neurosurgery
Gillette Children's Specialty Healthcare
St. Paul, Minnesota

Thieme
New York · Stuttgart

Thieme Medical Publishers, Inc.
333 Seventh Ave.
New York, NY 10001

Executive Editor: Kay Conerly
Managing Editor: Judith Tomat
Editorial Assistant: Lorina Lana
Senior Vice President, Editorial and Electronic Product Development: Cornelia Schulze
Production Editor: Kenneth L. Chumbley
International Production Director: Andreas Schabert
Vice President, Finance and Accounts: Sarah Vanderbilt
President: Brian D. Scanlan
Compositor: Prairie Papers Inc.
Printer: Everbest Printing Co.

**Library of Congress Cataloging-in-Publication Data**

Neurosurgical infectious disease : surgical and nonsurgical management / [edited by] Walter A. Hall, Peter D. Kim.
    p. ; cm.
 Includes bibliographical references.
 ISBN 978-1-60406-805-4 (alk. paper)—ISBN 978-1-60406-821-4 (eISBN)
 I. Hall, Walter A., 1957- II. Kim, Peter D.
 [DNLM: 1. Central Nervous System Infections—therapy. 2. Anti-Infective Agents—therapeutic use. 3. Central Nervous System Infections—diagnosis. 4. Communicable Diseases—therapy. WL 301]
 RC386.5
 616.8′3—dc23

2013003829

**Important note:** Medical knowledge is ever-changing. As new research and clinical experience broaden our knowledge, changes in treatment and drug therapy may be required. The authors and editors of the material herein have consulted sources believed to be reliable in their efforts to provide information that is complete and in accord with the standards accepted at the time of publication. However, in view of the possibility of human error by the authors, editors, or publisher of the work herein or changes in medical knowledge, neither the authors, editors, nor publisher, nor any other party who has been involved in the preparation of this work, warrants that the information contained herein is in every respect accurate or complete, and they are not responsible for any errors or omissions or for the results obtained from use of such information. Readers are encouraged to confirm the information contained herein with other sources. For example, readers are advised to check the product information sheet included in the package of each drug they plan to administer to be certain that the information contained in this publication is accurate and that changes have not been made in the recommended dose or in the contraindications for administration. This recommendation is of particular importance in connection with new or infrequently used drugs.

Some of the product names, patents, and registered designs referred to in this book are in fact registered trademarks or proprietary names even though specific reference to this fact is not always made in the text. Therefore, the appearance of a name without designation as proprietary is not to be construed as a representation by the publisher that it is in the public domain.

Printed in China

5 4 3 2 1

ISBN 978-1-60406-805-4

Also available as an e-book:
eISBN 978-1-60404-821-4

This book is dedicated to Madeleine and Stanley Smalley for their unwavering support, encouragement, and love over three decades.

*Walter A. Hall*


This book is dedicated, with love and gratitude, to my parents, Kenneth and Susan Kim.

*Peter D. Kim*

# Contents

Contents

# Foreword

This book of nineteen chapters, edited by Drs. Walter A. Hall and Peter D. Kim, is a comprehensive exposition of the major aspects of common and rare central nervous system (CNS) infections in neurosurgical patients, their diagnosis, and surgical and nonsurgical management.

It is characterized by a finely tuned balance between basic information and scholarly documentation of the entities described. Chapters 1 and 2, on the Immunology of the CNS and Microbiological Diagnosis of CNS Infections, are of special interest. These are unique examples because of the fine details that are provided and their applications to patient management. The bibliography in each chapter is up to date and documents the newest developments in the diagnosis of common and more unusual infectious agents and the complication(s) that may occur.

Chapter 9, on meningeal infections, presents the most common pathogens for acute bacterial meningitis by age group, the recommended empirical therapy, and provides helpful epidemiological information on these infections. A chapter focusing on the pediatric patient population and infections of the CNS is especially welcome, with its discussion and management of cerebrospinal fluid ventricular shunt infections. The imaging scans presented are of excellent resolution both here and in other chapters, for example, Chapter 8 on brain abscesses. The details on complications, sequelae, and prognosis are very complete.

In summary, this book should be of interest to many different professionals: medical students, graduate health professional students, medical and surgical residents, neurosurgical residents, pediatricians, internists, neurosurgeons, and consultants in adult/pediatric neurology and infectious diseases.

Patricia Ferrieri, MD
*Professor*
*Chairman's Fund Endowed Chair in*
*Laboratory Medicine and Pathology*
*Professor*
*Department of Pediatrics,*
*Division of Infectious Diseases*
*University of Minnesota Medical School*
*Minneapolis, Minnesota*
*Director, Clinical Microbiology Laboratory*
*University of Minnesota Medical Center,*
*Fairview*
*Fairview, Minnesota*

# Preface

Infections involving the central nervous system (CNS) can cause significant neurological morbidity and mortality. Evolving threats such as insect-borne encephalitides make news headlines, while familiar diseases such as bacterial meningitis and postoperative infection continue to burden society with significant morbidity. The clinical outcome in these patients with CNS infection is often related to the speed with which the diagnosis is made and appropriate surgical and medical management is initiated. Expeditious identification of an infectious process is now possible through enhanced radiological screening through magnetic resonance imaging, while advanced microbiological techniques, such as the polymerase chain reaction, allow for earlier identification of the responsible infectious agents. All the while, an ever expanding arsenal of antimicrobial agents exists in tenuous balance with the rapid spread of resistant bacterial strains. All of these advancements are discussed in this compilation, making it an appropriate resource for medical students, residents, internists, microbiologists, neurologists, neurosurgeons, and infectious disease specialists.

In order to inform the medical community of the advances in the treatment of these once dreaded infections, this work was conceived due to the last in-depth coverage of this topic being introduced more than a decade ago. The format of the material presented is categorized into five sections that include background information, such as immunology of the CNS, microbiological diagnosis of CNS infection, antibiotic resistance, and imaging of CNS infections. The second section identifies specific etiological agents that result in infection, including viruses, fungi, parasites, and bacteria. The various anatomical locations (meninges, epidural and subdural spaces, intracranial vasculature, vertebral column, and the spinal canal) where CNS infections are manifest are addressed in the third section. Distinctly neurosurgical issues, such as antibiotic prophylaxis, postoperative intracranial infection, and the infection of implanted devices, constitute the fourth section. Unique patient populations are discussed in the fifth and last section and include pediatric patients, immunocompromised hosts, and those that experience systemic infection while in the neurocritical care unit.

Having been involved in the formulation of two previous texts on this extremely important topic, the senior author (WAH) felt compelled to update the current level of knowledge of the surgical and nonsurgical management of these disease entities by recruiting an array of expects with a global depth to share their cumulative experience and insight with the reading audience.

Walter A. Hall
*Syracuse, New York*

Peter D. Kim
*St. Paul, Minnesota*

# Contributors

**Ali Akhaddar, MD**
Full Professor of Neurosurgery
Department of Neurosurgery
Mohammed V Military Teaching Hospital
Mohammed V Souissi University–Hay Riyad
Rabat, Morocco

**Christopher D. Baggott, MD**
Resident
Department of Neurological Surgery
University of Wisconsin School of
    Medicine and Public Health
Madison, Wisconsin

**Mohamed Boucetta, MD**
Full Professor of Neurosurgery
Department of Neurosurgery
Mohammed V Military Teaching Hospital
Mohammed V Souissi University–Hay Riyad
Rabat, Morocco

**Karin Byers, MD, MS**
Clinical Director
Division of Infectious Diseases
University of Pittsburgh Medical Center
Pittsburgh, Pennsylvania

**Hoon Choi, MD**
Resident
Department of Neurosurgery
SUNY Upstate Medical University
Syracuse, New York

**Zvi R. Cohen, MD**
Staff Neurosurgeon
Chaim Sheba Medical Center
Tel Hashomer, Israel
Lecturer
The Sackler School of Medicine
Tel Aviv, Israel

**Eric M. Deshaies, MD**
Director
SUNY Upstate Neurovascular Center
Assistant Professor of Neurosurgery
Assistant Professor of Neuroscience and
    Physiology
Department of Neurosurgery
SUNY Upstate Medical University
Syracuse, New York

**Joseph B. Domachowske, MD**
Professor of Pediatrics, Microbiology, and
    Immunology
Department of Pediatrics
SUNY Upstate Medical University
Syracuse, New York

**Barry C. Fox, MD**
Clinical Professor of Medicine
Division of Infectious Diseases
University of Wisconsin Hospital and
    Clinics
Madison, Wisconsin

**Yuriko Fukuta, MD**
Infectious Diseases and Internal Medicine
Wheeling Clinic
Wheeling, West Virginia

**Ramesh Grandhi, MD**
Resident
Department of Neurological Surgery
University of Pittsburgh School of Medicine
Pittsburgh, Pennsylvania

**Gahl Greenberg, MD**
Staff Neurosurgeon
Department of Neurosurgery
Chaim Sheba Medical Center
Tel Hashomer, Israel

**Stephen J. Haines, MD**
Lyle A. French Chair
Professor and Head
Department of Neurosurgery
University of Minnesota
Minneapolis, Minnesota

**Walter A. Hall, MD, MBA**
Professor of Neurosurgery
Department of Neurological Surgery
SUNY Upstate Medical University
Syracuse, New York

**Gillian Harrison, BS**
Medical Student
University of Pittsburgh School of Medicine
Pittsburgh, Pennsylvania

**Daraspreet Singh Kainth, MD**
Resident
Department of Neurosurgery
University of Minnesota
Minneapolis, Minnesota

**Peter D. Kim, MD, PhD**
Neurosurgeon
Department of Neurosurgery
Gillette Children's Specialty Healthcare
St. Paul, Minnesota

**Frederike Knerlich-Lukoschus, MD**
Clinic of Neurosurgery
University Medical Center
  Schleswig-Holstein–Kiel
Kiel, Germany

**Sandi Lam, MD, MBA**
Assistant Professor
Section of Neurosurgery
Department of Surgery
University of Chicago
Chicago, Illinois

**Maciej S. Lesniak, MD, MHCM, FACS**
Professor of Neurosurgery, Neurology, and
  Cancer Biology
Director
Neurosurgical Oncology and the
  Neuro-Oncology Research Laboratories
University of Chicago
Chicago, Illinois

**Ian E. McCutcheon, MD**
Professor
Department of Neurosurgery
The University of Texas M. D. Anderson
  Cancer Center
Houston, Texas

**Joshua E. Medow, MD, MS, FAANS**
Endovascular Neurosurgeon and
  Neurointensivist
Director of Neurocritical Care
Assistant Professor of Neurosurgery and
  Biomedical Engineering
University of Wisconsin School of
  Medicine and Public Health
Madison, Wisconsin

**Thomas M. Moriarty, MD, PhD**
Chief
Department of Pediatric Neurosurgery
Kosair Children's Hospital
Norton Neuroscience Institute
Louisville, Kentucky

**Ian Mutchnick, MD, MS**
Attending Physician
Department of Pediatric Neurosurgery
Kosair Children's Hospital
Norton Neuroscience Institute
Louisville, Kentucky

**Arya Nabavi, MD, PhD, MaHM**
Professor of Neurosurgery
Vice Chairman
Department of Neurosurgery
University Medical Center
 Schleswig-Holstein–Kiel
Kiel, Germany

**Pragati Nigam, PhD**
Postdoctoral Fellow
The Brain Tumor Center
University of Chicago
Chicago, Illinois

**Ouzi Nissim, MD**
Staff Neurosurgeon
Department of Neurosurgery
Chaim Sheba Medical Center
Tel Hashomer, Israel

**Kunal M. Patel, MD**
Neuroradiology Fellow
Department of Radiology
University of California–San Diego
San Diego, California

**Michael F. Regner, BA**
Medical Student
Department of Neurosurgery
University of Wisconsin School of
 Medicine and Public Health
Madison, Wisconsin

**Daniel K. Resnick, MD, MS**
Professor and Vice Chairman
Department of Neurosurgery
University of Wisconsin School of
 Medicine and Public Health
Madison, Wisconsin

**Roberto Spiegelmann, MD**
Head, Stereotactic Radiosurgery Unit and
 Functional Neurosurgery Service
Department of Neurosurgery
Chaim Sheba Medical Center
Senior Lecturer
The Sackler School of Medicine
Tel Aviv, Israel

**Andreas M. Stark, MD, PhD**
Professor of Neurosurgery
Department of Neurosurgery
University Medical Center
 Schleswig-Holstein–Kiel
Kiel, Germany

**Manika Suryadevara, MD**
Assistant Professor of Pediatrics
Department of Pediatrics
SUNY Upstate Medical University
Syracuse, New York

**Kyle I. Swanson, MD**
Resident
Department of Neurosurgery
University of Wisconsin School of
 Medicine and Public Health
Madison, Wisconsin

**Dino Terzic, MD**
Resident
Department of Neurosurgery
University of Minnesota
Minneapolis, Minnesota

**Charles L. Truwit, MD**
Professor and Chief of Radiology
Hennepin County Medical Center
Minneapolis, Minnesota

**Elizabeth Tyler-Kabara, MD, PhD**
Assistant Professor
Department of Neurological Surgery and
 Bioengineering
Director
Department of Pediatric Epilepsy Surgery
University of Pittsburgh Medical Center
Pittsburgh, Pennsylvania

**Peter C. Warnke, MD**
Associate Professor of Surgery
Director
Department of Stereotactic and Functional
 Neurosurgery
University of Chicago
Chicago, Illinois

# I

# Background Information

# 1

# Immunology of the Central Nervous System

**Pragati Nigam and Maciej S. Lesniak**

The brain is an organ with unique characteristics that function to restrain immunologic responses that could potentially damage tissue. In this chapter, we describe how the immune responses in the central nervous system (CNS) are modulated and regulated. We also discuss the resident immune cells in the CNS, the trafficking of lymphocytes across the blood–brain barrier (BBB), and the chemokines that function to recruit lymphocytes in the CNS microvasculature.

## ■ Immunosurveillance of the Central Nervous System

Certain organs, such as the brain, eyes, and testicles, are particularly sensitive to damage due to inflammation. Thus, these tissues have developed singular properties that limit the immunologic responses to antigenic challenge—a phenomenon that has been termed *immunologic privilege*.[1] In agreement with this hypothesis, Sir Peter Medawar observed that the brain does not reject foreign tissue grafts.[2] The rationale for the existence of the phenomenon of immunologic privilege is that activation of the immune system in these organs can be extremely deleterious to the organism. The brain is susceptible to increases in tissue volume because of limitations in space imposed by the dura mater and the cranium. Once neurons are damaged, they cannot be replaced. It is well established

that the brain and eyes harbor specialized microvasculature where events such as lymphocyte adhesion to the endothelium and the free exchange of solutes are highly regulated.[3–5] Furthermore, the CNS lacks classic antigen-presenting cells (APCs), as well as constitutive expression of major histocompatibility complex I and II (MHC I, II). Similarly, the CNS is devoid of lymphatic vessels.

Currently, it is recognized that the CNS immune privilege phenomenon is not complete, and that foreign materials implanted within the CNS can elicit an immune response, although it is delayed and tightly controlled.[6] It has also been observed that tissue grafts implanted within the CNS are eventually rejected, and delayed-type hypersensitivity reactions can occur. Pathogenic autoimmune diseases of the CNS exist as well, as demonstrated by experimental autoimmune encephalomyelitis (EAE). Thus, the CNS is more appropriately described as an immunologically specialized organ than as an immunologically privileged one.

## ■ Vascular Anatomy

The CNS microvessels are designed to perform two major tasks: (1) prevent ions and other solutes in the blood from entering the parenchyma and (2) enhance regional blood flow wherever needed. The anatomic structures consist of a series of barriers; these include the blood–cerebrospinal fluid (CSF) barrier, which prevents the free exchange of solutes between the blood and the CSF, and the BBB, which is the most prominent interface between the immune and nervous systems. The blood–CSF barrier results from the presence of the choroid plexus epithelium, in which the cells are connected by tight junctions and are responsible for secreting CSF into the brain ventricles. The BBB consists of endothelial cells of the cerebral microvasculature, pericytes, and astrocytes, which have been well characterized in terms of their morphology and biochemistry. The transcellular passage of molecules across the BBB is inhibited as a result of low pinocytotic activity. The elaborate network of tight junctions between the endothelial cells of BBB[7] limits the paracellular diffusion of hydrophilic molecules. It is also known that blood molecules are prevented from entering the parenchyma by several permanently active transportation mechanisms.[8]

The first evidence that T cells can migrate across the healthy BBB into the CNS came from animal models of neurodegenerative diseases, including multiple sclerosis and EAE. Here, it was demonstrated that autoreactive CD4+ T cells recently activated in vitro could migrate into the CNS and initiate a series of events culminating in inflammation, loss of barrier restriction, edema formation, and demyelination.[9] T cells were found to reside in the CNS perivascular spaces, allowing encounter with antigen presented by MHC class II–positive perivascular macrophages.[10] T cells in the resting state were unable to migrate across the BBB and could not transfer the disease. This indicated an active role for the BBB in regulating the entry of lymphocytes into the CNS by restricting migration to activated T cells. It is interesting to observe that CD3+ T cells can also be found in postmortem samples of choroid plexus in individuals with no known neurologic disorders, indicating that some lymphocytes may enter the CNS during steady state.[11]

## Immune Cells in the Central Nervous System Environment

Even under normal physiologic conditions, the CNS is not an environment that lacks cells of hematopoietic origin. Various cells reside in the CNS that constitute a resident, quiescent immune system. The distribution of hematopoietic cells resident in the CNS is compartmentalized, indicative of specific functions attributed to cells present in distinct microenvironments. The major cells of hematopoietic origin present in the CNS are microglia and APCs. Microglia are localized predominantly in the parenchyma of the CNS (although also present in the perivascular area) and function in the maintenance of neuronal homeostasis as well as tissue surveillance, whereas APCs reside predominantly in the interface between the CNS and the blood–CSF space.[12–17]

### Antigen-Presenting Cells

#### Perivascular Antigen-Presenting Cells

Perivascular APCs consist of a heterogeneous population that includes perivascular macrophages, perivascular microglia, and dendritic cells (DCs).[18,19] It is thought that perivascular APCs act as sentinels at the BBB, their endocytic and phagocytic activity scanning for both the presence of pathogens and neuronal damage.[20] These cells localize to the perivascular spaces around cerebral vessels of small to medium size.[21] Perivascular cells are continuously replenished from the bone marrow, and it is estimated that one-third of these cells are replaced during a trimester period in rats, indicating that precursor cells of perivascular APCs (most likely monocytes) can cross the intact BBB.[22]

Perivascular macrophages have a role in the recruitment of lymphocytes across the BBB and can also promote the invasion of activated T cells into the parenchyma of the CNS.[23,24] In addition, it has been shown that these cells have an essential role in the activation of recently immigrated pathogenic CD4+ T cells.[18,25] Macrophages and DCs are enriched in the meninges and choroid plexus, probably because of proximity to the CSF space.[26] It has been hypothesized that perivascular macrophages sample the CSF for the presence of pathogens, tissue debris, tumor cells, and red blood cells.

## Microglia

Microglia are the predominant cell type of the innate immune system within the CNS parenchyma. The distribution of microglial cells varies in the different areas of the CNS, ranging from approximately 5% in the cortex and corpus callosum to 12% in the substantia nigra of the murine brain,[27] and from 0.5% in the gray matter of the cerebellum and cerebral cortex to greater than 16% in the pons and medulla in a noninflamed human brain.[28,29] Microglia belong to the cell class of hematopoietic mononuclear phagocytic lineage; however, they are less efficient at antigen presentation than DCs. Microglia share many features with other myeloid cells, as they express Fc and complement receptors CD11b and F4/80.[30,31] However, some of the molecular differences between microglia and other dedicated phagocytic APCs include secretion of significantly lower levels of superoxide dismutase (SOD) in comparison with macrophages from the spleen or bone marrow.[32] Additionally, much of the interaction between microglia and T cells in the parenchyma occurs at a distance and is mediated via cytokine secretion, not antigen specificity.

Microglia appear to survey the microenvironment with highly motile fine protrusions.[33] It has been suggested that microglial protrusions survey the environment for inflammatory molecules, thus having an immunologic function. Recent studies, however, have shown that microglia play a role in synaptogenesis,[34] and in the monitoring and maintenance of synaptic functions[35] as well as the apoptosis of Purkinje cells.[36] Thus, microglia appear to have a key function during the development and maintenance of the CNS.[37] During embryogenesis, massive developmental apoptosis occurs in the nervous system; twice the number of neurons are generated than is present in the adult organism. Microglial functions have been implicated in the phagocytosis of apoptotic cells. They also promote the death of developing neurons[36,38] and are active at synaptic stripping during pathologic processes[39] and in synaptic remodeling.[29]

Another key difference between the function of microglia and that of other APCs is the interaction between microglia and neurons that leads to the inhibition of microglial cell activation. Microglia are the only mononuclear phagocytes that express neurotransmitter receptors, and they are rich in purinoceptors (e.g., dopamine receptors and adrenoreceptors). In the normal, healthy CNS, experiments using two-photon imaging have shown that microglia inspect neuronal synapses in vivo in the adult cerebral cortex.[35] Neuron–microglial cell inhibitory signaling can be mediated via several mechanisms; these include contact-dependent inhibitory influences, such as CD172A-CD47,[40] CD200-CD200R,[41,42] CD22-CD45,[42,43] and ICAM5-LFA1,[44] as well as soluble inhibitory cytokines, such as CX3CL1-CX3CR1 interactions.[45] Microglia sense damage once neuronal inhibition is removed or silenced (**Fig. 1.1**).

In their homeostatic resting state, microglia express very low levels of MHC class II molecules[46] and CD45.[47] In the presence of inflammation or pathologic events, microglia become activated and undergo morphological and immunophenotypic alterations, including the upregulation of MHC class II molecules.[48] Under these conditions, microglia secrete a diversity of chemokines, such as CCL1, CCL2, CCL5, and CXCL10, that function in the recruitment of lymphocytes and other APCs, such as macrophages and DCs. Evidence for the role of chemokines secreted by microglia in T-cell migration into the CNS parenchyma was provided by a study involving macro-

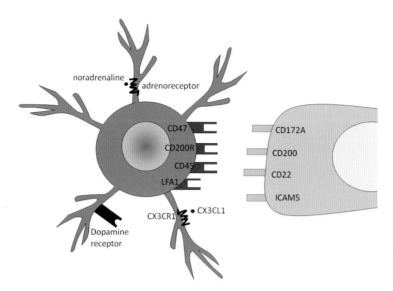

**Fig. 1.1** Neuron–microglia interactions lead to the inhibition of microglial activity via cell contact–dependent mechanisms or soluble inhibitory molecules.

phage colony–stimulating factor (M-CSF). Microglial activation is impaired in M-CSF–deficient mice, which significantly reduced T-cell migration but did not affect axonal repair.[49] Corroborating evidence for the importance of microglia-derived chemokines in T-cell migration was also provided by a study conducted by Heppner et al, which revealed that microglial paralysis inhibits the development and maintenance of inflammatory CNS lesions in the EAE mouse model.[50]

### T Cells

Under normal physiologic conditions, the CNS tightly regulates cell entry into the parenchyma and localizes immunosurveillance to the perivascular and subarachnoid spaces. The CSF of normal healthy individuals contains approximately $0.15 \times 10^6$ T cells, of which greater than 80% are central memory CD4+ T cells (which express CD45RO+/CD27+/CCR7+/CXCR3+ and L-selectin).[51] It has been suggested that the central memory CD4+ T cells present in the CSF are responsible for the routine immunosurveillance of the CNS, by searching for recall antigens presented by macrophages.[26] It has been estimated that the T cells present in the CSF are replaced by newly immigrating lymphocytes approxi-

mately twice per day; this provides a continuous influx of lymphocytes that have different T-cell-receptor (TCR) specificities, which allows a rapid reaction to antigens that are present within the subarachnoid space.[51-53]

In various different neuropathologic conditions, T cells cross the BBB and participate in inflammatory reactions that are deleterious to the individual. One example is multiple sclerosis (MS), in which the presence of CD4+ T cells that display a proinflammatory Th1 or Th17 profile (along with other inflammatory factors) results in an autoimmune disease characterized by recurrent episodes of demyelination and axonal lesions. The cytokines secreted by Th1 (interferon-γ [INF-γ]) and Th17 (interleukin-17 [IL-17]) result in the different clinical forms of MS.[54,55] In the EAE model, although Th1- and Th17-mediated lesions differ in their composition, there is no difference in the localization of lesions within the CNS. The Th17 cells present in lesions can convert to IFN-γ–producing Th1-like cells. There is also a difference between the lytic potential of Th1 and Th17 cells present at EAE lesions; the Th1 cells lysed astrocytes and fibroblasts that presented autoantigen, whereas the Th17 cells acquired cytotoxic potential only after conversion to the IFN-γ-producing Th1 phenotype.[56] The presence of Th17 cell infiltrates in the brain has also been shown in the experimental mouse model of malignant glioma and in human gliomas.[57]

CD4+ regulatory T cells have also been shown to cross over the BBB and infiltrate the CNS in human glioblastoma multiforme,[58] other astrocytomas,[59] and viral infections such as West Nile virus infection,[60] and their presence has been reported in the CSF of patients with MS.[61] The presence of regulatory T cells in the peripheral tissues can serve to generate tolerance against self-antigens and thus control autoimmune reactions. The presence of high levels of CD4+ Tregs within the CNS in mouse models of glioma is indicative of poor survival, as shown by the increase in life span after the depletion of Tregs in this model.[62] This finding remains to be corroborated for gliomas in humans.

Cytotoxic T lymphocytes (CTLs) facilitate the killing of specific target cells via the formation of the immunologic synapse, in which after antigen recognition, CD3/TCR complex is recruited to the area of contact between the CTL and the target cell and forms a central cluster. The T-cell cytoskeleton and the TCR-rich area undergo a series of alterations that result in the directed secretion of cytotoxic granules. A recent study demonstrates that infiltrating CTLs in glioblastoma can generate immunologic synapses with tumor cells.[63] CD8+ T cells that establish immunologic synapses with glioma cells and express polarized granzyme B as an effector molecule may be critical for antitumor-mediated immunologic responses within the CNS in human glioblastoma.

### Natural Killer (NK) Cells

Natural killer (NK) cells are recruited to the CNS in response to tissue injury. NK-cell depletion induces severe EAE.[64] Impaired recruitment of NK cells is associated with increased mortality related to EAE, as well as spastic paraplegia and inflammatory lesions with hemorrhage. Some studies indicate that NK cells may limit autoimmune responses by killing DCs, regulating T-cell proliferation, or secreting regulatory cytokines, although it seems likely that NK cells differentially regulate inflammatory responses at various anatomic sites.

## ■ T-Cell Recruitment into the Central Nervous System

T cells can enter the CNS via several routes, including migration from the blood to the CSF across the choroid plexus or meningeal vessels into the subarachnoid space, migration from the blood to the parenchymal perivascular spaces of the brain, and migration from the blood to the parenchymal perivascular space of the spinal cord. These different migration routes involve the transport of the T cells across various barriers: the blood–CSF barrier, the BBB, and the blood–spinal cord barrier.[51–53] Under inflammatory conditions, the expression of adhesion molecules and chemokines is induced on the endothelium at the BBB. This provides trafficking signals for circulating leukocytes to enter the CNS. When the endothelial BBB allows transendothelial migration, T-cell recruitment into the CNS is still highly regulated because the lymphocytes found in the perivascular spaces have a homogeneous effector memory phenotype that distinguishes them from lymphocytes found in other inflamed tissues.[51,65,66] T-cell migration into the CNS involves a three-step interaction between the leukocytes and the endothelium: (1) tethering and rolling of leukocytes on the BBB, (2) activation and firm adhesion, and (3) diapedesis (transendothelial migration). Each of these steps is described in detail below.

### Tethering and Rolling of Leukocytes on Endothelium

The contact between vascular endothelium and circulating lymphocytes is the result of fluid dynamics within the blood vessel. The term *leukocyte margination* describes the phenomenon in which cells flowing within the blood vessel are positioned closer to the vascular wall than to the center of the vessel.[67] Here, lymphocytes make a transient and reversible contact with the vascular endothelium. This contact is mediated by adhesion molecules of the selectin family and their carbohydrate ligands, initiating the rolling of leukocytes on the endothelial surface. This interaction, although not strong enough to anchor cells against the force of blood flow, allows cells to roll along the endothelium, continually making and breaking contact (**Fig. 1.2**).

The microvessels of a healthy brain and spinal cord of SJL/N mice constitutively express vascular cell adhesion molecule-1 (VCAM-1), platelet endothelial cell adhesion molecule-1 (PECAM-1), and intercellular adhesion molecule-2 (ICAM-2). (The latter two molecules are also expressed on vascular endothelial cells at other sites.[68])

During inflammatory diseases such as EAE, tethering and rolling of leukocytes can be observed in superficial brain and meningeal microvessels by performing intravital microscopy.[69] In inflamed murine vessels, CD8+ T cells have been shown to roll by adhering to the endothelium via P-selectin glycoprotein ligand-1 (PSGL-1), whereas CD4+ T cells roll via α4-integrin.[70] P- and E-selectin can also mediate lymphocyte rolling in inflamed brain vessels.[71,72] During EAE, there is upregulation of both VCAM-1 and ICAM-1 on the CNS endothelium, but not of P- or E-selectin.[73] It has been suggested that the α4-integrin/VCAM-1 interactions mediate the steps of adhesion of lymphocytes to the BBB because antibodies that block α4-integrins or endothelial

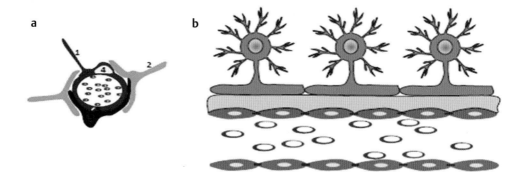

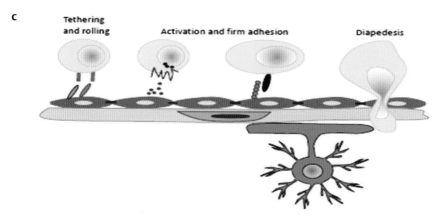

**Fig. 1.2** Structure of the blood–brain barrier (BBB) and T-cell recruitment into the central nervous system (CNS). **(a)** BBB: *1*, neuron; *2*, astrocyte; *3*, pericyte; *4*, endothelial capillary cell; *5*, tight junction. **(b)** Structure of normal, noninflamed BBB: lymphocytes and red blood cells flow through the blood vessel. **(c)** Recruitment of T cells across the inflamed BBB. Figure depicts the multistep process leading to the transendothelial migration of T cells into the CNS parenchyma.

VCAM-1 significantly reduce the adhesion of lymphocytes to the brain vascular endothelium; however, they have little effect on transendothelial migration of autoreactive lymphocytes.[74]

### Activation and Firm Adhesion

For leukocytes to adhere to the endothelium, it is essential for integrin activation to occur. This is mediated via G-protein-coupled receptors (GPCRs). Intravital microscopy studies of T-cell interactions with microvasculature in the brain and spinal cord have shown that GPCR signaling is essential for the firm adhesion of autoreactive T cells on endothelium of CNS.[72,75] Prior rolling of lymphocytes along the endothelium allows sampling of the surface of endothelial cells, resulting in activation of integrins on lymphocytes and subsequent adhesion and firm arrest.[76-78] Chemokines secreted by the inflamed BBB bind their receptors, resulting in increased affinity of integrin binding and clustering at the cell surface; this in turn leads to the enhanced avidity of the adhesion molecules for their ligands.[79,80] The inflamed BBB endothelium in EAE secretes the homeostatic chemokines CCL19 and CCL21,[81,82] which allows the binding of B cells, T cells, and mature DCs that express the CCR7 (see **Fig. 1.2**).

The upregulation of ICAM-1 and VCAM-1 on endothelial cells of the CNS microvasculature during EAE allows the binding of inflammatory cells expressing the respective ligands lymphocyte function–associated antigen-1 (LFA-1, also known as α1β2-integrin) and α4β1-integrin, but not L-selectin or α4β7-integrin.[73,83] The G-protein–dependent activation of LFA-1 on lymphocytes allows the firm adhesion on endothelial ICAM-1 and arrests the rolling of lymphocytes along the endothelium. Only activated integrins can mediate the firm adhesion of leukocytes to the vascular endothelium.

### Diapedesis (Transendothelial Migration)

During diapedesis, leukocytes migrate across an inflamed BBB through endothelial cells, leaving tight junctions intact.[84] In vitro studies confirm that diapedesis across the BBB is a process that involves LFA-1 and ICAM-1.[85] Blocking LFA-1 on autoreactive T cells resulted in a significantly reduced number of T cells migrating across the vascular endothelium into the spinal cord parenchyma, demonstrating that LFA-1 is used for transendothelial migration, but not for capture and adhesion in microvessels. Furthermore, other studies show that endothelioma cells that lack both ligands for LFA-1 (ICAM-1 and ICAM-2) can mediate adhesion of T cells to activated endothelium, but no longer mediate transendothelial migration[86] (see **Fig. 1.2**).

## ■ Expression and Function of Chemokines and Their Receptors at the Blood–Brain Barrier

The CNS endothelium secretes a diversity of chemokines, each with distinct effects on circulating lymphocytes. The expression and regulation of inflammatory chemokines in the CNS microvasculature have been less studied than in the peripheral lymphoid tissues or other organs. As a result, the number of studies that have characterized the in vivo expression of inflammatory cytokines in the brain is limited. However, several studies have characterized inflammatory chemokines in in vitro preparations of brain microvasculature endothelium. This section focuses on homeostatic chemokines that have a role during the occurrence of inflammation within the CNS.

### CCL19 and CCL21

The chemokines CCL19, also known as macrophage inflammatory protein-3β (MIP-3β), and CCL21, also known as secondary lymphoid tissue chemokine (SLC), function under physiologic conditions to recruit naïve T cells and B cells and mature DCs, which bind to the chemokine via its receptor CCR7 into lymphoid tissues.[87-90] The expression of these cytokines has been studied in the CNS microvasculature under normal physiologic conditions, as well as in neuroinflammatory conditions such as MS and its mouse model, EAE. Messenger RNA (mRNA) transcripts of CCL19 are constitutively expressed in both normal and inflamed endothelium of postcapillary venules; however, mRNA transcripts of CCL21 are induced during the course of EAE.

One study demonstrated that the expression of CCL21 but not CCL19 by oligodendrocytes in transgenic mice leads to inflammation within the CNS. The mice expressing CCL19 displayed normal development, whereas the mice that expressed CCL21 in oligodendrocytes did not survive past 4 weeks post partum[91] because of deficiency in motor function. The inflammation of the CNS was caused predominantly by neutrophil and eosinophil infiltration and by reactive microglia and astrocytes; however, the expression of CCL21 alone did not lead to lymphocytic infiltration. Another study examined the expression of these chemokines and the receptor in brain and CSF samples from patients with MS.[92] The authors found a large number of CCR7+ cells and the expression of MHC II and CD86 (markers of antigen presentation by DCs) within MS lesions. It is interesting to note that T cells localized to the lesions did not express CCR7; however, T cells and DCs in the CSF expressed CCR7. The authors proposed that activated microglia and macrophages express signals associated with maturing DCs, including CCR7, that are capable of stimulating central memory T cells locally.

## CXCL12

The chemokine CXCL12 (also known as stromal cell–derived factor-1) functions as a potent chemoattractant for lymphocytes and monocytes.[93] In addition, CXCL12 aids in angiogenesis by recruiting endothelial precursor cells from the bone marrow.[94] CXCL12 is implicated in carcinogenesis because of its role in the neovascularization of tumors.[95] It has also been shown to have a role in tumor metastasis.[96]

In the CNS, CXCL12 is expressed as three different isoforms: CXCL12α (expressed by neurons), CXCL12β, and CXCL12γ (expressed

by endothelial cells).[97] The CXCL12-CXCR4 signaling pathway has been shown to be involved in the development and modulation of synapse formation within the CNS. There is widespread expression of CXCL12 and CXCR4 within the CNS, including the endothelium of the BBB, hippocampus, cortex, olfactory bulb, meninges, and cerebellum.[98] Similarly, the expression of CXCR4 is readily detectable on many cells in the CNS, including microglia, endothelial cells of the BBB, astrocytes, oligodendrocytes, and neurons.[99]

In MS lesions, the expression of CXCL12 along the blood vessels of the BBB and in astrocytes is increased. In studies conducted in the EAE mouse model, the levels of CXCL12 were significantly increased at the peak of the disease, and the expression of this chemokine was localized to the microvessels along the parenchymal surface of endothelial cells, as opposed to the abluminal surface in the noninflamed endothelium. Similarly, CXCL12 was expressed predominantly along the parenchymal surface of BBB endothelium in the arterioles and venules of the CNS in normal individuals and in the noninflamed areas of the MS brain, whereas the expression of this chemokine in venules shifted to the luminal side of the endothelial surface in patients with MS.[100,101]

## CCL2

Studies in CCL2 knockout mice demonstrate that this chemokine has a nonredundant role in regulating monocyte infiltration of the CNS during inflammatory processes. Similarly, mice deficient in CCR2 (receptor for CCL2) have impaired recruitment of monocytes to tissues.[102] Patients with MS have lower levels of CCL2 in the CSF in comparison with patients who have other noninflammatory neurologic diseases. Levels of CCL2 decrease in the CSF during the active phase of MS.[53,103] The lower levels of CCL2 in the CSF of these patients have been attributed to the consumption of CCL2 by CCR2+ monocytes and T cells. It is also possible that CCR2 is downregulated in migrating cells.[104,105] Transgenic mice that constitutively express low levels of CCL2 in the CNS have a reduced severity of EAE in comparison with littermate controls, possibly because of the effects of CCL2 on circulating lymphocytes.[106]

## CXCL9 and CXCL10

It has been suggested that CXCR3 (receptor for CXCL9, CXCL10, and CXCL11) has a role in the trafficking of leukocytes into the CNS during neuroinflammatory pathologic conditions. CXCR3 is expressed on B cells, NK cells, activated T cells, and some monocytes.[107] The chemokines CXCL9 and CXCL10 are readily detected in the brain during EAE.[53] The presence of neutralizing antibodies specific for CXCL10 leads to a reduced severity of EAE and lower levels of inflammatory T cells in the CNS.[108] Thus, it is surprising to observe that mice deficient in CXCL10 are more susceptible to EAE. It is possible that the absence of CXCL10 is associated with the upregulation of CXCL11 in the CNS and the downregulation of CXCL9 in lymph nodes. Although CXCR3 is important for T-cell trafficking into the CNS, its role is not pivotal for the transendothelial migration of memory CD4+ T cells into the BBB.[109] This is further demonstrated by the fact that CXCR3 knockout mice have an enhanced severity of EAE, which may be due to the lack of CXCR3-mediated INF-γ secretion.[110]

## CX3CL1

CX3CL1 is a type 1 transmembrane glycoprotein chemokine that is present at high levels in the neurons of the normal CNS,[111] but not on blood vessels.[112,113] It functions as an adhesion molecule or as a chemoattractant once proteolytically cleaved. Its receptor CX3CR1 is expressed by NK cells, lymphocytes, and monocytes, and in the CNS it is also expressed by microglia.[33,114] The absolute number of NK cells is significantly reduced in the inflamed CNS of mice with EAE that are CX3CR1-deficient in comparison with wild-type mice. This impaired recruitment of NK cells into the CNS is associated with increased severity of disease and decreased survival.[64]

## ◾ Conclusion

As depicted in this chapter, the brain is an immunologically specialized organ in which surveillance is tightly regulated. Under normal physiologic conditions, the passage of molecules across the BBB is limited by the presence of tight junctions between its endothelial cells. The main immune cells present in the CNS under normal conditions are perivascular APCs and microglia. The latter have immunologic functions as well as a role in the monitoring and maintenance of synaptic functions. However, in various inflammatory and neurodegenerative diseases, other immune cells, such as CD4+ T cells, NK cells, and CTLs, cross the BBB and infiltrate the CNS parenchyma, with deleterious results to the individual. These cells infiltrate the CNS because of the chemoattractant properties of molecules secreted by the brain endothelium. The chemokines displayed on the endothelium bind to the receptors on circulating leukocytes and initiate reactions that result in integrin activation, arrest, firm adhesion, and finally extravasation to within the CNS. The degree to which these processes occur ultimately determines the degree of the immune response.

### References

1. Barker CF, Billingham RE. Immunologically privileged sites. Adv Immunol 1977;25:1–54
2. Medawar PB. Immunity to homologous grafted skin; the fate of skin homografts transplanted to the brain, to subcutaneous tissue, and to the anterior chamber of the eye. Br J Exp Pathol 1948;29(1):58–69
3. Pachter JS, de Vries HE, Fabry Z. The blood-brain barrier and its role in immune privilege in the central nervous system. J Neuropathol Exp Neurol 2003;62(6):593–604
4. Rubin LL, Staddon JM. The cell biology of the blood-brain barrier. Annu Rev Neurosci 1999;22:11–28
5. Schlosshauer B. The blood-brain barrier: morphology, molecules, and neurothelin. Bioessays 1993;15(5):341–346
6. Ransohoff RM, Kivisäkk P, Kidd G. Three or more routes for leukocyte migration into the central nervous system. Nat Rev Immunol 2003;3(7):569–581
7. Reese TS, Karnovsky MJ. Fine structural localization of a blood-brain barrier to exogenous peroxidase. J Cell Biol 1967;34(1):207–217

8. Zlokovic BV. The blood-brain barrier in health and chronic neurodegenerative disorders. Neuron 2008;57(2):178–201

9. Hickey WF, Hsu BL, Kimura H. T-lymphocyte entry into the central nervous system. J Neurosci Res 1991;28(2):254–260

10. Cross AH, Cannella B, Brosnan CF, Raine CS. Homing to central nervous system vasculature by antigen-specific lymphocytes. I. Localization of [14]C-labeled cells during acute, chronic, and relapsing experimental allergic encephalomyelitis. Lab Invest 1990;63(2):162–170

11. Kivisäkk P, Mahad DJ, Callahan MK, et al. Human cerebrospinal fluid central memory CD4+ T cells: evidence for trafficking through choroid plexus and meninges via P-selectin. Proc Natl Acad Sci USA 2003;100(14):8389–8394

12. Aloisi F. Immune function of microglia. Glia 2001;36(2):165–179

13. Kreutzberg GW. Microglia: a sensor for pathological events in the CNS. Trends Neurosci 1996;19(8):312–318

14. Matyszak MK, Perry VH. The potential role of dendritic cells in immune-mediated inflammatory diseases in the central nervous system. Neuroscience 1996;74(2):599–608

15. Karman J, Ling C, Sandor M, Fabry Z. Initiation of immune responses in brain is promoted by local dendritic cells. J Immunol 2004;173(4):2353–2361

16. Fischer HG, Reichmann G. Brain dendritic cells and macrophages/microglia in central nervous system inflammation. J Immunol 2001;166(4):2717–2726

17. Streit WJ. Microglia as neuroprotective, immunocompetent cells of the CNS. Glia 2002;40(2):133–139

18. Greter M, Heppner FL, Lemos MP, et al. Dendritic cells permit immune invasion of the CNS in an animal model of multiple sclerosis. Nat Med 2005;11(3):328–334

19. Mrass P, Weninger W. Immune cell migration as a means to control immune privilege: lessons from the CNS and tumors. Immunol Rev 2006;213:195–212

20. Williams K, Alvarez X, Lackner AA. Central nervous system perivascular cells are immunoregulatory cells that connect the CNS with the peripheral immune system. Glia 2001;36(2):156–164

21. Bechmann I, Priller J, Kovac A, et al. Immune surveillance of mouse brain perivascular spaces by blood-borne macrophages. Eur J Neurosci 2001;14(10):1651–1658

22. Hickey WF, Vass K, Lassmann H. Bone marrow-derived elements in the central nervous system: an immunohistochemical and ultrastructural survey of rat chimeras. J Neuropathol Exp Neurol 1992;51(3):246–256

23. Tran EH, Hoekstra K, van Rooijen N, Dijkstra CD, Owens T. Immune invasion of the central nervous system parenchyma and experimental allergic encephalomyelitis, but not leukocyte extravasation from blood, are prevented in macrophage-depleted mice. J Immunol 1998;161(7):3767–3775

24. Agrawal S, Anderson P, Durbeej M, et al. Dystroglycan is selectively cleaved at the parenchymal basement membrane at sites of leukocyte extravasation in experimental autoimmune encephalomyelitis. J Exp Med 2006;203(4):1007–1019

25. McMahon EJ, Bailey SL, Castenada CV, Waldner H, Miller SD. Epitope spreading initiates in the CNS in two mouse models of multiple sclerosis. Nat Med 2005;11(3):335–339

26. McMenamin PG. Distribution and phenotype of dendritic cells and resident tissue macrophages in the dura mater, leptomeninges, and choroid plexus of the rat brain as demonstrated in wholemount preparations. J Comp Neurol 1999;405(4):553–562

27. Lawson LJ, Perry VH, Dri P, Gordon S. Heterogeneity in the distribution and morphology of microglia in the normal adult mouse brain. Neuroscience 1990;39(1):151–170

28. Mittelbronn M, Dietz K, Schluesener HJ, Meyermann R. Local distribution of microglia in the normal adult human central nervous system differs by up to one order of magnitude. Acta Neuropathol 2001;101(3):249–255

29. Kofler J, Wiley CA. Microglia: key innate immune cells of the brain. Toxicol Pathol 2011;39(1):103–114

30. Perry VH, Hume DA, Gordon S. Immunohistochemical localization of macrophages and microglia in the adult and developing mouse brain. Neuroscience 1985;15(2):313–326

31. Hanisch UK. Microglia as a source and target of cytokines. Glia 2002;40(2):140–155

32. Enose Y, Destache CJ, Mack AL, et al. Proteomic fingerprints distinguish microglia, bone marrow, and spleen macrophage populations. Glia 2005;51(3):161–172

33. Nimmerjahn A, Kirchhoff F, Helmchen F. Resting microglial cells are highly dynamic surveillants of brain parenchyma in vivo. Science 2005;308(5726):1314–1318

34. Roumier A, Béchade C, Poncer JC, et al. Impaired synaptic function in the microglial KARAP/DAP12-deficient mouse. J Neurosci 2004;24(50):11421–11428

35. Wake H, Moorhouse AJ, Jinno S, Kohsaka S, Nabekura J. Resting microglia directly monitor the functional state of synapses in vivo and determine the fate of ischemic terminals. J Neurosci 2009;29(13):3974–3980

36. Marín-Teva JL, Dusart I, Colin C, Gervais A, van Rooijen N, Mallat M. Microglia promote the death of developing Purkinje cells. Neuron 2004;41(4):535–547

37. Prinz M, Mildner A. Microglia in the CNS: immigrants from another world. Glia 2011;59(2):177–187

38. Bessis A, Béchade C, Bernard D, Roumier A. Microglial control of neuronal death and synaptic properties. Glia 2007;55(3):233–238

39. Trapp BD, Wujek JR, Criste GA, et al. Evidence for synaptic stripping by cortical microglia. Glia 2007;55(4):360–368

40. Junker A, Krumbholz M, Eisele S, et al. MicroRNA profiling of multiple sclerosis lesions identifies modulators of the regulatory protein CD47. Brain 2009;132(Pt 12):3342–3352

41. Hoek RM, Ruuls SR, Murphy CA, et al. Downregulation of the macrophage lineage through

interaction with OX2 (CD200). Science 2000; 290(5497):1768–1771

42. Barclay AN, Wright GJ, Brooke G, Brown MH. CD200 and membrane protein interactions in the control of myeloid cells. Trends Immunol 2002;23(6):285–290

43. Ransohoff RM, Cardona AE. The myeloid cells of the central nervous system parenchyma. Nature 2010;468(7321):253–262

44. Gahmberg CG, Tian L, Ning L, Nyman-Huttunen H. ICAM-5—a novel two-facetted adhesion molecule in the mammalian brain. Immunol Lett 2008;117(2):131–135

45. Hundhausen C, Misztela D, Berkhout TA, et al. The disintegrin-like metalloproteinase ADAM10 is involved in constitutive cleavage of CX3CL1 (fractalkine) and regulates CX3CL1-mediated cell-cell adhesion. Blood 2003;102(4):1186–1195

46. de Haas AH, Boddeke HW, Biber K. Region-specific expression of immunoregulatory proteins on microglia in the healthy CNS. Glia 2008;56(8): 888–894

47. Ford AL, Goodsall AL, Hickey WF, Sedgwick JD. Normal adult ramified microglia separated from other central nervous system macrophages by flow cytometric sorting. Phenotypic differences defined and direct ex vivo antigen presentation to myelin basic protein-reactive CD4+ T cells compared. J Immunol 1995;154(9):4309–4321

48. Perry VH. A revised view of the central nervous system microenvironment and major histocompatibility complex class II antigen presentation. J Neuroimmunol 1998;90(2):113–121

49. Kalla R, Liu Z, Xu S, et al. Microglia and the early phase of immune surveillance in the axotomized facial motor nucleus: impaired microglial activation and lymphocyte recruitment but no effect on neuronal survival or axonal regeneration in macrophage-colony stimulating factor-deficient mice. J Comp Neurol 2001;436(2):182–201

50. Heppner FL, Greter M, Marino D, et al. Experimental autoimmune encephalomyelitis repressed by microglial paralysis. Nat Med 2005;11(2): 146–152

51. Engelhardt B, Ransohoff RM. The ins and outs of T-lymphocyte trafficking to the CNS: anatomical sites and molecular mechanisms. Trends Immunol 2005;26(9):485–495

52. Ubogu EE, Cossoy MB, Ransohoff RM. The expression and function of chemokines involved in CNS inflammation. Trends Pharmacol Sci 2006;27(1):48–55

53. Rebenko-Moll NM, Liu L, Cardona A, Ransohoff RM. Chemokines, mononuclear cells and the nervous system: heaven (or hell) is in the details. Curr Opin Immunol 2006;18(6):683–689

54. El-behi M, Rostami A, Ciric B. Current views on the roles of Th1 and Th17 cells in experimental autoimmune encephalomyelitis. J Neuroimmune Pharmacol 2010;5(2):189–197

55. Brucklacher-Waldert V, Stuerner K, Kolster M, Wolthausen J, Tolosa E. Phenotypical and functional characterization of T helper 17 cells in multiple sclerosis. Brain 2009;132(Pt 12):3329–3341

56. Domingues HS, Mues M, Lassmann H, Wekerle H, Krishnamoorthy G. Functional and pathogenic differences of Th1 and Th17 cells in experimen-tal autoimmune encephalomyelitis. PLoS ONE 2010;5(11):e15531

57. Wainwright DA, Sengupta S, Han Y, Ulasov IV, Lesniak MS. The presence of IL-17A and T helper 17 cells in experimental mouse brain tumors and human glioma. PLoS ONE 2010;5(10):e15390

58. El Andaloussi A, Lesniak MS. An increase in CD4+CD25+FOXP3+ regulatory T cells in tumor-infiltrating lymphocytes of human glioblastoma multiforme. Neuro Oncol 2006;8(3):234–243

59. El Andaloussi A, Lesniak MS. CD4+ CD25+ FoxP3+ T-cell infiltration and heme oxygenase-1 expression correlate with tumor grade in human gliomas. J Neurooncol 2007;83(2):145–152

60. Stewart BS, Demarest VL, Wong SJ, Green S, Bernard KA. Persistence of virus-specific immune responses in the central nervous system of mice after West Nile virus infection. BMC Immunol 2011;12:6

61. Fritzsching B, Haas J, König F, et al. Intracerebral human regulatory T cells: analysis of CD4+ CD25+ FOXP3+ T cells in brain lesions and cerebrospinal fluid of multiple sclerosis patients. PLoS ONE 2011;6(3):e17988

62. El Andaloussi A, Han Y, Lesniak MS. Prolongation of survival following depletion of CD4+CD25+ regulatory T cells in mice with experimental brain tumors. J Neurosurg 2006;105(3):430–437

63. Barcia C Jr, Gómez A, Gallego-Sanchez JM, et al. Infiltrating CTLs in human glioblastoma establish immunological synapses with tumorigenic cells. Am J Pathol 2009;175(2):786–798

64. Huang D, Shi FD, Jung S, et al. The neuronal chemokine CX3CL1/fractalkine selectively recruits NK cells that modify experimental autoimmune encephalomyelitis within the central nervous system. FASEB J 2006;20(7):896–905

65. Zeine R, Owens T. Direct demonstration of the infiltration of murine central nervous system by Pgp-1/CD44high CD45RB(low) CD4+ T cells that induce experimental allergic encephalomyelitis. J Neuroimmunol 1992;40(1):57–69

66. Engelhardt B, Martin-Simonet MT, Rott LS, Butcher EC, Michie SA. Adhesion molecule phenotype of T lymphocytes in inflamed CNS. J Neuroimmunol 1998;84(1):92–104

67. Goldsmith HL, Spain S. Margination of leukocytes in blood flow through small tubes. Microvasc Res 1984;27(2):204–222

68. Engelhardt B. Molecular mechanisms involved in T cell migration across the blood-brain barrier. J Neural Transm 2006;113(4):477–485

69. Kerfoot SM, Kubes P. Overlapping roles of P-selectin and alpha 4 integrin to recruit leukocytes to the central nervous system in experimental autoimmune encephalomyelitis. J Immunol 2002;169(2):1000–1006

70. Battistini L, Piccio L, Rossi B, et al. CD8+ T cells from patients with acute multiple sclerosis display selective increase of adhesiveness in brain venules: a critical role for P-selectin glycoprotein ligand-1. Blood 2003;101(12):4775–4782

71. Carvalho-Tavares J, Hickey MJ, Hutchison J, Michaud J, Sutcliffe IT, Kubes P. A role for platelets and endothelial selectins in tumor necrosis factor-alpha-induced leukocyte recruitment in the

brain microvasculature. Circ Res 2000;87(12): 1141–1148

72. Piccio L, Rossi B, Scarpini E, et al. Molecular mechanisms involved in lymphocyte recruitment in inflamed brain microvessels: critical roles for P-selectin glycoprotein ligand-1 and heterotrimeric G(i)-linked receptors. J Immunol 2002;168(4):1940–1949

73. Steffen BJ, Butcher EC, Engelhardt B. Evidence for involvement of ICAM-1 and VCAM-1 in lymphocyte interaction with endothelium in experimental autoimmune encephalomyelitis in the central nervous system in the SJL/J mouse. Am J Pathol 1994;145(1):189–201

74. Laschinger M, Vajkoczy P, Engelhardt B. Encephalitogenic T cells use LFA-1 for transendothelial migration but not during capture and initial adhesion strengthening in healthy spinal cord microvessels in vivo. Eur J Immunol 2002;32(12): 3598–3606

75. Vajkoczy P, Laschinger M, Engelhardt B. Alpha4-integrin-VCAM-1 binding mediates G protein-independent capture of encephalitogenic T cell blasts to CNS white matter microvessels. J Clin Invest 2001;108(4):557–565

76. Ley K. Molecular mechanisms of leukocyte recruitment in the inflammatory process. Cardiovasc Res 1996;32(4):733–742

77. Johnston B, Butcher EC. Chemokines in rapid leukocyte adhesion triggering and migration. Semin Immunol 2002;14(2):83–92

78. Ley K, Laudanna C, Cybulsky MI, Nourshargh S. Getting to the site of inflammation: the leukocyte adhesion cascade updated. Nat Rev Immunol 2007;7(9):678–689

79. Adamson P, Wilbourn B, Etienne-Manneville S, et al. Lymphocyte trafficking through the blood-brain barrier is dependent on endothelial cell heterotrimeric G-protein signaling. FASEB J 2002; 16(10):1185–1194

80. Alon R, Feigelson S. From rolling to arrest on blood vessels: leukocyte tap dancing on endothelial integrin ligands and chemokines at sub-second contacts. Semin Immunol 2002;14(2):93–104

81. Columba-Cabezas S, Serafini B, Ambrosini E, Aloisi F. Lymphoid chemokines CCL19 and CCL21 are expressed in the central nervous system during experimental autoimmune encephalomyelitis: implications for the maintenance of chronic neuroinflammation. Brain Pathol 2003;13(1): 38–51

82. Alt C, Laschinger M, Engelhardt B. Functional expression of the lymphoid chemokines CCL19 (ELC) and CCL 21 (SLC) at the blood-brain barrier suggests their involvement in G-protein-dependent lymphocyte recruitment into the central nervous system during experimental autoimmune encephalomyelitis. Eur J Immunol 2002;32(8): 2133–2144

83. Baron JL, Madri JA, Ruddle NH, Hashim G, Janeway CA Jr. Surface expression of alpha 4 integrin by CD4 T cells is required for their entry into brain parenchyma. J Exp Med 1993;177(1):57–68

84. Engelhardt B, Wolburg H. Mini-review: Transendothelial migration of leukocytes: through the front door or around the side of the house? Eur J Immunol 2004;34(11):2955–2963

85. Carman CV, Springer TA. A transmigratory cup in leukocyte diapedesis both through individual vascular endothelial cells and between them. J Cell Biol 2004;167(2):377–388

86. Lyck R, Reiss Y, Gerwin N, Greenwood J, Adamson P, Engelhardt B. T-cell interaction with ICAM-1/ICAM-2 double-deficient brain endothelium in vitro: the cytoplasmic tail of endothelial ICAM-1 is necessary for transendothelial migration of T cells. Blood 2003;102(10):3675–3683

87. Robbiani DF, Finch RA, Jäger D, Muller WA, Sartorelli AC, Randolph GJ. The leukotriene C(4) transporter MRP1 regulates CCL19 (MIP-3beta, ELC)-dependent mobilization of dendritic cells to lymph nodes. Cell 2000;103(5):757–768

88. Reif K, Ekland EH, Ohl L, et al. Balanced responsiveness to chemoattractants from adjacent zones determines B-cell position. Nature 2002;416(6876):94–99

89. Bromley SK, Thomas SY, Luster AD. Chemokine receptor CCR7 guides T cell exit from peripheral tissues and entry into afferent lymphatics. Nat Immunol 2005;6(9):895–901

90. Yoshida R, Nagira M, Kitaura M, Imagawa N, Imai T, Yoshie O. Secondary lymphoid-tissue chemokine is a functional ligand for the CC chemokine receptor CCR7. J Biol Chem 1998;273(12): 7118–7122

91. Chen SC, Leach MW, Chen Y, et al. Central nervous system inflammation and neurological disease in transgenic mice expressing the CC chemokine CCL21 in oligodendrocytes. J Immunol 2002;168(3):1009–1017

92. Kivisäkk P, Mahad DJ, Callahan MK, et al. Expression of CCR7 in multiple sclerosis: implications for CNS immunity. Ann Neurol 2004;55(5): 627–638

93. Bleul CC, Fuhlbrigge RC, Casasnovas JM, Aiuti A, Springer TA. A highly efficacious lymphocyte chemoattractant, stromal cell-derived factor 1 (SDF-1). J Exp Med 1996;184(3):1101–1109

94. Zheng H, Fu G, Dai T, Huang H. Migration of endothelial progenitor cells mediated by stromal cell-derived factor-1alpha/CXCR4 via PI3K/Akt/eNOS signal transduction pathway. J Cardiovasc Pharmacol 2007;50(3):274–280

95. Kryczek I, Wei S, Keller E, Liu R, Zou W. Stroma-derived factor (SDF-1/CXCL12) and human tumor pathogenesis. Am J Physiol Cell Physiol 2007;292(3):C987–C995

96. Müller A, Homey B, Soto H, et al. Involvement of chemokine receptors in breast cancer metastasis. Nature 2001;410(6824):50–56

97. Stumm RK, Rummel J, Junker V, et al. A dual role for the SDF-1/CXCR4 chemokine receptor system in adult brain: isoform-selective regulation of SDF-1 expression modulates CXCR4-dependent neuronal plasticity and cerebral leukocyte recruitment after focal ischemia. J Neurosci 2002;22(14):5865–5878

98. van der Meer P, Ulrich AM, González-Scarano F, Lavi E. Immunohistochemical analysis of CCR2, CCR3, CCR5, and CXCR4 in the human brain: potential mechanisms for HIV dementia. Exp Mol Pathol 2000;69(3):192–201

99. Krumbholz M, Theil D, Cepok S, et al. Chemokines in multiple sclerosis: CXCL12 and CXCL13

up-regulation is differentially linked to CNS immune cell recruitment. Brain 2006;129(Pt 1): 200–211

100. McCandless EE, Piccio L, Woerner BM, et al. Pathological expression of CXCL12 at the blood-brain barrier correlates with severity of multiple sclerosis. Am J Pathol 2008;172(3):799–808

101. Holman DW, Klein RS, Ransohoff RM. The blood-brain barrier, chemokines and multiple sclerosis. Biochim Biophys Acta 2011;1812(2): 220–230

102. Charo IF, Ransohoff RM. The many roles of chemokines and chemokine receptors in inflammation. N Engl J Med 2006;354(6):610–621

103. Sørensen TL, Ransohoff RM, Strieter RM, Sellebjerg F. Chemokine CCL2 and chemokine receptor CCR2 in early active multiple sclerosis. Eur J Neurol 2004;11(7):445–449

104. Kivisäkk P, Trebst C, Liu Z, et al. T-cells in the cerebrospinal fluid express a similar repertoire of inflammatory chemokine receptors in the absence or presence of CNS inflammation: implications for CNS trafficking. Clin Exp Immunol 2002;129(3): 510–518

105. Mahad D, Callahan MK, Williams KA, et al. Modulating CCR2 and CCL2 at the blood-brain barrier: relevance for multiple sclerosis pathogenesis. Brain 2006;129(Pt 1):212–223

106. Elhofy A, Wang J, Tani M, et al. Transgenic expression of CCL2 in the central nervous system prevents experimental autoimmune encephalomyelitis. J Leukoc Biol 2005;77(2):229–237

107. Liu L, Callahan MK, Huang D, Ransohoff RM. Chemokine receptor CXCR3: an unexpected enigma. Curr Top Dev Biol 2005;68:149–181

108. Sorensen TL. Targeting the chemokine receptor CXCR3 and its ligand CXCL10 in the central nervous system: potential therapy for inflammatory demyelinating disease? Curr Neurovasc Res 2004;1(2):183–190

109. Callahan MK, Williams KA, Kivisäkk P, Pearce D, Stins MF, Ransohoff RM. CXCR3 marks CD4+ memory T lymphocytes that are competent to migrate across a human brain microvascular endothelial cell layer. J Neuroimmunol 2004;153(1-2):150–157

110. Liu L, Huang D, Matsui M, et al. Severe disease, unaltered leukocyte migration, and reduced IFN-gamma production in CXCR3-/- mice with experimental autoimmune encephalomyelitis. J Immunol 2006;176(7):4399–4409

111. Bazan JF, Bacon KB, Hardiman G, et al. A new class of membrane-bound chemokine with a CX3C motif. Nature 1997;385(6617):640–644

112. Sunnemark D, Eltayeb S, Nilsson M, et al. CX3CL1 (fractalkine) and CX3CR1 expression in myelin oligodendrocyte glycoprotein-induced experimental autoimmune encephalomyelitis: kinetics and cellular origin. J Neuroinflammation 2005; 2:17

113. Harrison JK, Jiang Y, Chen S, et al. Role for neuronally derived fractalkine in mediating interactions between neurons and CX3CR1-expressing microglia. Proc Natl Acad Sci USA 1998;95(18):10896–10901

114. Nishiyori A, Minami M, Ohtani Y, et al. Localization of fractalkine and CX3CR1 mRNAs in rat brain: does fractalkine play a role in signaling from neuron to microglia? FEBS Lett 1998;429(2): 167–172

# 2

# Microbiological Diagnosis of Central Nervous System Infections

**Yuriko Fukuta and Karin Byers**

The central nervous system (CNS) may be infected by various organisms, including bacteria, viruses, fungi, and parasites. Numerous noninfectious etiologies may mimic CNS infections. The causative organisms in postoperative infections are quite different from those of nonsurgical infections. The patient's endogenous skin flora, primarily gram-positive bacteria, are a frequent cause of postoperative infection. Hospital-acquired pathogens, including *Staphylococcus aureus*, gram-negative bacilli, and fungi, are the other group of pathogens commonly encountered; the latter group are often resistant to multiple antimicrobial agents. CNS infections often necessitate emergent interventions because of high mortality and complications. This chapter reviews the microbiological diagnosis of CNS infections.

## ■ Specimen Selection and Collection

Selection of the appropriate specimens and tests for the detection of causative organisms is crucial in treating infectious diseases. Whenever possible, antimicrobial therapy should be held until appropriate specimens are collected unless delay in treatment poses an unacceptable risk to the patient.

## Cerebrospinal Fluid

Lumbar puncture with cerebrospinal fluid (CSF) analysis is usually essential to diagnose CNS infections. Typical CSF findings in meningitis are shown in **Table 2.1**.

### Opening Pressure and Appearance

The CSF opening pressure is measured with an air–water manometer. In adults, the normal CSF opening pressure ranges from 50 to 190 mm $H_2O$. Variation of pressure with deep respiration provides assurance that fluid flow into the manometer is unobstructed. Opening pressure in bacterial meningitis ranges from 200 to 500 mm $H_2O$.

The CSF is normally clear and colorless but may appear cloudy or turbid in patients with increased concentrations of white blood cells ($> 200/mm^3$), red blood cells ($> 400/mm^3$), bacteria ($> 10^5$ colony-forming units /mL), or protein. In patients with a traumatic tap, an initially bloody CSF should clear as the flow of CSF continues.

### Cell Count

The normal CSF white blood cell (WBC) count in children and adults is 0 to $5/mm^3$. The CSF WBCs may be slightly higher in neonates. In a study of uninfected neonates aged 0–28 days, the median count was 3 WBCs/$mm^3$, but it was up to $19/mm^3$ (95th percentile). It decreased to a median of 2 WBCs/

**Table 2.1** Typical cerebrospinal fluid findings in patients with selected infectious causes of meningitis

| | WBC count (cells/mm³) | Primary cell type | Glucose (mg/dL) | Protein (mg/dL) |
|---|---|---|---|---|
| Normal range | 0–5[a] | | 0.6[b] | < 50 |
| Acute viral meningitis | 50–1,000 | Mononuclear | > 45 | < 200 |
| Acute bacterial meningitis | 1,000–5,000 | Neutrophilic | < 40 | 100–500 |
| Neurosyphilis | >10 | Mononuclear | Decreased | Elevated |
| Lyme meningitis | < 500 | Mononuclear | Normal | < 620 |
| Primary amebic meningoencephalitis[c] | Elevated | Neutrophilic | Decreased | Elevated |
| *Angiostrongylus cantonensis* meningitis | Elevated | Eosinophilic (16–72%) | Normal | Elevated |
| Tuberculous meningitis | 50–300 | Mononuclear | < 45 | 50–300 |
| Cryptococcal meningitis | 20–500 | Mononuclear | < 40 | > 45 |
| Coccidioidal meningitis | < 700 | Mononuclear or eosinophilic | Decreased | Elevated |

*Abbreviations:* CSF, cerebrospinal fluid; RBC, red blood cell; WBC, white blood cell
[a]May be up to 10/mm³ in neonates.
[b]Ratio of CSF glucose to blood glucose. A value of less than 0.5 should be considered abnormal.
[c]A high RBC count in CSF is commonly seen.

mm³. The 95th percentile was 9 WBCs/mm³.[1] The CSF WBC count may be increased after neurosurgical procedures. Elevations of CSF WBC counts can occur in patients with traumatic lumbar puncture or in patients with intracerebral or subarachnoid hemorrhage. In these situations, the following formula should be used as a correction factor for the true WBC count in the presence of CSF red blood cells (RBCs):

Corrected WBC in CSF =
Total WBC in CSF – (WBC in Blood × RBC in CSF/RBC in Blood)

### Glucose and Protein

The actual CSF glucose concentration may be falsely low in the presence of hypoglycemia; therefore, the CSF glucose should always be compared with a simultaneous serum glucose; the normal ratio of CSF glucose to serum glucose is approximately 0.6, and ratios of less than 0.5 should be considered abnormal. Lumbar CSF protein concentrations greater than 50 mg/dL and ventricular CSF concentrations greater than 15 mg/dL are considered abnormal.

A CSF glucose concentration of less than 34 mg/dL, a ratio of CSF glucose to blood glucose of less than 0.23, a CSF protein concentration greater than 220 mg/dL, a CSF leukocyte count of more than 2,000/mm³, or a CSF neutrophil count of more than 1,180/mm³ is highly predictive of bacterial meningitis.[2]

### CSF Culture

From 1 to 2 mL of CSF specimen should be sent for bacterial culture, and optimally from 5 to 10 mL for mycobacterial and fungal culture.

### Other Diagnostic Methods

Many immunologic tests and nucleic acid amplification tests are useful for the evaluation of CNS infections. Please refer to each section for details.

## Acute Meningitis/Ventriculitis

### Microbiology

Common organisms and useful diagnostic tests are shown in **Table 2.2**.

### Viral Meningitis

Enteroviruses (primarily echoviruses and coxsackieviruses) are the most common cause of viral meningitis. HSV can also cause a viral meningitis. HSV-2 meningitis is generally seen with a primary genital outbreak. HSV-1 may also cause viral meningitis. When this is recurrent it is thought to be a cause of Mollaret's meningitis, which is defined as a benign, recurrent lymphocytic meningitis. Other herpesviruses, including HSV-1, varicella-zoster virus (VZV), cytomegalovirus (CMV), Epstein-Barr virus (EBV), and human herpesviruses types 6, 7, and 8 (HHV-6, -7, -8), cause aseptic meningitis and encephalitis. Aseptic meningitis and encephalitis due to mumps are commonly seen in unimmunized patients. From 5 to 10% of patients infected with human immunodeficiency virus (HIV) develop acute viral meningitis either when the virus is acquired or during the seroconversion phase.[4] Arthropod-borne viruses, such as West Nile virus, cause meningoencephalitis in areas of endemicity.

### Bacterial Meningitis

*Streptococcus pneumoniae* is the most common organism. *S. pneumoniae*, *Neisseria meningitidis*, *S. aureus*, other streptococci, *Listeria monocytogenes*, and *Haemophilus* species account for most of the community-acquired meningeal pathogens.[5] Hospital-acquired meningitis typically occurs after neurosurgical procedures. Postoperative CSF leak and traumatic CSF leak are known risk factors for meningitis. About half of cases are caused by gram-negative bacilli (primarily *Pseudomonas aeruginosa*, *Klebsiella* species, and *Escherichia coli*). *S. aureus* and coagulase-negative staphylococci are also common.

### Spirochetal Meningitis

*Treponema pallidum* invades the CNS during early infection. Early infections may result in cranial nerve palsies and particularly a facial nerve palsy. Clinical neurosyphilis is divided into four distinct syndromes: syphilitic meningitis and meningovascular syphilis usually occur within 5 years of infection, whereas parenchymatous neurosyphilis and gummatous neurosyphilis occur 10 to 20 years after infection.

*Borrelia burgdorferi* usually disseminates to the CNS early in infection. From 10 to 15% of patients with Lyme disease have nervous system involvement, including lymphocytic meningitis, in the third stage, several months to years after initial infection.[6]

### Amebic Meningitis

*Naegleria fowleri* and *Acanthamoeba* species are the common organisms. *N. fowleri* usually lives in freshwater. It causes a rapidly fatal meningoencephalitis in healthy persons with recreational freshwater exposure. Granulomatous amebic encephalitis with *Acanthamoeba* species occurs in immunocompromised patients subacutely.

### Helminthic Meningitis

*Angiostrongylus cantonensis* and *Gnathostoma spingerum* are the most common organisms of eosinophilic meningitis outside Europe and North America.[7] They are acquired by eating infected hosts (i.e., snails or freshwater prawns for *A. cantonensis*, undercooked freshwater fish or chicken for *G. spingerum*).

### Diagnosis

Tests that should be sent routinely when acute meningitis is suspected are summarized in **Table 2.3**. Additional tests should be considered based on suspected organisms.

### Viral Meningitis

*Cerebrospinal Fluid*

Viral meningitis usually causes a lymphocytic pleocytosis with mildly elevated protein and decreased glucose concentrations; however, one study reported that about half of patients with viral meningitis had a neutrophil predominance in the CSF for more than 24 hours after the onset

**Table 2.2** Common organisms of acute meningitis and useful diagnostic tests

| Organisms | Risk factors/ areas of endemicity | Tests CSF | Tests Blood |
|---|---|---|---|
| **Viruses** | | | |
| Nonpolio enteroviruses | | PCR | |
| HSV-1, HSV-2, VZV | | PCR | |
| CMV | Immunocompromised | PCR | |
| Epstein-Barr virus | Immunocompromised | PCR | |
| Mumps virus | Unimmunized | | Complement fixation, hemagglutination inhibition |
| West Nile virus | United States | WNV-specific IgM by ELISA, PCR | |
| St. Louis encephalitis virus | United States | Anti-St. Louis encephalitis virus IgM antibodies | Anti-St. Louis encephalitis virus IgM antibodies |
| HIV | Sexual contact, intravenous drug use | | HIV ELISA (negative in acute phase), PCR |
| **Bacteria** | | | |
| Streptococcus pneumoniae | | Bacterial culture | Blood culture |
| Neisseria meningitidis | | Bacterial culture | Blood culture |
| Streptococcus agalactiae | | Bacterial culture | |
| Haemophilus influenzae | | Bacterial culture | |
| Listeria monocytogenes | | Bacterial culture | Blood culture |
| Staphylococcus aureus | Surgical procedures | Bacterial culture | |
| Coagulase-negative staphylococci | Surgical procedures | Bacterial culture | |
| Gram-negative rods | Surgical procedures | Bacterial culture | |
| Propionibacterium acnes | Surgical procedures | Bacterial culture | |
| Mycobacterium tuberculosis | Prior residence or travel in a country with a high prevalence of TB, known contact, IVDA | AFB culture | |
| **Spirochetes** | | | |
| Treponema pallidum | Sexual contact | VDRL | |
| Borrelia burgdorferi | Tick bite | Western blot | ELISA (screening) |
| **Amebae, helminths** | | | |
| Naegleria fowleri | Swimming in freshwater | CSF wet mount, PCR | |
| Angiostrongylus cantonensis | Travel history to the South Pacific and Southeast Asia | Microscopic exam | |

*Abbreviations:* AFB, acid-fast bacillus; CMV, cytomegalovirus; CSF, cerebrospinal fluid; ELISA, enzyme-linked immunosorbent assay; HIV, human immunodeficiency virus; HSV, herpes simplex virus; IgM, immunoglobulin M; PCR, polymerase chain reaction; VDRL, Venereal Disease Research Laboratory; VZV, varicella-zoster virus; WNV, West Nile virus

**Table 2.3** Routine tests for cerebrospinal fluid in patients with suspected acute meningitis

| |
|---|
| White blood cell count with differential |
| Red blood cell count |
| Glucose concentration |
| Protein concentration |
| Gram stain |
| Bacterial culture |

of symptoms.[8] A CSF neutrophil predominance is not useful as a sole criterion in distinguishing between aseptic and bacterial meningitis. Viral culture is not clinically useful because it takes too long for identification and the sensitivity is low.[9]

*Immunology*

Paired serology is diagnostic for herpes simplex encephalitis and enterovirus infections but is not useful clinically as seroconversion typically takes weeks, emphasizing the importance of polymerase chain reaction (PCR) in the detection of viruses in CSF specimens. Complement fixation and hemagglutination inhibition in serum specimens are the most reliable for mumps meningitis because the viral culture is not practically useful. Testing of paired acute and convalescent sera, collected 2–3 weeks apart, should demonstrate a diagnostic fourfold rise in mumps antibody titer.

*Nucleic Acid Amplification Tests*

PCR is the standard test for the detection of enteroviruses and HSV, VZV, EBV, CMV, or HHV-6 meningoencephalitis. The sensitivity of PCR for HSV encephalitis were 98% and the specificity were 94%.[10] PCR may become positive only a few days after the onset of symptoms.

**Bacterial Meningitis**

*Cerebrospinal Fluid*

The CSF WBC count is usually elevated to 1,000 to 5,000/mm³; however, it can be normal in neonates and in patients with meningococcal or *L. monocytogenes* meningitis. Also, neutrophils usually predominate, although approximately 10% of patients present with a predominance of lymphocytes in the CSF. This is more common in neonatal gram-negative bacillary meningitis and meningitis caused by *L. monocytogenes*.[11] Patients with very low CSF WBC counts (0–20/mm³) despite high CSF bacterial concentrations tend to have a poor prognosis.[12]

Elevated CSF protein and decreased CSF glucose concentrations are seen in bacterial meningitis; however, normal CSF WBC and protein concentrations may be seen in patients with neonatal meningitis and severely immunocompromised patients and in specimens obtained at the onset of symptoms.

*Cerebrospinal Fluid Culture*

Gram stain of the CSF shows bacteria in 90% of *S. pneumoniae* and *Haemophilus influenzae* cases, 75% of *N. meningitidis* cases, 50% of gram-negative bacilli cases, and 24 to 50% of *L. monocytogenes* cases.[13,14] Prior antimicrobial therapy decreases the probability of identifying organisms by 50%.

CSF culture is considered a gold standard. The probability of identifying the organism may be decreased to less than 50% in patients with prior antimicrobial therapy. Fungal culture and acid-fast bacillus (AFB) culture need to be considered in immunocompromised patients or patients with subacute or chronic symptoms.

*Blood Culture*

Blood culture is also crucial to diagnose bacterial meningitis. The causative organism was recovered from 86% of pediatric patients.[15] Blood samples should be drawn at first, even if antimicrobial therapy needs to be started before lumbar puncture because of clinical deterioration.

*Markers of Inflammation*

C-reactive protein (CRP) and serum procalcitonin (PCT) levels were significantly higher in acute bacterial meningitis than in acute viral meningitis.[16,17] The high negative predictive value may be used to rule out bacterial meningitis when CSF analysis is inconclusive and Gram stain is negative.

### Nucleic Acid Amplification Tests

The use of broad-based bacterial PCR in CSF for community-acquired bacterial meningitis has been studied. One study showed 59% sensitivity and 97% specificity.[19] This test may be useful for excluding bacterial meningitis or when patients have received prior antimicrobial therapy.

## Spirochetal Meningitis

### Treponema pallidum

CSF abnormalities are common in syphilitic meningitis.

The sensitivity of CSF Venereal Disease Research Laboratory (VDRL) testing is 30 to 70%, but it is very specific. A reactive CSF VDRL test is sufficient to diagnose neurosyphilis, but a nonreactive result does not exclude the diagnosis.[20] Serum RPR for VDRL should be monitored for a fourfold decrease in titers over 6–12 months. CSF WBCs and VDRL should also improve and eventually return to normal after treatment.

### Borrelia burgdorferi

Lyme meningitis typically causes lymphocytic pleocytosis with elevated protein concentration. Enzyme-linked immunosorbent assay (ELISA) with *B. burgdorferi* antigen is recommended for the initial screening test. If it is positive, the diagnosis should be confirmed with Western blot of the CSF specimen because of the high number of false-positive reactions.[21] If the suspicion is high and Western blot is negative, this should be repeated in 2 weeks. If the Western blot confirms the diagnosis of Lyme disease and there is concern for Lyme meningitis, then a lumbar puncture should be performed. This usually causes a lymphocytic pleocytosis. CSF should be evaluated for intrathecal antibodies against *Borrelia burgdorferi*. CSF PCR could also support this diagnosis.

## Amebic Meningitis

Primary amebic meningoencephalitis usually reveals a neutrophilic pleocytosis with a low glucose level, high protein level, and red blood cells.

The Gram stain is not useful. The CSF specimen should be stained with Giemsa or Wright stain to identify trophozoites. The value of serologic testing is variable.

## Helminthic Meningitis

Fifty percent of cases of *A. cantonensis* meningitis show an eosinophilic pleocytosis with a high protein level. Larvae may sometimes be found on microscopy of the CSF in *A. cantonensis* meningitis. The sensitivity and specificity of serologic studies are variable.[7]

## ■ Shunt Infections

### Microbiology

Coagulase-negative staphylococci are the most common organisms.[22] *S. aureus*; gram-negative bacteria, including *Acinetobacter*, *E. coli*, *Klebsiella pneumoniae*, and *Pseudomonas aeruginosa*; diphtheroids, such as *Propionibacterium acnes*; and anaerobes are also seen.[23] Gram-negative organisms are commonly found in specimens from patients with shunts terminating in the peritoneal cavity.[24] Shunt infections due to *Candida* species may be seen in immunocompromised patients, patients receiving broad-spectrum antimicrobial therapy, and those with indwelling bladder or intravenous catheters.[25]

### Diagnosis

### Cerebrospinal Fluid

Leukocytosis is seen in 80% of shunt infections.[26] Leukocyte counts in CSF obtained by lumbar puncture or valve puncture tend to be higher than those in ventricular CSF. Progressively decreasing CSF glucose and increasing CSF protein accompanied by advancing CSF pleocytosis suggest infection even if all cultures are negative.

## Cultures

### Cerebrospinal Fluid Culture

Microorganisms are recovered more often from valve puncture CSF specimens and ventricular CSF specimens than from lumbar CSF specimens. The diagnosis may be more difficult when the distal portion of the shunt is infected.

### Blood Culture

Blood cultures should be obtained in patients with ventriculoatrial shunts because blood cultures are positive in more than 90% of cases.[27]

## Nucleic Acid Amplification Tests

Banks et al reported that CSF PCR was positive and cultures were negative in 49% of cases. Most of these cases had received prolonged intravenous antibiotics previously.[28] There was no positive culture result with negative CSF PCR. The PCR method has not yet been standardized; however, it can be considered when all cultures are negative despite suggestive symptoms and CSF cell analysis.

# ■ Hardware Infection

Many types of hardware are placed in neurosurgical procedures, including deep brain stimulation surgery, as well as in bone flaps and shunts.

## Microbiology

*S. aureus* is the most common organism.[29] *P. acnes* and gram-negative rods, including *Acinetobacter baumannii* and *P. aeruginosa*, are also reported.

## Diagnosis

The most useful cultures are intraoperative specimens. Superficial cultures may be difficult to interpret because the most common pathogens are also skin flora.

# ■ Chronic Meningitis/Ventriculitis

## Microbiology

Common organisms and diagnostic tests for chronic meningitis are shown in **Table 2.4**.

## Bacterial Meningitis

Tuberculous meningitis is the most common form of chronic meningitis. It is difficult to diagnose, sometimes requiring empiric treatment.

## Fungal Meningitis

Cryptococcal meningitis is the most common fungal meningitis. Coccidioidal meningitis is endemic in the American Southwest. Brief exposure of visitors from outside the area of endemicity can result in the acquisition of meningeal disease. The Midwest and Southeast in the United States are the major areas where histoplasmosis is endemic. Other forms of fungal meningitis are usually seen in immunocompromised patients.

## Amebic Meningitis

Granulomatous meningitis due to *Acanthamoeba* species may cause symptoms over a period of weeks to months. It is usually seen in those who are immunocompromised due to other diseases, such as diabetes, alcoholism, cirrhosis, HIV, chemotherapy, or transplantation.

## Diagnosis

### Bacterial Meningitis

#### Cerebrospinal Fluid

The CSF in tuberculous meningitis usually shows lymphocytic pleocytosis with a low glucose level. Adenosine deaminase (ADA) may be elevated, but it is not useful to distinguish tuberculous meningitis from bacterial meningitis.[30] The most common strains use the acid-fast properties of mycobacteria. These include the Ziehl-Neelson stain and the Kinyoun stain. The sensitivity of these stains is 25%. The sensi-

**Table 2.4** Common organisms of chronic meningitis and the diagnostic tests

| Organisms | Risk factors/ areas of endemicity | Tests | |
|---|---|---|---|
| | | CSF | Others |
| **Bacteria** | | | |
| Coagulase-negative staphylococci | Neurosurgery | Culture | |
| *Mycobacterium tuberculosis* | Microbacterial culture (5–10 mL), TB PCR[b] | AFB culture (5–10 mL) | PPD, interferon gamma release assays |
| *Actinomyces* | Immunocompromise, dental infection | Anaerobic culture | Pathology |
| *Nocardia*[a] | Immunocompromise | Culture | |
| **Fungi** | | | |
| *Cryptococcus neoformans* | HIV | Antigen, india ink, culture | Antigen |
| *Coccidioides immitis* | Arizona, California | Complement fixation test, culture | |
| *Histoplasma capsulatum* | Midwest, Southeast | Anti-*Histoplasma* antibodies, culture | Urine antigen, serum antigen |
| *Candida* species | Immunocompromise | Culture | |
| *Sporothrix schenckii* | Immunocompromise, skin injury | Culture | Skin biopsy |
| *Blastomyces dermatitidis* | Southeastern and central states | Antigen, culture | |
| **Virus** | | | |
| Echovirus | X-linked agammaglobulinemia | Viral culture | |
| **Parasites** | | | |
| *Angiostrongylus cantonensis* | Travel history | Microscopic exam | |

*Abbreviations:* AFB, acid-fast bacillus; CSF, cerebrospinal fluid; HIV, human immunodeficiency virus; PPD, purified protein derivative

[a]Usually occurs with brain abscesses. The microbiology laboratory should be informed when nocardial infection is suspected because the use of selective media is preferable and requires prolonged incubation.

[b]If a larger sample can be obtained and centrifuged, the pellet may have a higher yield.

tivity of culture for these organisms ranges from 18–83%.[31] Many studies of the use of PCR have been carried out; however, the method and the interpretation have not yet been standardized.

Organisms are not frequently recovered from lumbar CSF in patients with postoperative chronic meningitis; however, they may be found on implanted material when it is removed.

### Tuberculin Skin Test and Interferon Gamma Release Assay

These tests are appropriate to diagnose latent tuberculosis; however, neither can be used to support or exclude the diagnosis of meningitis because of insufficient sensitivity and specificity.[32]

## Fungal Meningitis

Generally, a large amount of CSF is required to increase the sensitivity of fungal CSF culture. Immunologic tests should be also considered based on the potential organisms.

In cryptococcal meningitis, the opening pressure is often elevated. If the opening pressure is ≥ 25 cm $H_2O$ and there are symptoms of elevated intracranial pressure, it may require serial drainage or even placement of a lumbar drain. Cryptococcal polysaccharide antigen testing in serum and CSF is widely used because of high accuracy.[33] The CSF is more often positive than the serum for antigen. India ink smears of CSF are positive in 50% of patients without acquired immunodeficiency syndrome (AIDS) and more than 80% of patients with AIDS. *Cryptococcus neoformans* is generally recovered from CSF cultures in 3 to 7 days in untreated patients.

In coccidioidal meningitis, the complement fixation test in CSF is very sensitive and specific. CSF culture and smear are not commonly positive.

In *Histoplasma* meningitis, anti-*Histoplasma* antibodies in the CSF are found in 80% of cases. At least 10 mL of CSF should be sent for culture to recover *Histoplasma*. The serum or urine *Histoplasma* antigen test is useful if patients have disseminated histoplasmosis.[34] If the result is positive, it would support this diagnosis.

## Amebic Meningitis

If there is a space-occupying lesion and evidence of intracranial pressure, a lumbar puncture should not be performed. If it can be done safely, then a wet mount should be performed. A Giemsa stain may reveal *Acanthamoeba*. If available, PCR may make the diagnosis of *Balamuthia*. However, if these are negative, a brain biopsy has the highest diagnostic yield.

## ■ Encephalitis

Distinguishing among encephalitis, encephalopathy, and postinfectious immune-mediated processes is challenging because of the nonspecific clinical presentations.

The common causes of infectious encephalitis are described in **Table 2.5**.

The CSF opening pressure, cell count with differential, and protein and glucose concentrations should be measured, and Gram stain, bacterial cultures, and PCR studies for HSV and VZV should be performed in immunocompetent patients. Lymphocytic pleocytosis with a normal glucose level and an elevated protein level are generally seen in the CSF of patients with viral encephalitis.

In immunocompromised patients, CSF PCR for CMV and HHV-6 should be performed. PCR for JC virus, HIV, and EBV should also be considered. The specificity of viral CSF cultures is very high, although the sensitivity is quite low.

## ■ Brain Abscess

### Microbiology

The causative organisms frequently depend on the predisposing conditions (**Table 2.6**). Brain abscess can occur after cranial operations, including craniotomy and brain biopsy.[35] The incidence of brain abscess after intracranial procedures ranges from 0.2% to 0.6%.[35,36]

Streptococci are the organisms most commonly cultured from patients with brain abscess.[37] They are frequently isolated in mixed infections. *S. aureus*, *P. acnes*, Enterobacteriaceae (e.g., *Proteus* species, *E. coli*, *Klebsiella* species, and *Pseudomonas* species), and *Clostridium* species are also commonly found in patients after neurosurgery.[35,38] Infection due to anaerobes and polymicrobial infection are commonly seen in brain abscess related to dental infection or otogenic infection.

Nocardial brain abscess may occur as an isolated CNS lesion or as part of disseminated infection in association with a pulmonary or cutaneous lesion. *Mycobacterium tuberculosis,* nontuberculous mycobacteria, and *Toxoplasma gondii* have been observed in HIV patients and non-HIV patients. *Candida* species have emerged as the most prevalent fungal agents.[39] Most cases of aspergillosis and mucormycosis occur in severely immu-

**Table 2.5** Common Organisms of Encephalitis and the Diagnostic Tests

| Organisms | Risk Factors/ Areas of Endemicity | Tests | |
|---|---|---|---|
| | | **CSF** | **Others** |
| **Viruses** | | | |
| HSV-1, VZV | | PCR | |
| HHV-6 | Immunocompromised | PCR | |
| Nonpolio enteroviruses | Neonates, hypogammaglobulinemia, summer | PCR | |
| CMV | Immunocompromised | PCR | |
| WNV | United States | WNV-specific IgM by ELISA | |
| JC virus | HIV | PCR | |
| EBV | Immunocompromised | PCR | |
| St. Louis encephalitis virus | North and South America | Anti-St. Louis encephalitis virus IgM antibodies | Anti-St. Louis encephalitis virus IgM antibodies, viral culture of brain tissue, 4-fold rise in serum antibodies |
| EEE virus | North and South America | Anti-EEE virus IgM antibodies | IgM antibodies, 4-fold rise in serum antibodies |
| California encephalitis group of viruses | North America | Anti-California encephalitis group of viruses IgM antibodies | IgM antibodies, 4-fold rise in serum antibodies |
| **Bacteria** | | | |
| *Mycoplasma pneumoniae* | | PCR | |
| *Mycobacterium tuberculosis*[a] | | PCR, AFB culture | |

*Abbreviations:* AFB, acid-fast bacillus; CMV, cytomegalovirus; CSF, cerebrospinal fluid; EBV, Epstein-Barr virus; EEE, Eastern equine encephalitis; ELISA, enzyme-linked immunosorbent assay; HHV, human herpesvirus; HIV, human immunodeficiency virus; HSV, herpes simplex virus; IgM, immunoglobulin M; PCR, polymerase chain reaction; VZV, varicella-zoster virus; WNV, West Nile virus

[a]Usually presents as meningoencephalitis.

nocompromised patients. Several protozoa and helminths, such *Trypanosoma cruzi*[40] and *Entamoeba histolytica*,[41] have been reported to produce brain abscess.

### Diagnosis

#### Cultures

Stereotactic computed tomography (CT)–guided aspiration facilitates the microbiological diagnosis and guides antimicrobial therapy.

At the time of aspiration, specimens should be sent for Gram stain, routine aerobic and anaerobic cultures, and fungal culture. If a fungal infection is strongly suspected, special stains (e.g., mucicarmine, Grocott-Gomori methenamine-silver nitrate) should be performed. Acid-fast stains with cultures for mycobacteria and *Nocardia* should be sent to the lab if these organisms are suspected. The microbiology laboratory should always be informed when nocardiosis is suspected because

**Table 2.6**  Predisposing conditions and common organisms of brain abscess

| Predisposing conditions | Common organisms |
|---|---|
| Neurosurgery or trauma | *Staphylococcus aureus*, streptococci, *Propionibacterium acnes*, Enterobacteriaceae, *Clostridium* species |
| Otogenic infection or sinusitis | Streptococci, Enterobacteriaceae, *Haemophilus* species, *Bacteroides* species, *Prevotella* species |
| Dental infection | Streptococci, *Fusobacterium* species, *Prevotella* species, *Actinomyces* species, *Bacteroides* species |
| Lung abscess or empyema | Streptococci, *Nocardia* species, *Fusobacterium* species, *Bacteroides* species, *Prevotella* species |
| Bacterial endocarditis | Streptococci, *Staphylococcus aureus* |
| Human immunodeficiency virus infection | *Toxoplasma gondii*, *Cryptococcus neoformans*, *Mycobacterium* species |
| Immunosuppressant use | *Aspergillus* species, *Candida* species, *Scedosporium* species, gram-negative rods, *Nocardia* species |

the diagnosis may be missed using routine laboratory methods. Fungi can often be identified by the appearance in tissue even if the cultures are negative. Ideally, both culture and histologic examination should be done together.

Multiple sequenced 16S ribosomal DNA PCR amplification revealed more types of bacteria than routine cultures in one study.[42] The detection of fastidious organisms, such as *Mycoplasma hominis* and *Fusobacterium necrophorum*, was more rapid with molecular detection. Molecular techniques can be used for patients with negative cultures likely due to prior antibiotic use.

### Immunology

Elevated anti-*Toxoplasma* immunoglobulin G antibody aids the diagnosis in an immunosuppressed host (mainly with AIDS) who has characteristic neuroradiographic abnormalities.

## ■ Subdural Empyema/ Cranial Epidural Abscess/ Suppurative Intracranial Thrombophlebitis

### Microbiology

#### Subdural Empyema

The most common conditions predisposing to cranial subdural empyema are otorhinologic infections.[43] Subdural empyema also occurs after head trauma or neurosurgery.

Common organisms include streptococci, staphylococci, aerobic gram-negative bacilli, and anaerobes.[44] Polymicrobial infections are common. Postoperative and posttraumatic infections are more commonly caused by staphylococci and aerobic gram-negative bacilli.[45] Also, *P. acnes* is isolated after trauma and neurosurgical procedures.

## Cranial Epidural Abscess/Suppurative Intracranial Thrombophlebitis

Cranial epidural abscess is often accompanied by cranial subdural empyema because cranial epidural abscess can cross the cranial dura along emissary veins. Suppurative intracranial thrombophlebitis frequently occurs in association with subdural empyema, epidural abscess, or bacterial meningitis. Therefore, the causative organisms of cranial epidural abscess and suppurative intracranial thrombophlebitis are usually similar to those of cranial subdural empyema. Cranial epidural abscess may also occur after fetal scalp monitoring and halo pin penetration.[46]

### Diagnosis

### Cultures

Cranial subdural empyema and epidural abscesses usually require neurosurgical exploration in addition to antimicrobial agents. Aerobic and anaerobic cultures of purulent material are needed to direct the specific antimicrobial therapy.

### Cerebrospinal Fluid

A lumbar puncture with CSF analysis is contraindicated in patients with subdural empyema because it may precipitate cerebral herniation.[47] Also, CSF cultures are negative unless subdural empyema is complicated by bacterial meningitis.

## ■ Vertebral Osteomyelitis/ Spondylodiskitis/ Spinal Epidural Abscess/ Spinal Subdural Empyema

### Microbiology

Vertebral osteomyelitis and spondylodiskitis, infection of the intervertebral disk, can be hematogenous or continuous to a soft tissue infection. Spinal epidural abscess usually occurs hematogenously or by local extension from vertebral osteomyelitis. It can also occur postoperatively.

*S. aureus* is overall the most common microorganism.[48] Coagulase-negative staphy-lococci and gram-negative rods, including *E. coli* and *P. aeruginosa*, are sometimes recovered from patients with prolonged bacteremia.[48,49] Isolation of coagulase-negative staphylococci, *P. acnes*, gram-negative rods, and *Candida* species is frequently associated with spinal surgeries. Anaerobes and gram-negative rods are recovered when infections are adjacent to soft tissue, such as in a sacral decubitus ulcer. The possibility of tuberculous spondylitis (Pott disease), usually a result of past hematogenous foci, should be considered, especially in areas of endemicity.

Spinal subdural empyema is very uncommon. It occurs hematogenously or contiguously.[50] The most frequent microbial isolate is *S. aureus*.

### Diagnosis

### Cultures

#### Blood Culture

Blood cultures are crucial when vertebral osteomyelitis is suspected. Positive blood cultures occur in 30 to 78% of cases.[51]

#### Tissue Culture

A biopsy is warranted if blood cultures are negative or when polymicrobial osteomyelitis is suspected. Biopsy specimens should be cultured for aerobic and anaerobic bacteria and for fungi. Cultures for mycobacteria or *Brucella* should be performed if the patient has risk factors. For mycobacteria this would include immunosuppression or a mycobacterial infection at another site. For *Brucella*, this would include exposure to domestic farm animals or consumption of raw meat or unpasteurized milk products. Open biopsy has a sensitivity ranging from 75% to 93%.[52,53] On the other hand, the sensitivity of CT-guided percutaneous biopsy is 50%.

### Markers of Inflammation

The erythrocyte sedimentation rate and C-reactive protein level are increased in 98 and 100% of cases, respectively.[52,54] Therefore, a negative value is helpful to rule out vertebral osteomyelitis when cultures are negative.

# References

1. Kestenbaum LA, Ebberson J, Zorc JJ, Hodinka RL, Shah SS. Defining cerebrospinal fluid white blood cell count reference values in neonates and young infants. Pediatrics 2010;125(2):257–264
2. Spanos A, Harrell FE Jr, Durack DT. Differential diagnosis of acute meningitis. An analysis of the predictive value of initial observations. JAMA 1989;262(19):2700–2707
3. Kupila L, Vuorinen T, Vainionpää R, Hukkanen V, Marttila RJ, Kotilainen P. Etiology of aseptic meningitis and encephalitis in an adult population. Neurology 2006;66(1):75–80
4. de Almeida SM, Letendre S, Ellis R. Human immunodeficiency virus and the central nervous system. Braz J Infect Dis 2006;10(1):41–50
5. McMillan DA, Lin CY, Aronin SI, Quagliarello VJ. Community-acquired bacterial meningitis in adults: categorization of causes and timing of death. Clin Infect Dis 2001;33(7):969–975
6. Halperin JJ. Neurologic manifestations of Lyme disease. Curr Infect Dis Rep 2011;13(4):360–366 [epub ahead of print]
7. Ramirez-Avila L, Slome S, Schuster FL, et al. Eosinophilic meningitis due to *Angiostrongylus* and *Gnathostoma* species. Clin Infect Dis 2009; 48(3):322–327
8. Negrini B, Kelleher KJ, Wald ER. Cerebrospinal fluid findings in aseptic versus bacterial meningitis. Pediatrics 2000;105(2):316–319
9. Polage CR, Petti CA. Assessment of the utility of viral culture of cerebrospinal fluid. Clin Infect Dis 2006;43(12):1578–1579
10. Lakeman FD, Whitley RJ; National Institute of Allergy and Infectious Diseases Collaborative Antiviral Study Group. Diagnosis of herpes simplex encephalitis: application of polymerase chain reaction to cerebrospinal fluid from brain-biopsied patients and correlation with disease. J Infect Dis 1995;171(4):857–863
11. Mylonakis E, Hohmann EL, Calderwood SB. Central nervous system infection with *Listeria monocytogenes*. 33 years' experience at a general hospital and review of 776 episodes from the literature. Medicine (Baltimore) 1998;77(5):313–336
12. Pagliano P, Fusco U, Attanasio V, et al. Pneumococcal meningitis in childhood: a longitudinal prospective study. FEMS Immunol Med Microbiol 2007;51(3):488–495
13. Gray LD, Fedorko DP. Laboratory diagnosis of bacterial meningitis. Clin Microbiol Rev 1992;5(2):130–145
14. Brouwer MC, van de Beek D, Heckenberg SG, Spanjaard L, de Gans J. Community-acquired *Listeria monocytogenes* meningitis in adults. Clin Infect Dis 2006;43(10):1233–1238
15. Coant PN, Kornberg AE, Duffy LC, Dryja DM, Hassan SM. Blood culture results as determinants in the organism identification of bacterial meningitis. Pediatr Emerg Care 1992;8(4):200–205
16. Ibrahim KA, Abdel-Wahab AA, Ibrahim AS. Diagnostic value of serum procalcitonin levels in children with meningitis: a comparison with blood leukocyte count and C-reactive protein. J Pak Med Assoc 2011;61(4):346–351
17. Alkholi UM, Abd Al-Monem N, Abd El-Azim AA, Sultan MH. Serum procalcitonin in viral and bacterial meningitis. J Glob Infect Dis 2011;3(1): 14–18
18. Saha SK, Darmstadt GL, Yamanaka NP, et al. Rapid diagnosis of pneumococcal meningitis: implications for treatment and measuring disease burden. Pediatr Infect Dis J 2005;24(12):1093–1098
19. Welinder-Olsson C, Dotevall L, Hogevik H, et al. Comparison of broad-range bacterial PCR and culture of cerebrospinal fluid for diagnosis of community-acquired bacterial meningitis. Clin Microbiol Infect 2007;13(9):879–886
20. Hook EW III, Marra CM. Acquired syphilis in adults. N Engl J Med 1992;326(16):1060–1069
21. Wormser GP, Dattwyler RJ, Shapiro ED, et al. The clinical assessment, treatment, and prevention of Lyme disease, human granulocytic anaplasmosis, and babesiosis: clinical practice guidelines by the Infectious Diseases Society of America. Clin Infect Dis 2006;43:1086–1134
22. Naradzay JF, Browne BJ, Rolnick MA, Doherty RJ. Cerebral ventricular shunts. J Emerg Med 1999;17(2):311–322
23. Sacar S, Turgut H, Toprak S, et al. A retrospective study of central nervous system shunt infections diagnosed in a university hospital during a 4-year period. BMC Infect Dis 2006;6:43
24. Shapiro S, Boaz J, Kleiman M, Kalsbeck J, Mealey J. Origin of organisms infecting ventricular shunts. Neurosurgery 1988;22(5):868–872
25. Montero A, Romero J, Vargas JA, et al. *Candida* infection of cerebrospinal fluid shunt devices: report of two cases and review of the literature. Acta Neurochir (Wien) 2000;142(1):67–74
26. Conen A, Walti LN, Merlo A, Fluckiger U, Battegay M, Trampuz A. Characteristics and treatment outcome of cerebrospinal fluid shunt-associated infections in adults: a retrospective analysis over an 11-year period. Clin Infect Dis 2008;47(1):73–82
27. Kaufman BA. Infections of cerebrospinal fluid shunts. In: Scheld WM, Whitley RJ, Durack DT, eds. Infections of the Central Nervous System. 2nd ed. Philadelphia, PA: Lippincott–Raven Publishers; 1997:555–577
28. Banks JT, Bharara S, Tubbs RS, et al. Polymerase chain reaction for the rapid detection of cerebrospinal fluid shunt or ventriculostomy infections. Neurosurgery 2005;57(6):1237–1243, discussion 1237–1243
29. Boviatsis EJ, Stavrinou LC, Themistocleous M, Kouyialis AT, Sakas DE. Surgical and hardware complications of deep brain stimulation. A seven-year experience and review of the literature. Acta Neurochir (Wien) 2010;152(12):2053–2062
30. Tuon FF, Higashino HR, Lopes MI, et al. Adenosine deaminase and tuberculous meningitis—a systematic review with meta-analysis. Scand J Infect Dis 2010;42(3):198–207
31. van Well GT, Paes BF, Terwee CB, et al. Twenty years of pediatric tuberculous meningitis: a retrospective cohort study in the western cape of South Africa. Pediatrics 2009;123(1):e1–e8
32. Park SY, Jeon K, Um SW, Kwon OJ, Kang ES, Koh WJ. Clinical utility of the QuantiFERON-TB Gold

In-Tube test for the diagnosis of active pulmonary tuberculosis. Scand J Infect Dis 2009;41(11-12):818–822

33. Goodman JS, Kaufman L, Koenig MG. Diagnosis of cryptococcal meningitis. Value of immunologic detection of cryptococcal antigen. N Engl J Med 1971;285(8):434–436

34. Wheat LJ, Musial CE, Jenny-Avital E. Diagnosis and management of central nervous system histoplasmosis. Clin Infect Dis 2005;40(6):844–852

35. McClelland S III, Hall WA. Postoperative central nervous system infection: incidence and associated factors in 2111 neurosurgical procedures. Clin Infect Dis 2007;45(1):55–59

36. Korinek AM; Service Epidémiologie Hygiène et Prévention. Risk factors for neurosurgical site infections after craniotomy: a prospective multicenter study of 2944 patients. The French Study Group of Neurosurgical Infections, the SEHP, and the C-CLIN Paris-Nord. Neurosurgery 1997;41(5):1073–1079, discussion 1079–1081

37. Prasad KN, Mishra AM, Gupta D, Husain N, Husain M, Gupta RK. Analysis of microbial etiology and mortality in patients with brain abscess. J Infect 2006;53(4):221–227

38. Lu CH, Chang WN, Lin YC, et al. Bacterial brain abscess: microbiological features, epidemiological trends and therapeutic outcomes. QJM 2002;95(8):501–509

39. Cortez KJ, Walsh TJ. Space-occupying fungal lesions. In: Scheld WM, Whitley RJ, Marra CM, eds. Infections of the Central Nervous System. 3rd ed. Philadelphia, PA: Lippincott Williams & Wilkins; 2004:713–734

40. Yoo TW, Mlikotic A, Cornford ME, Beck CK. Concurrent cerebral American trypanosomiasis and toxoplasmosis in a patient with AIDS. Clin Infect Dis 2004;39(4):e30–e34

41. Morishita A, Yamamoto H, Aihara H. A case of amebic brain abscess. No Shinkei Geka 2007;35(9):919–925

42. Al Masalma M, Armougom F, Scheld WM, et al. The expansion of the microbiological spectrum of brain abscesses with use of multiple 16S ribosomal DNA sequencing. Clin Infect Dis 2009;48(9):1169–1178

43. Silverberg AL, DiNubile MJ. Subdural empyema and cranial epidural abscess. Med Clin North Am 1985;69(2):361–374

44. Dill SR, Cobbs CG, McDonald CK. Subdural empyema: analysis of 32 cases and review. Clin Infect Dis 1995;20(2):372–386

45. Dashti SR, Baharvahdat H, Spetzler RF, et al. Operative intracranial infection following craniotomy. Neurosurg Focus 2008;24(6):E10

46. Papagelopoulos PJ, Sapkas GS, Kateros KT, Papadakis SA, Vlamis JA, Falagas ME. Halo pin intracranial penetration and epidural abscess in a patient with a previous cranioplasty: case report and review of the literature. Spine (Phila Pa 1976) 2001;26(19):E463–E467

47. Nathoo N, Nadvi SS, van Dellen JR, Gouws E. Intracranial subdural empyemas in the era of computed tomography: a review of 699 cases. Neurosurgery 1999;44(3):529–535, discussion 535–536

48. Zimmerli W. Clinical practice. Vertebral osteomyelitis. N Engl J Med 2010;362(11):1022–1029

49. Bhavan KP, Marschall J, Olsen MA, Fraser VJ, Wright NM, Warren DK. The epidemiology of hematogenous vertebral osteomyelitis: a cohort study in a tertiary care hospital. BMC Infect Dis 2010;10:158

50. De Bonis P, Anile C, Pompucci A, Labonia M, Lucantoni C, Mangiola A. Cranial and spinal subdural empyema. Br J Neurosurg 2009;23(3):335–340

51. Mylona E, Samarkos M, Kakalou E, Fanourgiakis P, Skoutelis A. Pyogenic vertebral osteomyelitis: a systematic review of clinical characteristics. Semin Arthritis Rheum 2009;39(1):10–17

52. Jensen AG, Espersen F, Skinhøj P, Frimodt-Møller N. Bacteremic *Staphylococcus aureus* spondylitis. Arch Intern Med 1998;158(5):509–517

53. Nolla JM, Ariza J, Gómez-Vaquero C, et al. Spontaneous pyogenic vertebral osteomyelitis in nondrug users. Semin Arthritis Rheum 2002;31(4):271–278

54. Khan MH, Smith PN, Rao N, Donaldson WF. Serum C-reactive protein levels correlate with clinical response in patients treated with antibiotics for wound infections after spinal surgery. Spine J 2006;6(3):311–315

# 3

# Antibiotics and the Development of Resistance

Peter D. Kim and Walter A. Hall

Since their introduction into medical practice, antibiotics have played an enormous role in decreasing morbidity from bacterial infection and have therefore been invaluable in neurosurgical practice. Entities such as meningitis and brain abscess, which were associated with high mortality rates before antibiotic therapy, are now frequently cured with appropriate combinations of surgery and antibiotic therapy. Because of the immune-privileged nature of the central nervous system (CNS), the common use of implanted devices, and the frequent use of steroids, infection is of great concern in neurosurgical practice; therefore, the rational, effective use of antibiotics is of great importance. An understanding of antibiotic mechanisms of action and the mechanisms with which microbes develop resistance is essential for the neurosurgeon.

The intelligent use of antibiotics is crucial for the successful prevention and management of infections. The principle of using the agent with the narrowest spectrum for the least amount of time to eradicate a particular infection is well recognized, but not universally practiced. The lack of a definitive culture is often an impediment to successful treatment. Additionally, the incorrect assumption that antibiotics with broad coverage are more effective than an appropriate narrow-spectrum antibiotic against a particular microbial species can lead to antibiotic misuse. Vancomycin, for example, is no more effective against methicillin-sensitive *Staphylococcus aureus* than either cephazolin or oxacillin.

A second key principle for therapeutic success is that, although the excessive use of antibiotics should be avoided, complete eradication of an infection is necessary for a successful clinical outcome. Therefore, surgical treatment is necessary if hardware is involved (that may be removed), such as a cerebrospinal fluid (CSF) shunt or an intrathecal catheter. Similarly, if a suppurative collection exists, such as a bacterial brain abscess, subdural empyema, or cranial epidural abscess that is too large for antibiotic penetration, surgical evacuation is necessary. Attempting to treat an infection through medical management only, such as in the case of a partially drained abscess[1] or an infected CSF shunt that is not removed,[2] can often result in a recurrent infection.

In the practice of surgery, antibiotics have played an enormous role in preventing surgical site infections and in the provision of effective surgical treatment. Antibiotic prophylaxis, which is discussed in Chapter 14, is standard practice in neurosurgery. Postoperative infections, when they do occur, are treatable with antibiotics, although reoperation is often essential. Of course, antibiotic prophylaxis will not compensate for poor sterile technique, and in the case of contamination from a breach or from penetrating cerebral trauma, infections are likely to occur. Failure of wound healing due to lapses in surgical technique, poor nutritional status, or CSF fistula offers a portal for bacterial invasion that will occur despite antibiotic prophylaxis. In these circumstances, the identification of the infectious agent and its sensitivities is critical for the successful eradication of the infection, as is the removal of any modifiable risk factors for the development of infection.

In treating infections of the CNS, the concept of the blood–brain barrier (BBB) plays an important role. Antibiotic penetration into the central nervous system (CNS) is variable, which can influence antibiotic selection, although the BBB may be compromised during infection, allowing hydrophilic antibiotics to enter the CSF. Vancomycin and the fluoroquinolones, which are lipophilic molecules, cross the BBB particularly well. Aminoglycosides and β-lactam antibiotics are hydrophilic and therefore do not penetrate the BBB very easily. Intraventricular or intrathecal administration of antibiotics can provide direct entry into the CSF space; however, the presence of external ventricular drainage or a lumbar drain is required for drug instillation. Intraventricular antibiotics have been suggested both as treatment for ventriculitis[3] and for prophylaxis at the time of surgery to prevent shunt infection.[4] β-Lactam antibiotics can be epileptogenic and are therefore generally not administered via an intraventricular route despite their relatively poor penetration of the BBB.[5]

Allergies may also play a role in the choice of which antibiotic to use. Patients with chronic diseases may have had exposure to multiple antibiotics, with the opportunity to develop multiple sensitivities to the drugs. The specifics of a patient's reaction to a particular allergy are important to note because some reactions may not be true allergies, and others, such as "red man syndrome" from vancomycin, may not preclude the use of the agent if it is given in concert with diphenhydramine.

Antibiotic resistance has been extensively discussed both in the scientific literature and the popular media, and its importance cannot be overstated. The rise in the prevalence of methicillin-resistant *Staphylococcus aureus* (MRSA) has been well documented. In the United States from 1975 to 1991, the rate of MRSA infections in the hospital setting rose from 2.4 to 29%.[6] Additionally, the incidence of community-associated MRSA infections has been on the rise.[7] By the following decade, MRSA infections were estimated to account for approximately 2% of all hospital admissions.[8] Vancomycin was developed with the intention that it would be highly resistant to the development of bacterial resistance, and its name is based on the fact that its developers thought that the resistant bacteria might be vanquished. Despite these high hopes, strains of vancomycin-resistant enterococci (VRE) and some strains of *S. aureus* that are vancomycin intermediate (VISA) or vancomycin resistant (VRSA) have been isolated. The newer drug linezolid is the first line in the treatment of infections resistant to vancomycin; however, the increased use of linezolid will no doubt ultimately lead to the development of strains resistant to this antibiotic.

Antibiotics are categorized into classes based on their structure and mechanisms of action. Antibiotics can further be classified as bacteriocidal or bacteriostatic. Bacteriostatic agents depend on the functional immune system to destroy the bacteria but may be as effective as bacteriocidal drugs in the right setting. The mechanisms and spectra of commonly used antibiotics are listed in **Table 3.1**.

Antibiotic resistance occurs via multiple mechanisms (see **Table 3.1**). Resistance to β-lactam antibiotics occurs when bacteria express β-lactamase, an enzyme that simply breaks down the drug. Bacterial circumvention of the toxicity of several antibiotics occurs when the bacteria synthesize altered proteins that do not bind the drugs. This phenomenon occurs in resistance to aminoglycoside and macrolide antibiotics. A third mechanism of resistance involves the use of efflux pumps, such as in tetracycline resistance.

Genes for antibiotic resistance are often encoded on plasmids, which are extrachromosomal elements that replicate stably in bacterial hosts.[9] Many plasmids are capable of conjugation, a process in which rapid transfer of the plasmid occurs between bacteria. Conjugation can occur

**Table 3.1** Antibiotics commonly used in central nervous system infections

| Class | Examples | Spectrum | Mechanism of action | Mechanism of resistance |
|-------|----------|----------|---------------------|------------------------|
| Aminoglycosides | Gentamycin, tobramycin | Gram-negative | Protein synthesis | Altered protein |
| Macrolides | Azithromycin | Gram-positive (including intracellular) | Protein synthesis | Altered protein |
| Fluoroquinolones | Levofloxacin, gatifloxacin, ciprofloxacin | Broad | DNA replication | Altered protein |
| β-Lactams | Penicillins, cephalosporins, meropenem | Gram-positive→broad | Cell wall formation | β-Lactamase |
| Glycopeptide | Vancomycin | Gram-positive (including MRSA) | Cell wall formation | Altered peptide |
| Oxazoladinones | Linezolid | Gram-positive (including VRE) | Protein synthesis | Altered rRNA, efflux pump |
| Nitroamidazole | Metronidazole | Anaerobic | DNA breakdown | Decreased activation |

*Abbreviations*: MRSA, methicillin-resistant *Staphylococcus aureus*; rRNA, ribosomal RNA; VRE, vancomycin-resistant enterococci

across a wide array of species and can even occur from gram-negative to gram-positive bacteria and vice versa.

Because of the ease with which antibiotic resistance can spread from site to site within the body and between patients, the control of reservoirs of antibiotic resistance can be helpful in reducing hospital-acquired infections and those at the surgical site. Of utmost importance is rigorous adherence to protocols aimed at reducing the spread of antibiotic-resistant bacteria from patient to patient. Hand washing and gel-based decontamination, when practiced, reduce the prevalence of MRSA and other antibiotic-resistant bacterial strains within the hospital setting.[10] Intranasal mupirocin administered preoperatively for decolonization of MRSA has been demonstrated in the orthopedic literature to reduce the rate of surgical site infections[11] and may be useful in neurosurgical procedures. In settings with a high risk for MRSA infection, vancomycin is probably a better choice for preoperative prophylaxis than is cefazolin.[12]

The timing of antibiotic administration is another important consideration. In general, antibiotic administration should be delayed until a culture of the suspected site of infection has been obtained. The rate at which antibiotic administration decreases culture sensitivity is not known for most situations; however, unless the patient is critically ill and culture cannot be obtained in a timely fashion, it is reasonable in most situations to wait for the culture results. A frustrating situation arises when a known infection is being treated but positive cultures are not available from which to tailor antibiotic treatment. The length of treatment with antibiotics is also important because the premature cessation of treatment will often lead to the recurrence of infection and may place the patient at risk for antibiotic resistance. The timing of antibiotic administration in presurgical prophylaxis has been intensively scrutinized, and many institutions have protocols in place to maximize the effectiveness of pre-surgical antibiotics.

Antibiotic-impregnated materials have also been used in an attempt to prevent colonization and the subsequent infection of hardware. Shunt tubing impregnated with rifampin and clindamycin (Bactiseal; Codman, Raynham, Massachusetts) has been used with reports of success in lowering the rate of device-associated infection.[13-16] Increased antibiotic resistance in isolates from infections that do occur have not been reported, but that possibility is at least a theoretical consideration. Data regarding similar antibiotic-impregnated external ventricular drains are less clear in revealing a therapeutic benefit.[17] Antibiotic-coated sutures (Vicryl Plus; Ethicon, San Angelo, Texas ) are also available, and they may decrease the rate of postoperative infection.[18]

## ■ Conclusion

The prevention and treatment of infections are an important part of neurosurgical practice. The optimal use of antibiotics is important in managing patients and in preventing the development and spread of antibiotic-resistant strains. Despite the availability of multiple classes of antimicrobial agents with diverse mechanisms of action, resistance will invariably develop with extensive antibiotic use and can spread rapidly within the hospital environment. Strict attention to hygiene, with pre- and postoperative protocols, can reduce surgical site infections. Appropriate treatment when infections do occur lowers the risk for recurrence and the spread of antibiotic-resistant pathogens.

Obviously, the neurosurgeon will not have the background of the microbiologist or pharmacologist when choosing an antibiotic regimen. For that reason, it is important for the neurosurgeon to work in concert with the infectious disease specialists and the pharmacist when necessary to devise treatment regimens for patients with infections of the CNS.

## References

1. Kondziolka D, Duma CM, Lunsford LD. Factors that enhance the likelihood of successful stereotactic treatment of brain abscesses. Acta Neurochir (Wien) 1994;127(1-2):85–90
2. Simon TD, Hall M, Dean JM, Kestle JR, Riva-Cambrin J. Reinfection following initial cerebrospinal fluid shunt infection. J Neurosurg Pediatr 2010;6(3):277–285
3. Tängdén T, Enblad P, Ullberg M, Sjölin J. Neurosurgical gram-negative bacillary ventriculitis and meningitis: a retrospective study evaluating the efficacy of intraventricular gentamicin therapy in 31 consecutive cases. Clin Infect Dis 2011;52(11):1310–1316
4. Gruber TJ, Riemer S, Rozzelle CJ. Pediatric neurosurgical practice patterns designed to prevent cerebrospinal fluid shunt infection. Pediatr Neurosurg 2009;45(6):456–460
5. Nau R, Sörgel F, Eiffert H. Penetration of drugs through the blood-cerebrospinal fluid/blood-brain barrier for treatment of central nervous system infections. Clin Microbiol Rev 2010;23(4):858–883
6. Panlilio AL, Culver DH, Gaynes RP, et al. Methicillin-resistant *Staphylococcus aureus* in U.S. hospitals, 1975-1991. Infect Control Hosp Epidemiol 1992;13(10):582–586
7. David MZ, Daum RS. Community-associated methicillin-resistant *Staphylococcus aureus*: epidemiology and clinical consequences of an emerging epidemic. Clin Microbiol Rev 2010;23(3):616–687 Review
8. David MZ, Medvedev S, Hohmann SF, Ewigman B, Daum RS. Increasing burden of methicillin-resistant *Staphylococcus aureus* hospitalizations at US academic medical centers, 2003-2008. Infect Control Hosp Epidemiol 2012;33(8):782–789
9. Firshein W, Kim P. Plasmid replication and partition in *Escherichia coli*: is the cell membrane the key? Mol Microbiol 1997;23(1):1–10
10. Sakamoto F, Yamada H, Suzuki C, Sugiura H, Tokuda Y. Increased use of alcohol-based hand sanitizers and successful eradication of methicillin-resistant *Staphylococcus aureus* from a neonatal intensive care unit: a multivariate time series analysis. Am J Infect Control 2010;38(7):529–534
11. Rao N, Cannella BA, Crossett LS, Yates AJ Jr, McGough RL III, Hamilton CW. Preoperative screening/decolonization for *Staphylococcus aureus* to prevent orthopedic surgical site infection: prospective cohort study with 2-year follow-up. J Arthroplasty 2011;26(8):1501–1507
12. Tacconelli E, Cataldo MA, Albanese A, et al. Vancomycin versus cefazolin prophylaxis for cerebrospinal shunt placement in a hospital with a high prevalence of meticillin [sic]-resistant *Staphylococcus aureus*. J Hosp Infect 2008;69(4):337–344
13. Eymann R, Chehab S, Strowitzki M, Steudel WI, Kiefer M. Clinical and economic consequences of antibiotic-impregnated cerebrospinal fluid shunt catheters. J Neurosurg Pediatr 2008;1(6):444–450

14. Hayhurst C, Cooke R, Williams D, Kandasamy J, O'Brien DF, Mallucci CL. The impact of antibiotic-impregnated catheters on shunt infection in children and neonates. Childs Nerv Syst 2008;24(5):557–562
15. Parker SL, Attenello FJ, Sciubba DM, et al. Comparison of shunt infection incidence in high-risk subgroups receiving antibiotic-impregnated versus standard shunts. Childs Nerv Syst 2009;25(1):77–83, discussion 85
16. Sciubba DM, Stuart RM, McGirt MJ, et al. Effect of antibiotic-impregnated shunt catheters in decreasing the incidence of shunt infection in the treatment of hydrocephalus. J Neurosurg 2005;103(2, Suppl)131–136
17. Sonabend AM, Korenfeld Y, Crisman C, Badjatia N, Mayer SA, Connolly ES Jr. Prevention of ventriculostomy-related infections with prophylactic antibiotics and antibiotic-coated external ventricular drains: a systematic review. Neurosurgery 2011;68(4):996–1005
18. Rozzelle CJ, Leonardo J, Li V. Antimicrobial suture wound closure for cerebrospinal fluid shunt surgery: a prospective, double-blinded, randomized controlled trial. J Neurosurg Pediatr 2008;2(2):111–117

# 4

# Radiology of Central Nervous System Infections

**Kunal M. Patel and Charles L. Truwit**

Imaging plays a central role in the evaluation of patients with central nervous system (CNS) infections. This is particularly true in the neurosurgical patient, in whom postoperative infections, although rare, can be fatal if not promptly identified and treated.[1] Computed tomography (CT) often serves as a key first test in the critically ill patient. Magnetic resonance (MR) imaging is the modality of choice in the evaluation of suspected CNS infection because of its superior contrast resolution and increased sensitivity in detecting meningeal disease, infarction, and posterior fossa pathology. Ultrasound (US) has a very limited role and is applicable only in infants with an open anterior fontanelle; however, it can provide valuable information in the right setting without the ionizing radiation of CT or sedation requirement of MR.[2]

## ▪ Diffuse Central Nervous System Infections

### Meningitis

Acute bacterial meningitis is inflammation of the meninges caused by bacterial microorganisms that seed the leptomeninges through hematogenous spread (most common mechanism), local spread from an adjacent nidus of infection, retrograde perineural spread, or direct introduction from a recent procedure, surgery, or trauma. Cerebrospinal fluid (CSF) studies from a lumbar puncture (LP) are often diagnostic, but neuroimaging is useful to exclude other pathologies, identify complications, and confirm the diagnosis in an equivocal setting.

CT is usually pursued in the evaluation of an acutely comatose patient, but scans are often normal in the setting of acute bacterial meningitis. Specific signs of meningitis include high density in the subarachnoid space (similar to hemorrhage) and effacement of the basilar cisterns.[3] On contrast-enhanced CT scans, leptomeningeal enhancement may be seen.[3] In addition to enhancement of the basal cisterns, occasionally enhancement of the subarachnoid space between the horizontal folia of the vermis may lead one to the diagnosis. CT can also be diagnostic of the complications of meningitis, such as hydrocephalus, subdural effusions (often seen in infants) and empyema, infarction (venous or arterial), and abscess formation.[3] Before LP, CT should be performed to identify the cause of increased intracranial pressure, such as diffuse cerebral edema, hydrocephalus, and cerebral herniation.

MR imaging is far superior to CT in visualizing the abnormalities of bacterial meningitis. The inflammatory exudate of meningitis is often isointense on T1-weighted images and hyperintense on T2-weighted images compared with adjacent parenchyma. Unenhanced fluid-attenuated inversion recovery (FLAIR) images may be abnormal, reflecting altered protein content of the CSF and/or inflammation of the leptomeninges; however, they are unfortunately often normal. Contrast-enhanced FLAIR images are extremely sensitive, and likely more so than conventional T1-weighted post-contrast images, in detecting early leptomeningeal inflammation. Contrast-enhanced T1-weighted images are, however, more specific in detecting associated parenchymal abnormalities and should be retained in MR protocols focused on CNS infection.[4] Diffuse pachymeningeal enhancement should be interpreted with caution in the post-LP setting because this finding has been reported in 1% of all patients after uncomplicated LP procedures.[5]

Diffusion-weighted imaging (DWI) is extremely sensitive in the early detection of arterial infarction from meningitis-induced vasospasm, or subdural empyema (**Fig. 4.1**), and venous infarction secondary to venous or dural sinus thrombosis. The area of infarction develops increased signal on FLAIR and T2-weighted images 12 to 24 hours later. In the acute stage, subcortical T2-hyperintensity is the key finding in meningitis-induced cortical venous infarction.

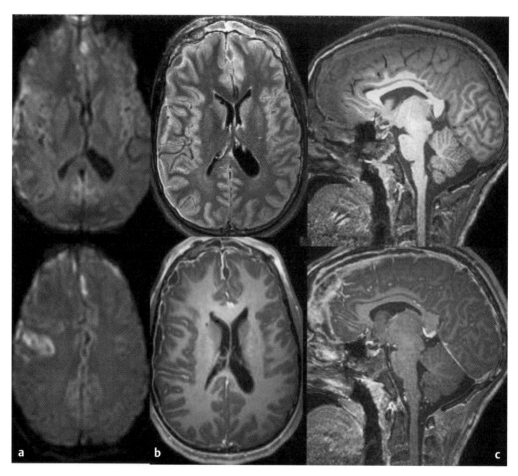

**Fig. 4.1a–c** Subdural empyema with venous infarction. Diffusion-weighted images **(a)** show foci of restricted diffusion that reflect bacterial meningitis, subdural empyema, and venous infarction related to cortical venous thrombosis. Axial fluid-attenuated inversion recovery (FLAIR) and contrast-enhanced T1-weighted **(b)** magnetic resonance images show multiloculate rim-enhancing subdural fluid collections with extension to interhemispheric fissure. Sagittal T1-weighted images pre- and post-contrast **(c)** show isointense thrombus, as well as filling defect within contrast enhancement of the anterior aspect of the superior sagittal sinus. (Images courtesy of C. Truwit, MD.)

MR angiography and MR venography may be considered when arterial or venous infarction is suggested on standard MR pulse sequences. Spread of subdural empyema into the interhemispheric fissure presages a potentially ominous course of the disease.

Viral or "aseptic" meningitis is typically caused by enteroviruses, and neurologic deficits are uncommon. Because imaging studies are usually normal, they are not part of routine work-up. Occasionally, subtle meningeal enhancement can be detected on post-contrast turboFLAIR MR images (**Fig. 4.2**).

Tuberculous (TB) meningitis is increasing in incidence in the United States because of immigration from areas of endemicity, acquired immunodeficiency syndrome (AIDS), and multidrug resistance. This infection is typically a secondary infection from a primary pulmonary source and is the most common form of CNS TB. High rates of morbidity and mortality from TB meningitis and its predilection for infants and children make early diagnosis and treatment imperative. CT has a limited role in detecting TB meningitis.

The classic MR finding of TB meningitis (**Fig. 4.3**) is marked nodular thickening and enhancement of the meninges at the base of the brain (in distinction to bacterial meningitis, which involves the convexities to a greater extent). This MR finding is often difficult to distinguish from the MR appearance of neurosarcoidosis, carcinomatous meningitis, and fungal meningitis. Associated tuberculomas are often seen and are characterized by single or multiple intraparenchymal masses with variable enhancement. Nodular meningeal thickening in addition to tuberculomas is highly suggestive of CNS TB. Vasculitis and subsequent infarction can result from infiltration of the exudate into the perivascular spaces. DWI is invaluable in the early detection of this complication.[3]

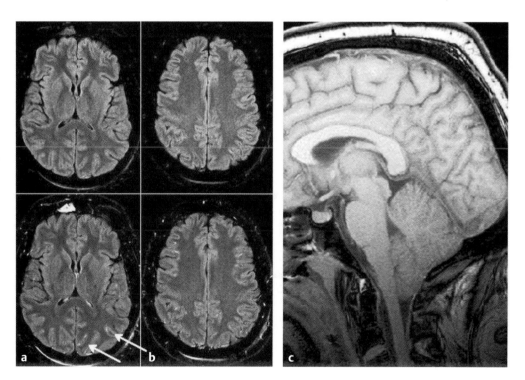

**Fig. 4.2a–c** Meningitis. Pre-contrast **(a)** and post-contrast **(b)** fluid-attenuated inversion recovery (FLAIR) images show subtle leptomeningeal enhancement (*arrows*). Subsequent lumbar puncture (LP) revealed aseptic meningitis. Low-lying cerebellar tonsils were incidentally noted on sagittal T1-weighted image **(c)**, indicating a Chiari I malformation. Patient did not have an adverse outcome after LP. (Images courtesy of C. Truwit, MD.)

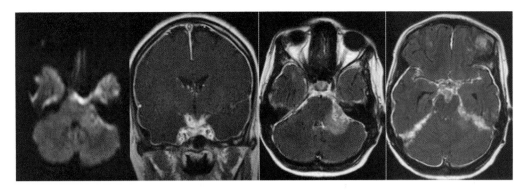

**Fig. 4.3** Tuberculous meningitis. Diffusion-weighted image (far left) shows mildly restricted diffusion in the left cerebellopontine angle cistern. Coronal and axial contrast-enhanced T1-weighted images reveal marked nodular enhancement of the meninges in the basilar cisterns with extension into the left middle cerebellar peduncle. No discrete tuberculoma was present in this patient, who had recently emigrated from Mexico. (Images courtesy of C. Truwit, MD.)

Fungal meningitis, like TB meningitis, must be considered in immunocompromised patients. Numerous organisms are included under this umbrella term, and imaging findings are often nonspecific. In cryptococcal meningitis, dilated perivascular spaces in the deep gray nuclei maybe seen on MR. With time, these may evolve into gelatinous pseudocysts. Absence of enhancement is typical in an AIDS patient. As the patient's immune status improves after initiation of antiretroviral therapy, enhancement may appear in the areas of signal abnormality. In the angioinvasive form of zygomycosis (mucormycosis), a stroke protocol MR with MR angiography may be useful in evaluating complications such as arteritis, arterial occlusion with or without infarction, and mycotic aneurysms.[6] CT has no established diagnostic role in the specific diagnosis of fungal meningitis.

### Encephalitis

Encephalitis is most commonly caused by viruses. The location of parenchymal abnormality depends on the specific pathogen.

Herpes encephalitis results from reactivation of the herpes simplex virus in immunocompetent patients, has a predilection for the limbic system, and carries a high mortality rate (50–70%). CT is often normal, especially early in the disease course. In the late acute or subacute stage, CT may show low attenuation in the temporal lobes and insula. Hemorrhage on CT is often a late finding and is associated with a poor prognosis.

The best imaging clue on MR is increased signal on T2 and FLAIR images in the limbic system cortical and subcortical areas (particularly medial temporal and inferior frontal), with relative sparing of the white matter and basal ganglia (**Fig. 4.4**). Limbic encephalitis can have a similar MR appearance, although a history of primary malignancy (often lung) and subacute onset of symptoms distinguish it from herpes encephalitis. Additionally, the constellation of DWI restriction, cingulate gyrus involvement, and contralateral temporal lobe involvement is highly suggestive of herpes encephalitis.[7] Although bilateral signal abnormalities are present in 60% of cases in the acute stage, findings are often more prominent on one side.[6] In the setting of hemorrhage, susceptibility-weighted sequences (such as T2* images) show "blooming" of decreased signal in the areas of edematous brain.[7] Atrophy is a typical finding in the chronic or treated stage of herpes encephalitis.

Human immunodeficiency virus (HIV) encephalitis and progressive multifocal leukoencephalopathy (PML) are discussed in the section of this chapter on immunocompromised patients.

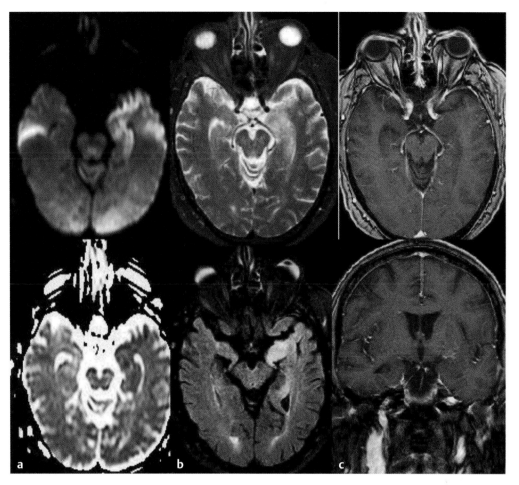

**Fig. 4.4a–c** Herpes encephalitis. Axial diffusion-weighted image, apparent diffusion coefficient (ADC) map **(a)**, and T2-weighted and fluid-attenuated inversion recovery (FLAIR) **(b)** images show asymmetric restricted diffusion and altered signal in the medial left temporal lobe and hippocampus. No significant enhancement is seen on post-contrast axial and coronal T1-weighted images **(c)**. Cerebrospinal fluid analysis confirmed herpes simplex virus. (Images courtesy of C. Truwit, MD.)

## Prion Diseases

Creutzfeldt-Jacob disease (CJD) is a rare, transmissible spongiform encephalopathy that is invariably fatal. On MR, symmetric FLAIR hyperintensity in the caudate and putamen with relative sparing of the pre- and postcentral gyri is typical in this condition. Thalamic involvement is less common in CJD than in variant CJD (vCJD), also known as bovine spongiform encephalopathy (BSE).

BSE, also known as mad cow disease, is a chronic neurodegenerative disease that affects the CNS of cattle. There is strong ev-

idence that vCJD is linked to the consumption of meat produced from BSE-infected cattle. In contrast to the classic form of CJD, vCJD affects younger patients (mean age, 28 years) and is characterized by prominent psychiatric and sensory symptoms.[8] Two classic findings are often present on the MR images of patients with vCJD (**Fig. 4.5**). The "pulvinar sign" arises from a relative T2 hyperintensity in the pulvinar of the thalamus compared with the anterior putamen, whereas the "hockey stick sign" is the result of symmetric pulvinar and dorsomedial thalamic nuclear hyperintensity.

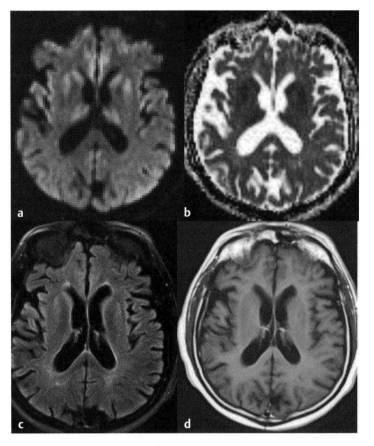

**Fig. 4.5a–d** Variant Creutzfeldt-Jakob disease (vCJD). "Hockey" sign is characterized by symmetric pulvinar and dorsomedial thalamic restricted diffusion **(a,b)** and fluid-attenuated inversion recovery (FLAIR) hyperintensity **(c)**. Note absence of contrast enhancement **(d)**. This is highly suggestive of vCJD. (Images courtesy of C. Truwit, MD.)

## ◼ Focal Central Nervous System Infections

### Cerebritis/Abscess

The progression of focal unencapsulated cerebritis to a discrete abscess has been established in animal models.[6] Four typical stages (early and late cerebritis, early and late capsule) are recognized, although it is rare to see all four stages clinically. The imaging findings of each stage are unique and outlined below.

- *Early cerebritis.* This stage classically presents 3 to 5 days after the onset of infection and is char-

acterized pathologically by tissue edema, vascular congestion, microscopic hemorrhage, and early necrosis without tissue destruction.[9] MR imaging typically shows focal but ill-defined and poorly marginated areas of edema (T1-hypointense and T2-hyperintense signal abnormality) with mild or no contrast enhancement. If microhemorrhages are present, areas of "blooming" may be seen on susceptibility-weighted images. CT is often normal or may show areas of low attenuation and local mass effect evidenced by sulcal effacement or ventricular compression.

- *Late cerebritis.* This stage classically presents 4 to 14 days after onset and is characterized pathologically by necrosis with tissue destruction, inflammatory cells, and granulation tissue.[9] Compared with the findings in early cerebritis, the area involved now has a necrotic core on CT and MR, with an irregular and a thin enhancing rim and perilesional vasogenic edema.
- *Early capsule.* This stage classically presents 2 to 4 weeks after the onset of infection and is characterized pathologically by increased collagen deposition along the liquefied necrotic margin.[9] On CT and MR, a thick-walled rim is seen, as is nearly homogeneous enhancement. There is greater vasogenic edema and mass effect from the larger necrotic core;

smaller adjacent daughter abscesses may also be seen.
- *Late capsule.* This stage classically presents more than a month after the onset of infection and is characterized pathologically by three capsule layers: an inner layer of gelatinous material, a middle layer of collagen, and an outer layer of gliosis.[9] On CT and MR, the capsule appears thicker, but the central core is much smaller, with significant regression in adjacent mass effect and edema.

In the equivocal setting, DWI is often used to help distinguish between abscess and intracranial neoplasm (**Fig. 4.6**). The central core of most bacterial abscesses demonstrates restricted diffusivity attributed to the highly cellular macromolecular contents within the cavity. MR spectrosco-

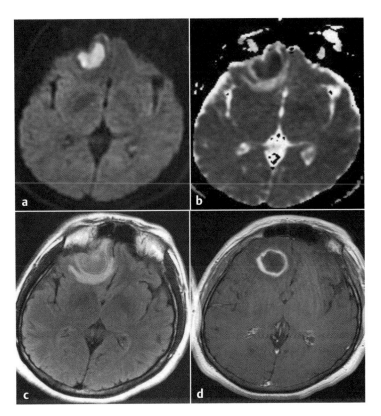

**Fig. 4.6a–d** Brain abscess. Axial diffusion weighted image **(a)** and apparent diffusion coefficient (ADC) map **(b)** reveal restricted diffusion in right frontal mass. TurboFLAIR **(c)** and contrast-enhanced T1-weighted **(d)** images show altered intralesional signal and rim enhancement, all of which are typical of bacterial abscess, as was confirmed at surgery. (Images courtesy of C. Truwit, MD.)

py can also be helpful because the central necrotic area of an abscess may show the presence of amino acids, such as succinate and acetate, that are not typically present in neoplasms.[4]

## ■ Special Conditions and Populations

### Immunocompromised Patients

HIV encephalitis is the most common CNS complication in HIV patients and is present in 30% of them. Diffuse, centrally located, nonenhancing periventricular white matter lesions are present. Detection of these white matter lesions and cortical atrophy on MR is highly suggestive of HIV encephalitis despite the absence of enhancement. MR spectroscopy can be helpful in the equivocal setting. Interrogation of the white matter abnormalities often reveals decreased N-acetyl-aspartate (NAA) levels as measured by reduced NAA-to-choline and NAA-to-creatine ratios; this is attributed to neuronal loss.[6] CT is often normal, although it may show volume loss and should be considered only to exclude other pathologies in an HIV patient.

PML is an opportunistic infection by the papovavirus (JC virus) that is seen almost exclusively in immunocompromised patients. MR findings include patchy, nonenhancing white matter lesions that can mimic the findings of HIV encephalitis. However, the abnormalities in PML (**Fig. 4.7**) are asymmetric and peripheral, as opposed to the bilateral and central abnormalities seen in HIV encephalitis.

Toxoplasmosis results from reactivation of the soil protozoan *Toxoplasma gondii* in the CNS of an immunocompromised host. On MR, it is characterized by a T2 centrally hypointense lesion with a nodular enhancing rim and significant adjacent edema (**Fig. 4.8**). The presence of an enhancing nodule within the enhancing rim (target sign) is highly suggestive of toxoplasmosis.[10] MR spectroscopy can show a prominent lipid peak, but this test is not typically necessary.

Cerebral aspergillosis is a serious infectious process that has an associated mortality rate approaching nearly 100% in immunocompromised patients. On MR, aspergillosis is characterized by multifocal lesions demonstrating a random distribution that relates to the angioinvasive character of the disease.[11] Intralesional hemorrhage (**Fig. 4.9**) is a key imaging finding in a significant percentage of cases. Although often evident on T2-weighted and gradient echo images, susceptibility-weighted imaging appears to be the most reliable test for elucidating such hemorrhage.

### Developing Nations and Immigrants

Neurocysticercosis is a CNS infection caused by the larval form of the pork tapeworm *Taenia solium*. Although this organism is endemic in Latin America, Asia, Africa, and Eastern Europe, its incidence in the United States is increasing as a consequence of immigration and travel. This infection is characterized by four pathologic stages.

- *Vesicular.* The viable larva forms a single cyst or a cluster of cysts within the ventricles or subarachnoid space of the brain and spinal cord (**Fig. 4.10**). When the larva is in the subarachnoid space (subarachnoid neurocysticercosis), viable cysts are seen. MR typically shows fluid collections with CSF-like intensity that may or may not reveal the scolex. When such lesions are no longer viable, grapelike clusters (racemose neurocysticercosis) can be seen. Foci of subjacent leptomeningeal enhancement may be seen, but intracystic scolices are not. Typical locations for racemose neurocysticercosis are the sylvian fissures and perimesencephalic and suprasellar cisterns.

- *Colloidal.* In this stage, the larva begins to degenerate, with increased surrounding edema and inflammation. T1 shortening (hyperintensity) is noted within the scolex on MR (**Figs. 4.11, 4.12**). Heterogeneous signal within the cyst may be present,

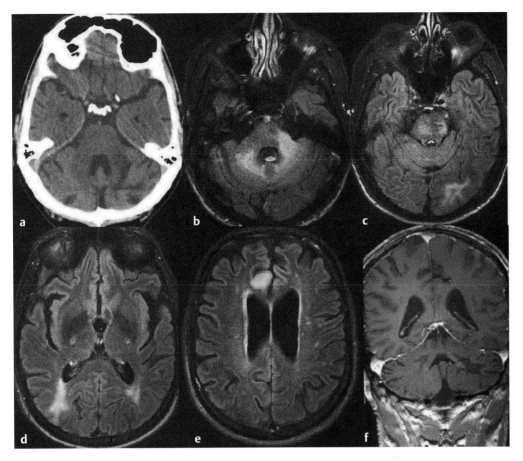

**Fig. 4.7a–f** Progessive multifocal leukoencephalopathy (PML). Axial unenhanced computed tomography **(a)** and fluid-attenuated inversion recovery (FLAIR) magnetic resonance **(b–e)** images show typical features of multifocal, asymmetric, predominantly white matter lesions of the cerebrum and cerebellum. Subtle gray matter hyperintensity is somewhat atypical. Contrast enhancement **(f)** is exceptional in PML. (Images courtesy of C. Truwit, MD.)

most likely reflecting increased turbidity within the cystic cavity. Many complications, such as the development of acute hydrocephalus and associated infarctions, occur during this stage (**Fig. 4.11**). Intraventricular cysts may be mobile, potentially complicating surgical interventions. In such cases, intraoperative CT or MR imaging in the surgical position is recommended.

- *Granular nodular.* This is the healing stage, in which the cyst begins to collapse, with regression of surrounding edema and inflammation. Intense enhancement of the cyst wall and occasional mass effect due to perilesional edema are seen on

MR. Adjacent daughter cysts are common as well.

- *Nodular calcified.* The lesion is completely mineralized in this stage. Appearance is best seen on CT: small calcified nodule with little or no surrounding edema.

Two other patterns are worth noting. Occasional overwhelming infection is seen, typically described as encephalitic neurocysticercosis. Lesions are seen at the gray–white junction of the brain and are typically "too numerous to count." Finally, patients with neurocysticercosis may have concomitant TB. In such cases, a calcified, granulomatous reaction of the basal meninges may be seen.

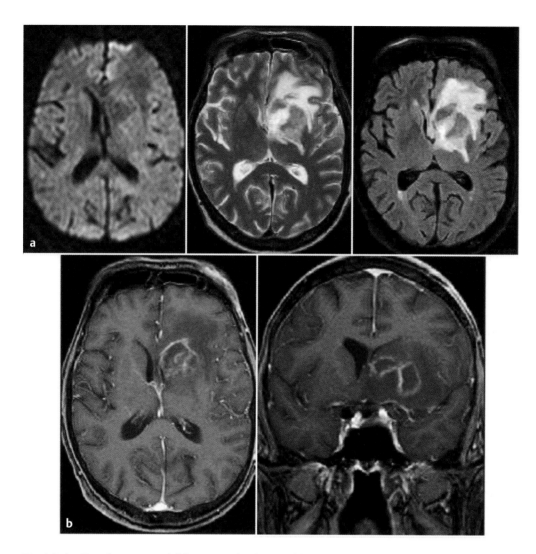

**Fig. 4.8a,b** Toxoplasmosis. Axial diffusion-weighted, T2, and fluid-attenuated inversion recovery (FLAIR) images **(a)** show left caudate head and lentiform nucleus lesions with perilesional vasogenic edema. Note absence of restricted diffusion. Contrast-enhanced axial and coronal T1-weighted images **(b)** show moderate rim enhancement. These features are highly suggestive of toxoplasmosis in this patient with human immunodeficiency virus (HIV) infection and acquired immunodeficiency syndrome (AIDS), although lymphoma could be considered on the basis of the location and imaging characteristics. (Images courtesy of C. Truwit, MD.)

### Pediatric Patients

Today's multidetector CT scanners allow the rapid and efficient imaging of pediatric patients, often without the need for sedation. However, one must consider the potentially harmful long-term side effects of ionizing radiation that CT delivers to young patients. MR offers superior images but typically requires sedation in infants and young children. US is a unique modality in the evaluation of CNS infection in infants that is not applicable in adults.

As in adults, the most common infection in pediatric patients is meningitis. Although the spectrum of pathogens var-

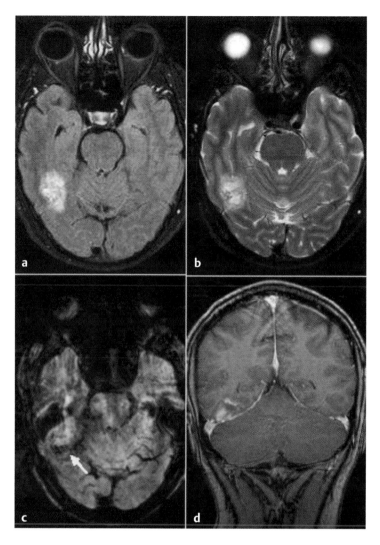

**Fig. 4.9a–d** Aspergillosis. Axial fluid-attenuated inversion recovery (FLAIR) **(a)** and T2-weighted **(b)** images show abnormal focus of hyperintensity within right posterior temporal lobe. Subtle hypointensity (*arrow*) is seen on susceptibility-weighted images **(c)**, reflecting intralesional hemorrhage, typical of aspergilloma. Contrast-enhanced T1-weighted images **(d)** show moderate enhancement. (Images courtesy of C. Truwit, MD.)

ies based on the age group, the CT and MR findings are usually similar to those in adult patients. US can be used to identify and follow ventriculomegaly in infants with hydrocephalus resulting from meningitis. Echogenic sulci, abnormal parenchymal echogenicity, meningeal thickening, and hyperemia have also been reported in infants with bacterial meningitis.[2] In complicated meningitis, subdural effusions are more common in infants than in older children and adults. Additionally, TB meningitis has a strong predilection for pediatric patients, but the imaging findings are similar for both age groups.

Because sinusitis is a very common condition in pediatric patients, intracranial complications from this ailment deserve special attention. These occur in 3.7 to 11% of pediatric patients hospitalized for sinus-

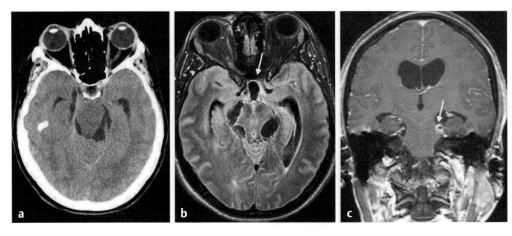

**Fig. 4.10a–c** Racemose neurocysticercosis. Axial computed tomography **(a)** and fluid-attenuated inversion recovery (FLAIR) **(b)** images show abnormal cerebrospinal fluid–like collections around the brainstem, as well as hydrocephalus. Note dilated third ventricle (*arrow*). Coronal contrast-enhanced T1-weighted **(c)** image shows focal enhancement (*arrow*) of the leptomeningeal process along left margin of the midbrain. (Images courtesy of C. Truwit, MD.)

itis and include meningitis, epidural or subdural empyema, cerebritis/abscess, mycotic aneurysm, and infarction.[12] The neuroimaging appearance of these abnormalities is typically similar in pediatric and adult patients. Additionally, orbital involvement by sinusitis can lead to cavernous sinus thrombosis, in which CT and MR imaging show an engorged ipsilateral superior ophthalmic vein, prominent extraocular muscles, and loss of the flow void in the cavernous sinus on T2-weighted images.[13]

### Neurosurgical Patients

### After Craniotomy/Craniectomy

Surgical site infections lead to increased morbidity and mortality and to prolonged hospitalization of the postoperative patient. Although uncomplicated cellulitis at the surgical site typically does not require imaging work-up, superficial surgical site infections may be complicated by osteomyelitis of the bone flap. Deeper extension of the infection may result in meningitis, cerebritis, and abscess.[14] CT is often the initial test of choice in suspected osteomyelitis and shows the lytic and sclerotic changes of the involved bone as well as focal osseous defects, calvarial thickening, and new bone formation. MR is also helpful in diagnosing osteomyelitis, with accuracy rates reported as high as 94%. MR findings of osteomyelitis include an intradiploic mass and heterogeneous T1 and T2 signal of the involved bone. Fat suppression is key in evaluating post-contrast images, which typically show strong but inhomogeneous enhancement of osteomyelitis. Focal absence of enhancement in the center of an avidly enhancing calvaria often suggests necrotic bone or developing abscess, which may prompt percutaneous or surgical management.[15]

### Implanted Devices

Foreign devices implanted into the CNS may also serve as nidi for infection. Because foreign material is known to reduce the host's capacity to resist pathogens, CNS infections in the setting of implanted devices can be rapidly fatal.[16] Permanent indwelling cath-

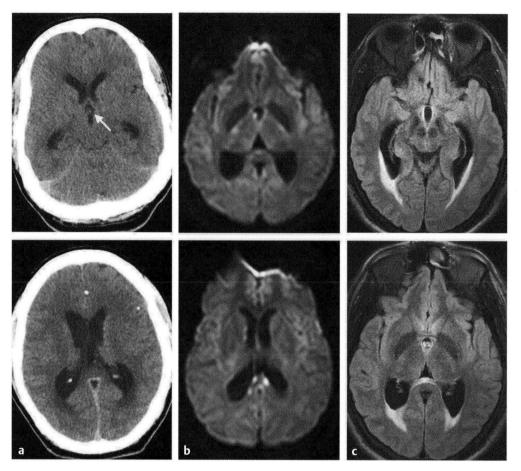

**Fig. 4.11a-c**   Colloidal phase, intraventricular neurocysticercosis. Axial unenhanced computed tomography **(a)** scans show subtle lesion at the foramen of Monro (*arrow*), calcification of the left frontal lobe, and hydrocephalus. Axial diffusion-weighted **(b)** images show abnormal foci of hyperintensity within the splenium, reflecting ischemia secondary to stretching of the corpus callosum in acute hydrocephalus. Focal hyperintensity of the scolex in the third ventricular lesion is seen as well. Axial fluid-attenuated inversion recovery (FLAIR) **(c)** images show interstitial edema secondary to hydrocephalus and hyperintensity of the neurocysticercosis cyst of the third ventricle. Hyperintensity of the scolex is seen only in colloidal phase. (Images courtesy of C. Truwit, MD.)

eters such as ventriculoperitoneal shunts can serve as a route for the spread of peritoneal space infection (e.g., from colonic perforation) into the cranial vault and resultant cerebritis or abscess.[17] Ventriculitis and other related conditions (ependymitis, intraventricular abscess, ventricular empyema, or pyocephalus) are uncommon but can be seen in patients with CSF shunts.[18]

CT is usually insensitive for evaluation, and MR is the test of choice. MR shows intraventricular debris or pus (often with fluid–fluid levels), abnormal periventricular and subependymal signal intensity, and enhancement of the ventricular lining. FLAIR imaging and DWI have been suggested as the most effective MR sequences to detect intraventricular debris.[19]

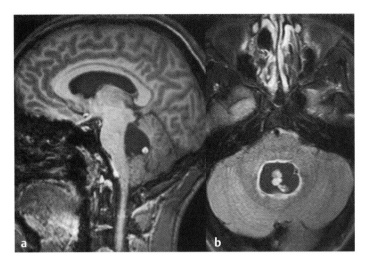

**Fig. 4.12a,b** Colloidal phase, intraventicular neurocysticercosis. Sagittal T1-weighted **(a)** image shows the hyperintense scolex within the encysted fourth ventricle. Contrast-enhanced fluid-attenuated inversion recovery (FLAIR) **(b)** image reveals the remainder of the lesion. As in the previous case, hyperintensity of the scolex is seen only in the colloidal phase. (Images courtesy of C. Truwit, MD.)

## References

1. McClelland S III, Hall WA. Postoperative central nervous system infection: incidence and associated factors in 2111 neurosurgical procedures. Clin Infect Dis 2007;45(1):55–59

2. Yikilmaz A, Taylor GA. Sonographic findings in bacterial meningitis in neonates and young infants. Pediatr Radiol 2008;38(2):129–137

3. Olsen WL. Central nervous system infections. In: Brant WE, Helms CA, eds. Fundamentals of Diagnostic Radiology. Philadelphia, PA: Lippincott Williams & Wilkins; 2007:156–181

4. Karagulle-Kendi AT, Truwit C. Neuroimaging of central nervous system infections. In: Roos KL, Tunkel AR, eds. Handbook of Clinical Neurology: Bacterial Infections of the Central Nervous System. New York, NY: Elsevier; 2010:239–255

5. Bakshi R, Mechtler LL, Kamran S, et al. MRI findings in lumbar puncture headache syndrome: abnormal dural-meningeal and dural venous sinus enhancement. Clin Imaging 1999;23(2):73–76

6. Hudgins P. Imaging of intracranial infections. In: Chung EM, Galvin JR, Glassman LM, et al, eds. Radiologic Pathology. 2011:451–459

7. Salzman KL. Herpes encephalitis. Salt Lake City, Utah: STATdx; 2011, 07 14

8. U.S. Department of Agriculture. Bovine spongiform encephalopathy–mad cow disease. 2005. http://www.fsis.usda.gov/factsheets/bovine_spongiform_encephalopathy_mad_cow_disease/index.asp. Accessed July 20, 2011

9. Osborne A. Diagnostic Radiology. St. Louis, MO: Mosby; 1994

10. Provenzale J. Toxoplasmosis. Salt Lake City, Utah: STATdx; 2011, 07 15

11. Tempkin AD, Sobonya RE, Seeger JF, Oh ES. Cerebral aspergillosis: radiologic and pathologic findings. Radiographics 2006;26(4):1239–1242

12. Zeifer B. Pediatric sinonasal imaging: normal anatomy and inflammatory disease. Neuroimaging Clin N Am 2000;10(1):137–159, ix

13. Reid JR. Complications of pediatric paranasal sinusitis. Pediatr Radiol 2004;34(12):933–942

14. Hosein IK, Hill DW, Hatfield RH. Controversies in the prevention of neurosurgical infection. J Hosp Infect 1999;43(1):5–11

15. Klisch JS, Spreer J, Bötefür I, et al. Calvarial sclerosing osteomyelitis. Pediatr Neurosurg 2002; 36(3):128–132

16. Nohra GK, Parks PJ. Reduction of surgical-site infections in neurosurgery–the advantage of antiseptics combined with a sterile surface. Eur Neurol Rev 2009;4(2):116–119

17. Vougioukas VI, Feuerhake F, Hubbe U, Reinacher P, Van Velthoven V. Latent abscess formation adjacent to a non-functioning intraventricular catheter. Childs Nerv Syst 2003;19(2):119–121

18. Cinalli GS, Spennato P, Ruggiero C, et al. Complications following endoscopic intracranial procedures in children. Childs Nerv Syst 2007;23(6): 633–644

19. Fujikawa AT, Tsuchiya K, Honya K, Nitatori T. Comparison of MRI sequences to detect ventriculitis. AJR Am J Roentgenol 2006;187(4):1048–1053

# II

# Etiologic Agents

# 5

# Viral Infections of the Central Nervous System

Joseph B. Domachowske, Manika Suryadevara, and Walter A. Hall

Viral infections of the central nervous system (CNS) can be divided into aseptic meningitis, encephalitis, meningoencephalitis, and infection-associated myelitis and myelopathies of the spinal cord. Substantial overlap exists among the agents that can cause each of these presentations, but some viral infections are predictably more severe than others. Aseptic viral meningitis is relatively common and usually self-limited, although exceptions are well described. Encephalitis and meningoencephalitis are less common, but because of parenchymal involvement, the illness is more severe and often life-threatening. Acute transverse myelitis, manifesting as progressive bilateral sensory, motor, or autonomic dysfunction of the spinal cord, has been associated with certain viral infections but carries a broader differential diagnosis that includes noninfectious causes.

## ■ Incidence and Demographics of Viral Meningitis and Meningoencephalitis

In temperate climates, most cases of aseptic meningitis occur during the summer months, reflecting the epidemiology and transmission of enteroviruses, the group of agents responsible for the vast majority of these cases. Similarly, most episodes of encephalitis occur during summer and fall, reflecting the transmission of arboviruses during peak mosquito breeding periods. Encephalitis outbreaks due to arboviruses can be geographically localized or epidemic, depending on the range of the mosquito vector(s) and the presence of natural animal reservoirs. Worldwide, arboviruses are the most important and most common causes of severe encephalitis. Since its emergence in the late 1800s, Japanese encephalitis virus, a mosquito-borne flavivirus, has spread throughout Asia to become the most common single agent of epidemic encephalitis, with up to 50,000 cases and 10,000 deaths annually.[1]

Before 1999, La Crosse virus was the most commonly identified arbovirus in the United States. Since 1999, this distinction has gone to West Nile virus (WNV). Soon after its emergence in 1999 in New York City, WNV spread rapidly across the country and into Mexico and Canada.[2] Between 1999 and 2005, more than 18,000 cases were documented, including approximately 700 deaths. Although it is estimated that fewer than 1% of WNV infections are severe, up to 20% of pediatric patients with this infection may present with encephalitis.[3]

During the prevaccination era, mumps virus was the leading cause of meningoencephalitis in the United States. Presently, mumps infection (caused by a member of the Paramyxoviridae family) is uncommon in developed countries where mumps vaccine coverage rates are high, although a large U.S. outbreak occurred in 2006, mostly in college students. During that outbreak, more than 6,000 cases of mumps were documented, and among those, at least 13 patients developed encephalitis (none died).[4] Historically, encephalitis complicated mumps in 0.75 per 1,000 cases, with a 14% case-fatality rate.[5] Of interest, other members of the Paramyxoviridae family, which have emerged globally, are also now known to cause outbreaks of encephalitis. One of these, Nipah virus, is a wide-scale epizootic viral agent of encephalitis identified in 1999 among Malaysian pig farmers, who were infected directly from animals. Subsequent outbreaks in humans have occurred in Singapore, Bangladesh, and India.[6] Human rabies encephalitis is very uncommon in developed countries but remains a major problem in resource-poor areas of the world, causing more than 55,000 deaths worldwide annually, almost always after the victim has been exposed to a rabid dog.[7] The infection is usually fatal, but recent advances and aggressive supportive care have led to a handful of individuals who survived infection.

In the United States, where arbovirus encephalitis is uncommon, mumps infection is largely controlled through vaccination programs, and rabies is rare, the herpesviruses remain the most frequently identified agents of encephalitis. Herpes simplex virus (HSV) encephalitis is the most common cause of acute sporadic fatal encephalitis in the United States, with approximately 50% of cases occurring in adults older than 50 years of age and 30% of all cases occurring in persons in the first two decades of life.[8] Epstein-Barr virus (EBV)–associated meningoencephalitis is seen in approximately 1% of primary EBV infections, usually in older children, adolescents, and young adults. Although this is an uncommon manifestation of EBV infection, the ubiquitous nature of infectious mononucleosis means that most primary care physicians who care for adolescents will encounter this complication in practice.

## Pathogenesis of Viral Meningitis and Meningoencephalitis

Most cases of viral meningitis and meningoencephalitis are secondary to a primary infection at a different anatomic site. Generally, after the virus is inhaled, ingested, or inoculated by an arthropod vector, it enters the lymphatic system, where it replicates, then seeds the bloodstream and solid organs. In most cases, virus is amplified at these sites, causing a secondary viremia. It is during this viremic phase that the CNS becomes infected. Infection of the brain can also occur when viruses infect peripheral or cranial nerves. This retrograde path of infection is important in the pathogenesis of encephalitis caused by rabies virus and HSV.

As a syndrome, acute transverse myelitis (ATM) is defined as progressive spinal cord dysfunction manifesting with sensory, motor, and/or autonomic signs and symptoms. This collection of findings can be caused by a heterogeneous group of infectious and noninfectious disorders. Although the broad diagnostic possibilities are beyond the scope of this chapter, it is included here because several viral infections can cause ATM, including herpes group viruses (HSV-1, HSV-2, EBV, cytomegalovirus [CMV], varicella-zoster virus [VZV], enteroviruses, WNV, human immunodeficiency virus type 1 or 2 [HIV-1 or -2], and human T-lymphotropic virus type 1 or 2 [HTLV-1 or -2]). These viruses can also cause meningoencephalitis, but the two conditions are only rarely seen in the same patient at the same time. The reasons why some patients develop ATM and others develop aseptic meningitis or encephalitis from the same viral etiology are unknown.

## Etiology of Viral Meningitis and Meningoencephalitis

### Herpesviruses

Most infections caused by the human herpesviruses HSV-1 and -2, EBV, CMV, and VZV are self-limited. Unfortunately, however, because of the neurotropism of herpesviruses, severe infections of the CNS are not uncommon, particularly in immunocompromised patients.

*Herpes simplex virus.* HSV accounts for 2 to 5% of encephalitis cases in the United States.[9] The case-fatality rate associated with untreated disease is as high as 70%, and survivors are almost always neurologically impaired. Both HSV-1 and HSV-2 cause encephalitis, but beyond the newborn period, most cases are caused by HSV-1. Although HSV is known to replicate in all areas of the brain, the infection has a predilection for the temporal lobes and the orbital regions of the frontal lobes (**Fig. 5.1**). HSV encephalitis must be differentiated from HSV meningitis, which is usually caused by HSV-2 and is a complication of primary genital herpes infection. In HSV meningitis, headache, photophobia, and meningismus appear before or shortly after the genital

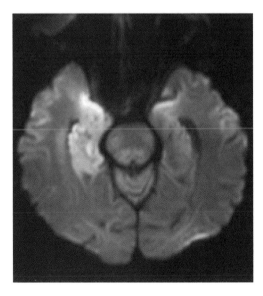

**Fig. 5.1** Axial magnetic resonance diffusion-weighted imaging showing an area of increased signal in the right medial temporal lobe that was confirmed to be herpes simplex encephalitis by polymerase chain reaction analysis of the cerebrospinal fluid.

lesions are noticed. Unlike in HSV encephalitis, recovery is almost always complete, even without antiviral therapy, although acyclovir is recommended to accelerate recovery. Therefore, HSV meningitis mimics other causes of viral "aseptic" meningitis and carries the same excellent prognosis. HSV encephalitis, on the other hand, is a highly lethal infection caused by HSV-1 in more than 90% of cases.[10] Infection can be either a result of primary HSV infection or associated with HSV reactivation.[11] Unlike most of the other, more common causes of viral meningoencephalitis, such as enterovirus and arbovirus infection, HSV disease is not seasonal. From a diagnostic standpoint, the cerebrospinal (CSF) reveals pleocytosis with a mononuclear cell predominance. The majority of cases are associated with hemorrhagic necrosis, so erythrocytes are found on CSF examination. As many as 25% of patients will have hypoglycorrhachia with an elevated CSF protein concentration (mean levels of approximately 80 mg/dL are seen in nearly all patients).[12] HSV is only rarely cultured from CSF, so historically, brain biopsy was required to confirm a suspected diagnosis. With the development of sensitive and specific DNA amplification assays over the past 15 years, the gold standard for diagnosis from CSF is now polymerase chain reaction (PCR).[13] Among available neurodiagnostic tests, only electroencephalography has proved somewhat useful. A typical pattern of uni- or bilateral periodic focal spikes against a background of slow activity, referred to as paroxysmal lateral epileptiform discharges (PLEDs), is suggestive of HSV encephalitis. For neuroimaging, magnetic resonance (MR) imaging is generally preferred over computed tomography (CT) during the initial evaluation because MR imaging findings are more likely to be abnormal.[14] Imaging studies performed later during the illness may reveal low-density, contrast-enhancing lesions, particularly in the temporal lobe. Patients with abnormalities like these, or who have already developed edema and/ or hemorrhage, have a poor prognosis.[15]

*Epstein-Barr virus.* Acute neurologic symptoms complicate between 1 and 5% of infectious mononucleosis cases. EBV encephalitis may present in the absence of infectious mononucleosis syndrome and should be considered as a cause of acute neurologic symptoms, particularly in teenagers. Typical CSF findings in cases of EBV encephalitis include a mild to moderate pleocytosis with mononuclear cells predominating, a slight elevation in CSF protein, and a normal glucose.[16] Serologic proof of acute EBV infection is strongly diagnostic, whereas CSF PCR specific for EBV provides a definitive diagnosis. The prognosis is generally favorable, but long-term sequelae are well described. EBV-associated cerebellitis is a rare occurrence that develops primarily in children.[17] Full recovery is expected but may require several weeks. Cranial nerve palsies, single or in combination, have also been described. Other manifestations of cranial nerve involvement with EBV infection include optic neuritis, deafness, and ophthalmoplegia. Some cases of brainstem encephalitis have also been reported.[18]

*Cytomegalovirus.* CNS involvement is common in infants with symptomatic congenital CMV infection, but in postnatal life, CMV meningoencephalitis is quite rare.[19] When it does occur, it may appear as a complication of CMV mononucleosis, as an isolated manifestation of primary CMV infection, or more likely as a primary or recurrent (reactivation) infection in an immunocompromised host.[20] Patients with solid-organ transplants may develop CMV encephalitis as a complication of their immunosuppression, and the recognition that patients with acquired immunodeficiency syndrome (AIDS) develop meningoencephalitis secondary to CMV infection is well established.[21]

*Varicella-zoster virus.* CNS complications of varicella, which may precede or follow the chickenpox, include transient cerebellar ataxia, encephalitis, aseptic meningitis, and transverse myelitis.[22] Encephalopathy as a sequela of Reye syndrome has become a rare complication because of the nearly complete elimination of aspirin use in pediatric patients. Patients who present with dermatologic findings consistent with varicella or zoster and who experience CNS symptoms should be evaluated and treated for the possibility that the infection has involved the CNS.

*Herpes B virus.* Herpes B virus, a pathogen indigenous in macaques, is a nonhuman herpesvirus that can cause encephalitis in humans. Transmission occurs by direct contact with the virus, usually from a monkey bite. The high prevalence of excretion of herpes B virus in the saliva of macaques has important implications for zoo handlers, veterinarians, and laboratory researchers. A vesicular rash may occur at the inoculation site, signaling a herpes-type infection. The virus has robust neurovirulence, causing rapidly progressive, often fatal hemorrhagic encephalitis. Guidelines for the prevention of herpes B viral infection emphasize proper and expert animal handling and assume that all macaques are shedding herpes B virus unless proven otherwise. For cases of macaque bites, post-exposure recommendations are available from the U.S. Centers for Disease Control and Prevention (Viral Exanthems and Herpesvirus Branch, Division of Viral Diseases [1-404-639-3595 or 1-888-232-6348]), including the use of acyclovir pending culture results.[23]

## Enteroviruses and Parechoviruses

Enteroviruses and parechoviruses comprise two genera of the family Picornaviridae and include more than 100 distinct human viruses. These small RNA viruses are responsible for frequent and often significant infections, including neurologic illness. By far, the most common neurologic manifestation of enterovirus infection is aseptic meningitis, which can occur either sporadically or in epidemics. In general, infection is more common in children, but during large outbreaks, substantial numbers of adults develop aseptic meningitis as well. Virtually all patients have fever and pharyngitis. Adolescents and adults often experience retrobulbar pain and photophobia, whereas young infants present with fever and irritability. Examination of the CSF will reveal a pleocytosis. Depending on the timing of the lumbar puncture, a neutrophil predominance may be observed, but neutrophils rarely account for more than 60% of the total number of cells (as is seen in bacterial meningitis). CSF protein levels are usually normal or slightly elevated, and CSF glucose concentrations, characteristically normal, may be slightly depressed. CSF PCR specific for enterovirus is available and should be used to confirm the etiology. The duration of illness is typically less than a week, although headaches may persist longer. The prognosis for enterovirus aseptic meningitis is excellent. Enteroviruses can also cause encephalitis, with echovirus 9 the most frequent cause of this more serious CNS infection. In general, patients with enteroviral encephalitis have a good prognosis, although fatalities do occur. Enterovirus 71 tends to infect the brainstem and since the 1980s has caused severe outbreaks in Asia. During some of those epidemics, mortality from enterovirus 71 encephalitis was as high as 30%.[24] Enteroviruses may also cause acute flaccid paralysis. The tropism of enteroviruses for the anterior horn cells is well appreciated in paralytic polio, but it should be mentioned that other enteroviuses, including coxsackievirus A7 and enteroviruses 70 and 71, have been linked to polio-like outbreaks.[25,26]

*Adenovirus.* Adenoviruses only rarely cause meningitis and meningoencephalitis, but when they do, the illness is generally more severe than infection caused by enteroviruses.[27]

## Arboviruses

Arboviruses are RNA viruses that are transmitted to humans through the bite of infected arthropods, such as mosquitoes, ticks, sand flies, and midges. Among the more than 400 distinct *ar*thopod-*bo*rne viruses, at least 150 are known to cause human disease. The medically important viruses that cause human CNS infections are listed in **Table 5.1,** along with their arthropod vectors and geographic distribution. Although most arbovirus infections are subclinical, symptomatic illness manifests in one of three ways: systemic febrile illness, hemorrhagic fever, or neuroinvasive disease. When neuroinvasion occurs, it may manifest as aseptic meningitis, encephalitis, or acute flaccid paralysis. Following a prodrome of fever, the neurologic symptoms begin, sometimes progressing rapidly. The severity and long-term outcome depend on the etiologic agent and several host factors, such as age, immune function, and underlying medical conditions.

In the United States, eight specific arboviruses that cause encephalitis have been isolated: the eastern equine encephalitis (EEE), western equine encephalitis (WEE), Venezuelan equine encephalitis (VEE), St. Louis encephalitis, Powassan, West Nile, California encephalitis, and Colorado tick fever viruses. EEE occurs throughout the eastern part of the United States. Most cases are sporadic and occur in the summer or fall in Florida and Georgia, although swampy areas as far north as New York State also harbor the virus, leading to rare human infections. The mosquito vector thrives only in swampy environments, limiting the spread of the infection much beyond these specific environs. Subclinical cases of EEE in humans are not common. Illness is abrupt, with high fever, headache, vomiting, seizures, and coma. The case-fatality rate is approximately 30%. WEE in the United States is slightly more common than EEE but geographically shifted west of the Mississippi River. Colorado leads the United States in the number of reported cases. The case-fatality rate is approximately 25%.[28] The VEE virus, named such because it was isolated first in that country, causes encephalitis, although infection is typically less severe, and with supportive care, fatalities are rare. Adults typically develop only an influenza-like illness, while encephalitis is confined to children. Outbreaks of VEE with epizootic spread to humans can be extensive. One such outbreak in 1971, extending from Central America into Texas, killed 200,000 horses and infected thousands of people.[29] St. Louis encephalitis virus is the most important mosquito-borne viral cause of epidemic encephalitis in the United States. The last

**Table 5.1** Medically significant arthropod-borne viruses causing human central nervous system infections

| Genus | Virus | Primary arthropod vector(s) | Endemicity in the United States | Global distribution |
|---|---|---|---|---|
| Flavivirus | West Nile | *Culex* mosquitoes | Widespread | Canada, Europe, Africa, Asia |
| Flavivirus | St. Louis encephalitis | *Culex* mosquitoes | Widespread | Entire western hemisphere |
| Flavivirus | Powassan | *Ixodes* ticks | Northeastern and north central states | Canada, Russia |
| Flavivirus | Tickborne encephalitis | *Ixodes* ticks | Imported only | Europe, northern Asia |
| Flavivirus | Japanese encephalitis | *Culex* mosquitoes | Imported only | Asia |
| Alphavirus | Eastern equine | *Aedes* and *Culiseta* mosquitoes | Eastern and Gulf states | Canada, Central and South America |
| Alphavirus | Western equine | *Culex* and *Culiseta* mosquitoes | Central and western states | Mexico, South America |
| Alphavirus | Venezuelan equine | *Aedes* and *Culex* mosquitoes | Imported only | Mexico, Central and South America |
| Bunyavirus | La Crosse (the most prevalent and pathogenic of the California serogroup viruses) | *Aedes* mosquitoes | Widespread in the Midwest and southeastern states (not California) | Canada |
| Coltivirus | Colorado tick fever | *Dermacentor* ticks | Western states, especially Colorado | Canada |

major outbreak occurred in the late 1970s, when thousands of individuals in the Midwest were infected. Cases are concentrated in the states of Indiana, Illinois, Ohio, Mississippi, Florida, and Texas, but nearly all states in the United States have reported some disease activity over the past 50 years. On average, approximately 200 cases are reported in a given year, with the vast majority occurring in the elderly population; however, only 10 cases were reported in 2010.[30] The overall case-fatality rate is between 5 and 15%. Powassan virus is a rare cause of meningoencephalitis in the northeastern United States and Canada that, unlike the other arthropod-borne infectious agents found in the United States, is transmitted by ticks, not by mosquitoes. There were no fatalities among the eight cases reported in 2010. Since WNV was first detected in the western hemisphere in 1999, it has become the leading cause of neuroinvasive arboviral illness in the United States. Among 629 cases reported in 2010, half of the patients had encephalitis, 38% had meningitis, and 8% had acute flaccid paralysis. Mortality was 9%. California serogroup viruses that cause encephalitis in the United States include the endemic La Crosse virus and the less commonly appreciated California encephalitis and Jamestown Canyon viruses. Most infections with La Crosse virus are subclinical. Typically, when clinical disease is seen, it occurs in young children. Infection can progress to fulminant encephalitis, but La Crosse virus encephalitis is only rarely fatal. Colorado tick fever virus is prevalent in the western mountainous region of the United States, where the tick vector resides. The typical infection caused by this virus is an influenza-like illness with fever, myalgia, and malaise. Neuroinvasive disease, although rare, can occur in young children. Like other viral infections of the CNS, illness can be self-limited to meningeal irritation or progress to encephalitis with coma. Fatalities from CNS complications are reported.[31]

## Rabies Virus

Rabies is an acute, progressive, and almost uniformly lethal viral infection of the CNS that is transmitted to humans from animals. Rabies is transmitted from an infected animal to a human through a bite, scratch, or aerosol. Domestic animals, especially dogs, account for nearly all rabies cases outside developed countries. In the United States and Canada, the raccoon has replaced the skunk as the most important potential source of rabies exposure. Humans who are scratched or bitten by wild mammals should be evaluated for post-exposure prophylaxis, which, when carried out properly, prevents rabies very effectively. Unlike bites from potentially rabid raccoons, skunks, foxes, and other medium-size wild mammals, the bite from a bat, especially during sleep, can go completely unnoticed. For this reason, bat bites can go unrecognized, resulting in a patient who does not seek post-exposure prophylaxis. Perhaps this explains why nearly all nonimported human cases of rabies in developed countries are caused by bat strain viruses.

The incubation period between the bite and the onset of symptoms is usually 20 to 90 days; however, well-documented cases have occurred 6 years following exposure.[32] Occasionally, symptoms occur sooner, with the shortest incubation periods being 7 to 10 days, usually when the animal has bitten or scratched the victim's face. The earliest symptoms are rather vague and insidious, but the most striking clinical clue may be pain, itching, burning, or tingling at the inoculation site. Together with fever and nausea, this prodrome lasts several days, after which time the more obvious neurologic symptoms result. Two broad presentations are seen. The more common presentation is referred to as furious rabies. Such patients exhibit extreme agitation, hyperactivity, fluctuating levels of consciousness, hypersalivation, and hydrophobia. Paralytic rabies is not associated with hydrophobia; instead, the patient develops acute flaccid paralysis, usually beginning in the limb that was bitten. The cranial nerves are involved, and rather than expressing agitation and fright, the patient appears expressionless. Paralytic rabies can be confused with Guillain-Barré syndrome. Distinguishing features supporting a diagnosis of rabies include fever, intact sensation, and urinary incontinence.[33] The majority of patients with rabies will have meningismus, with the CSF findings abnormal in a minority. When abnormal, the CSF shows a mild mononuclear cell pleocytosis. Rabies-specific diagnostic testing includes direct fluorescent antibody staining of corneal epithelial cells, which are easily obtained from corneal impressions on a glass slide, and of skin from a punch biopsy at the nape of the neck. These results are positive early because the virus migrates from the brain along the richly innervated cornea and hair follicles.[34] Additional testing to consider as the diagnosis is being established or confirmed includes CSF and saliva for rabies PCR and culture. The diagnosis can be confirmed post mortem by identifying the pathognomonic Negri bodies (cytoplasmic inclusions) in brain tissue.

The acute neurologic phase of infection continues for approximately a week until the patient develops coma. Before death, some patients are described as having acute, brief periods of lucidity fluctuating with periods of agitation and hopelessness. During the comatose period, complications to be expected include cerebral edema, syndrome of inappropriate antidiuretic hormone secretion, diabetes insipidus, and other manifestations of hypothalamic dysfunction. Cardiac arrhythmias are common. Survival after rabies infection has been documented in a very small number of patients, most of whom were previously vaccinated.[35] The first unvaccinated patient to survive rabies was a 15-year-old girl, who was treated with coma induction, midazolam, ribavirin, ketamine, and amantadine.[36] Multiple subsequent attempts at using this original Milwaukee protocol for rabies treatment have been discouraging, and two children who survived the initial phase died of complications during rehabilitation.[37] Details regarding the outcomes of 43 patients treated with evolving versions of the Milwaukee protocol can be found at http://www.mcw.edu/Pediatrics/InfectiousDiseases/PatientCare/Rabies.htm. Detailed metabolomics performed serially on CSF obtained from patients with rabies will likely allow further advances in treatment protocols. All human rabies cases should be managed with assistance from the U.S. Centers for Disease Control and Prevention so that the most current protocols can be implemented.

## Lymphocytic Choriomeningitis Virus

Lymphocytic choriomeningitis virus (LCMV) is an arenavirus that only rarely causes human infection. Illness usually follows exposure to rodents or rodent urine, as mice are the natural reservoir. Most infections are mild and self-limiting, but more serious infections can lead to meningitis and meningoencephalitis. The meningeal form of infection begins with an influenza-like systemic illness, followed by signs and symptoms of aseptic meningitis. Progression to meningoencephalitis leads to a more serious, life-threatening infection. CSF findings show a mild to moderate mononuclear cell pleocytosis with normal or slightly elevated protein and normal glucose levels. CSF PCR with LCMV-specific primers may yield the diagnosis. Serologic testing requires demonstrating a fourfold change in antibody titers when the acute and convalescent sera are compared. Other CNS manifestations that have been associated with LCMV infection include transverse myelitis, a Guillian-Barré–like syndrome, and transient or permanent hydrocephalus.[38]

## JC Virus

The human JC polyomavirus causes most cases of progressive multifocal leukoencephalopathy (PML). This clinical syndrome is characterized by progressive neurologic impairment in immunocompromised patients, without systemic symptoms such as fever. PML occurs when the host immune system fails to keep JC virus latent, and as it replicates in oligodendroglia, the cerebral white matter is destroyed in a multifocal pattern. Up to 25% of adults patients with AIDS will develop PML.[39] Other immunosuppressed patients are also at risk for PML, particularly those with primary T-cell deficiencies and those who have undergone a solid-organ or hematopoietic stem cell transplant. The clinical manifestations of PML vary and depend on the distribution of the patchy, multifocal areas of injury. Patients develop behavioral changes and cranial nerve dysfunction, which can lead to blindness, deafness, and/or lack of coordination.[40] The neurologic symptoms progress over a period of weeks to months. CSF analysis is usually normal. Viral culture and serology are not reliable for detecting the JC virus; however, the isolation of viral DNA from CSF with PCR is the diagnostic test of choice.[41] In adult patients with AIDS and neurologic symptoms, the detection of JC virus DNA in CSF has a predictive value of 99%, whereas the results from tissue obtained by brain biopsy are slightly lower.[42] Neuroimaging demonstrates patchy demyelination. Gray matter findings are subtle, if present at all. Histologic examination of the brain reveals foci of demyelination, enlarged oligodendrocytes, and giant astrocytes in a background of florid neutrophil infiltration.[43]

## Human T-Cell Lymphotropic Virus

HTLV-1 is a human retrovirus that is known to be associated with myelopathy. HTLV-1–associated myelopathy (HAM) is identical to the clinical syndrome of tropical spastic paraparesis (TSP), which was described in tropical areas of the world for many decades. HAM/TSP is now the accepted acronym to describe this disorder.[44] The disease occurs most commonly in areas of the world where HTLV-1 is endemic, including the Caribbean, southern Japan, equatorial and southern Africa, and Central and South America. In HTLV-1–seropositive persons, the incidence of HAM/TSP is estimated to be 3 to 22 per 100,000 HTLV-1–infected people per year.[45] The onset of symptoms usually occurs in the fourth decade of life. Clinical features include progressive spastic paraparesis and lower-extremity weakness, resulting in a fairly characteristic gait disturbance. Neurologic examination reveals hyperreflexia, clonus, extensor plantar reflexes, proximal muscle wasting, and spastic paresis with a slow, deliberate, scissoring gait. Although disease progression is variable, slow deterioration results in the inability to walk over a 10-year period in almost half of affected individuals. Treatments with systemic and/or intrathecal corticosteroids provide a transient benefit to some patients, and the combination of zidovudine with interferon-α has shown some promise in delaying disease progression.[46] Evidence suggests that the related retrovirus, HTLV-2, may also be associated with neurologic disorders ranging from spastic paraparesis that is indistinguishable from HAM/TSP to more widespread involvement of the CNS.[47]

## Transmissible Spongiform Encephalopathies

The neurodegenerative diseases of this group are referred to as prion disease. They are not caused by viruses, but rather by the accumulation of insoluble proteinaceous material in the CNS, leading to progressive cortical dysfunction. The abnormal deposition of an isoform of a cellular protein termed PrP$^c$ is thought to result in the characteristic neurologic dysfunction. Kuru was the first among the human transmissible spongiform encephalopathies (TSEs) to be described. The observation that kuru was seen only in members of the Fore tribe in Papua New Guinea, who practiced ritualistic cannibalism, including the consumption of human brain,[48] provided the clue that neurologic tissue was the source. Early studies of kuru and subsequent studies of the related TSEs known as Creutzfeldt-Jakob disease (CJD), Gerstmann-Sträussler-Scheinker disease, fatal familial insomnia, and variant CJD (vCJD) have demonstrated that brain homogenates from infected humans can transmit spongiform encephalopathy to primates. The emergence of bovine spongiform encephalopathy (BSE) in the United Kingdom during the mid 1980s received global attention. In the United Kingdom alone, more than 100 human cases of BSE were described, nearly a quarter of a million cattle died, and an additional 4.5 million were destroyed presumptively.[49] The natural history of TSE disease is best described for CJD. Three models of disease acquisition have been described: (1) sporadic, (2) genetic (inherited mutations in the PrP$^c$ gene), and (3) acquired disease following exposure to the protein. Sporadic CJD is the most common form,[50] occurring in approximately 1 per million population. Most patients present between 55 and 65 years of age, although several older teenagers have also been reported. In the late 1980s, CJD was reported in several children and young adults who had received human growth hormone prepared from human cadavers. Since then, more than 100 individuals have been given a diagnosis of CJD transmitted from growth hormone preparations predating the use of recombinant hormone.[51] Other sources of iatrogenic TSE reported have involved the use of dural grafts, corneal transplants, contaminated stereotactic neurosurgical equipment, and even blood transfusions. Transmission of BSE from cows to humans in the United Kingdom is now the known cause of vCJD, and although the origin of the problem remains somewhat controversial, most investigations have concluded that changes in the process used to render fat from cows and sheep for use in animal feeds contributed to the problem. The finding of BSE in U.S. cows has led to their exportation being banned in several important economic markets.[52]

Clinical signs and symptoms of sporadic CJD during the early stages are subtle, usually including motor and sensory disturbances. Headache and dizziness are common, and as the disease progresses, intellectual dysfunction with memory loss, speech disturbance, and anxiety have been described.[53] Neurologic abnormalities may include hyperreflexia and spasticity, indicating corticospinal tract dysfunction. Visual disturbances are common. Patients deteriorate into a persistent vegetative state and usually die within a year of symptom onset. The symptoms of vCJD differ in comparison. Psychiatric and sensory symptoms prevail. These patients are generally younger than those with sporadic CJD and more typically describe anxiety, depression, social withdrawal, and other nonspecific complaints. As the disease progresses, pyramidal tract dysfunction, rigidity, myoclonus, and cerebellar symptoms become apparent. The duration of illness is usually longer than a year before the patient succumbs to a complication of the vegetative state.

The diagnosis of TSE requires a high degree of clinical suspicion. A detailed history may reveal risk factors associated with beef consumption during the peak of BSE in the United Kingdom, and any potential transmission from an iatrogenic source should be immediately recognized from the patient's history. Routine laboratory tests, including a CSF examination, are nonspecific. CT findings on neuroimaging are not sufficiently specific to be helpful. On the other hand, MR imaging findings of increased T2 signals from the striatum and thalamus can offer a high index of suspicion for prion disease.[54] Definitive diagnosis requires brain biopsy. Histopathologic diagnosis should include immunocytochemical staining and Western blotting to detect the abnormal PrP$^c$ protein.[55] Instruments used during neurosurgical procedures in patients with suspected CJD or other TSE require strict decontamination protocols to eliminate the potential for transmission of the TSE agent during subsequent procedures on other individuals. Detailed procedures have been developed by the World Health Organization and are endorsed by the U.S. Centers for Disease Control and Prevention. This 35-page document addresses infection control procedures for surgical instruments, occupational exposure, handling of human tissue, and handling of bodies post mortem in the hospital and funeral home.[56] There are no known treatments for patients with any of the TSEs.

## ■ Specific Risk Factors for the Development of Central Nervous System Viral Infection

*Hypogammaglobulinemia.* Patients with X-linked agammaglobulinemia (Bruton disease) and those with hyperimmunoglobulin M syndrome secondary to CD40 ligand deficiency are susceptible to recurrent and severe enterovirus infection, including chronic meningoencephalitis.[57] Enterovirus-directed therapies are not available, and despite aggressive supportive care and high-dose enterovirus-specific immunoglobulin therapy, the most common cause of death in patients with Bruton disease is chronic enterovirus infection.[58]

*Toll-like receptor signaling defects.* Toll-like receptors (TLRs) are responsible for a myriad of innate immune responses that ultimately lead to recruitment and activation of antigen-specific B and T cells to sites of infection. Emerging evidence links defects in three different TLR signaling proteins with a predisposition to severe HSV encephalitis. Mutations in TLR-3, in UNC-93B1, a protein essential for signaling via TLR-3, -7, -8, and -9, and in TRAF3, a protein that functions downstream of UNC-93B1, have been described in children with recurrent and/or severe HSV encephalitis.[59]

## ■ Clinical Presentation

The patient's age, viral etiology, and the immune competence of the patient all influence the clinical manifestations of viral meningitis. Patients with enteroviral meningitis typically present with a prodrome of fever, malaise, and headache. The classic findings of meningismus and photophobia are seen in about half of adult patients with meningitis, but infants and young children only infrequently have nuchal rigidity. The index of suspicion for meningitis needs to be high for the very young, the very old, and those with compromised immune systems because these patients often present in an atypical manner. Patients with encephalitis will develop clinical evidence of parenchymal disease. Some viruses, like rabies virus and herpes B virus, produce encephalitis without significant meningeal involvement. Most other viral agents of encephalitis cause enough inflammation of the meninges that the clinical description for these infections is more accurately referred to as meningoencephalitis. Early in infection, during the primary viremia, the patient will exhibit symptoms of lethargy, fever, anorexia, and nausea. As the neurologic infection becomes established, headache, altered levels of consciousness, irritability, and seizures develop. Coma may ensue. Some patients exhibit bizarre behavior or describe vivid hallucinations. The Alice in Wonderland syndrome, described clearly by some patients with EBV-associated meningoencephalitis, represents visual hallucinations of geometric shapes changing in size and color.[60] Clinical manifestations also predictably reflect the anatomic location(s) of the virus replication, which can be focal or diffuse. For example, HSV-1 encephalitis tends to involve the inferotemporal frontal area of the cortex, resulting in focal seizures, personality changes, and aphasia, which reflect involvement of the internal capsule, limbic system, and Broca area.[61] Similarly, early on, rabies infects the limbic system, producing personality changes, while sparing the cortical regions. The result is a patient who has periods of complete lucidity, during which he or she describes the fear of impending death.

The clinical approach to a patient with presumed CNS viral infection depends on the severity of the illness and the extent of the neurologic findings. Invasive monitoring of the intracranial pressure (ICP) is helpful in patients with encephalitis who have signs of increased ICP. Once the cardiorespiratory status of the patient is stabilized, efforts to establish the etiologic diagnosis should be pursued. Infections for which specific antiviral therapy is available should be considered and empiric therapy initiated pending the results of diagnostic studies (**Table 5.2**). Attention to the possibility that a bacterial agent is causing the problem is crucial because early empiric antibiotic therapy can be lifesaving. Seizures can be secondary to neuroinvasion by the virus, inflammatory vasculitis, and/or electrolyte disturbances. Patients with cerebral edema may require ICP monitoring, osmotic therapy, and CSF removal in attempts to maintain an acceptable intracerebral pressure.[62]

HSV encephalitis can initially show low-density areas in the temporal lobes with mass effect on CT. These hypodense areas in the temporal lobes can become hemorrhagic with progression of the disease. On MR imaging, HSV encephalitis will involve the medial temporal lobe and will appear as an area of increased signal on diffusion-weighted imaging (**Fig. 5.1**) and fluid-attenuated inversion recovery (FLAIR) imaging (**Fig. 5.2**). Within days, the disease process can extend from the tem-

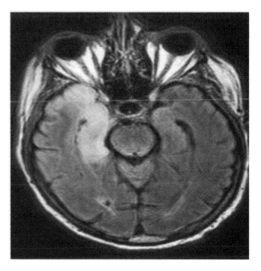

**Fig. 5.2** Axial fluid-attenuated inversion recovery (FLAIR) magnetic resonance image showing the same area of increased signal that was visible on the diffusion-weighted image in the right medial temporal lobe, representing herpes simplex encephalitis.

**Table 5.2** Preventive measures, diagnostic testing, and treatment for viral infections of the central nervous system

| Virus | Preventive measures | Diagnostic testing | Treatment |
|---|---|---|---|
| Herpes simplex type 1 or 2 virus | None | CSF PCR<br>Mucous membrane cultures and/or PCR | Acyclovir |
| Epstein-Barr virus | None | Epstein-Barr virus serology<br>CSF PCR | Supportive |
| Cytomegalovirus | None | CSF PCR | Ganciclovir |
| Varicella-zoster virus | Active immunization (Varivax; Merck, Whitehouse Station, NJ)<br>Passive protection (varicella immune globulin) | CSF PCR<br>Skin vesicle PCR and/or culture | Acyclovir |
| Herpes B virus | Monkey bite avoidance<br>Post-exposure prophylaxis with acyclovir | Contact CDC<br>CSF and mucous membrane samples for PCR and culture<br>http://www.cdc.gov/herpesbvirus/index.html | Acyclovir |
| Enterovirus | Polio vaccine<br>No vaccine for other enteroviruses | CSF PCR<br>Stool cultures for virus | Supportive |
| Adenovirus | None | CSF PCR<br>Respiratory virus culture and/or PCR | Supportive |
| Arboviruses | Mosquito deterrent<br>Vaccine for Japanese encephalitis virus | Virus-specific PCR testing of CSF<br>Serologic testing of paired sera obtained during acute infection and convalescence<br>Serum West Nile IgM more sensitive than CSF PCR during acute infection with WNV | Supportive |
| Rabies virus | Post-exposure prophylaxis with rabies vaccine and rabies immune globulin<br>Pre-exposure for high-risk occupations | Corneal impressions for DFA testing<br>Skin biopsy of nape of neck for DFA and/or PCR<br>Saliva for PCR and/or culture<br>Serology<br>CSF PCR<br>Brain biopsy for PCR and detection of pathognomonic Negri bodies | Largely supportive; see text for current protocols |
| Lymphocytic choriomeningitis virus | Rodent avoidance | CSF PCR<br>Paired serology | Supportive |
| JC virus | None | CSF PCR (blood PCR not helpful) | Supportive |
| HTLV-1 | None | Serology | Zidovudine with interferon-α |
| Prion disease | None | Brain biopsy to detect abnormal protein by immunocytochemistry and/or Western blotting | Supportive |

*Abbreviations:* CDC, Centers for Disease Control and Prevention; CSF, cerebrospinal fluid; DFA, direct fluorescent antibody; HTLV-1, human T-lymphotropic virus type 1; IgM, immunoglobulin M; PCR, polymerase chain reaction; WNV, West Nile virus poral lobe into the insula and subfrontal regions (**Figs. 5.3** and **5.4**). Because of the wide variety of diseases that can mimic HSV encephalitis, a brain biopsy should be considered for those patients in whom PCR of the CSF is negative for HSV DNA. It has been estimated that 45% of those who have a brain biopsy for a focal encephalopathic process will have HSV encephalitis.[10]

## ■ Treatment and Prevention

Prevention of infection by viruses that cause CNS infection is best accomplished through avoidance of exposure. Arbovirus infections, for example, are best prevented through the use of chemical and physical mosquito deterrents and for some viruses through public health–initiated mosquito abatement programs. Specific treatment is available for only a limited number of causative agents (**Table 5.2**), and post-exposure

prophylaxis is the mainstay of treatment for most cases of potential rabies exposure through the use of both rabies immune globulin and rabies vaccine.

Routine childhood immunizations have led to nearly complete elimination of mumps and measles as causes of meningoencephalitis in regions of the world where vaccine programs are robust. Vaccination has also dramatically changed the global challenge of poliomyelitis, with elimination of the infection in the western hemisphere[63] and dramatic reductions in polio infection in the rest of the world. Such progress offers hope for global eradication of polio in the coming decade. To date, the only enterovirus infection that is controlled through immunization programs is polio, which explains why enteroviral meningitis remains so common. Vaccines have also been developed for some arbovirus infections (**Table 5.2**). Vaccine programs for the prevention of Japanese encephalitis virus

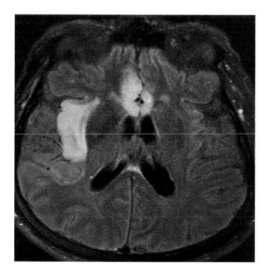

**Fig. 5.3** With continued progression of herpes simplex encephalitis, the insula is now involved, as demonstrated by the fluid-attenuated inversion recovery (FLAIR) signal in that location on this axial magnetic resonance image.

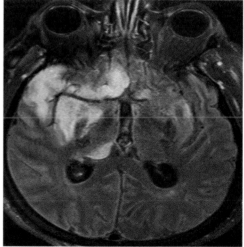

**Fig. 5.4** Axial fluid-attenuated inversion recovery (FLAIR) magnetic resonance image showing extension of herpes simplex encephalitis into the subfrontal region from the site of origin in the medial temporal lobe.

infection have reduced the disease burden in Asia, but problems still exist in China, with more than 10,000 cases of Japanese encephalitis virus infection annually.[64] To date, safe and effective HSV vaccines have remained elusive.

The treatment of CNS viral infections starts with identifying those agents for which specific antiviral therapy is available. Empiric therapy with acyclovir should be used in all cases of suspected HSV meningo-encephalitis until that virus is excluded or the responsible, alternative virus is found. Complications should be anticipated for every patient with viral meningitis or meningoencephalitis, and supportive therapy for those complications should be initiated early and aggressively. Dehydration and fever are easily treated. Patients may also require treatment of seizures, syndrome of inappropriate antidiuretic hormone secretion, hydrocephalus, and raised ICP.

Traditionally, neurosurgical intervention in patients suspected to have viral encephalitis due primarily to HSV has usually included either brain biopsy for diagnosis or the placement of an ICP monitor in the face of suspected elevated ICP. However, there is a role for emergency surgical decompression in the presence of uncal herniation.[65] Surgical decompression can be necessary more that 10 days after the onset of the clinical course because the estimated peak in ICP does not occur until the 12th day of the illness.[65]

Infections for which specific antiviral therapy is available include those caused by HSV-1 and -2, VZV, CMV, and herpes B virus. With the use of acyclovir, the morbidity and mortality from neonatal HSV encephalitis has declined from 70 to 40%. Varicella immune globulin and acyclovir have reduced the complications of primary VZV infection in immunocompromised patients, and although randomized trials have not evaluated the efficacy of acyclovir for VZV encephalitis, the medication is routinely used to treat this complication. Ganciclovir and foscarnet are antiviral medications that are used to treat CMV encephalitis, although their efficacy in this context is unknown.

## ■ Complications, Sequelae, and Prognosis

Encephalitis, unlike meningitis, has a high morbidity and mortality rate. Case-fatality rates differ based on the cause of the infection and the condition of the host. Among the arbovirus infections, St. Louis encephalitis carries a mortality rate of approximately 2% in children and 20% in the elderly,[66] while other viruses, such as WEE virus and EEE virus, produce higher morbidity and mortality in children than in adults. Rabies is almost always fatal, but progress in understanding the metabolic disturbances that occur during infection have provided some insights. Seizures are common during acute viral encephalitis. Among the sporadic viral encephalitides, HSV encephalitis is most frequently associated with epilepsy, which may often be severe. Seizures may be the presenting feature in 50% of patients with HSV encephalitis because of the involvement of the highly epileptogenic frontotemporal cortex. The occurrence of seizures in HSV encephalitis is associated with a poor prognosis. Among the arboviral encephalitides, Japanese encephalitis is most commonly associated with seizures, especially in children. Other viruses, like measles virus, varicella virus, mumps virus, influenza virus, and enteroviruses, may cause seizures, depending on the area of brain involved.[67] Details on the risk for epilepsy following recovery from each specific type of viral encephalitis have not been published. Prognosis once a diagnosis of viral encephalitis is confirmed depends on the infecting agent and on the extent of parenchymal involvement. The risk for death from rabies, PML, and EEE is extremely high, whereas mortality from EBV and La Crosse virus encephalitis is uncommon. The TSEs are uniformly fatal.

*Polio.* The most feared complication of infection with poliovirus is paralytic disease. The onset of paralysis may be abrupt, with complete loss of motor strength in one or more extremities. Bladder paralysis occurs in approximately 20% of patients. Bulbospinal poliomyelitis is an unusual complication. Involvement of cranial nerves VII and

X can manifest as facial, pharyngeal, and vocal cord paralysis. Hypoxia and hypercapnia requiring mechanical ventilation can occur secondary to pharyngeal paralysis, cervical cord involvement with respiratory muscle weakness or paralysis, or rarely parenchymal involvement with true polio encephalitis. The initial presentation of paralytic polio infection can mimic Guillain-Barré syndrome.[68]

*Subacute sclerosing panencephalitis (SSPE).* SSPE is an uncommon, slowly progressive disease of the CNS that is almost universally fatal. The most consistent risk factor for the development of SSPE is natural measles infection before the age of 2 years.[69] The decrease in cases of SSPE after the introduction of measles vaccination programs helped to establish the measles virus as the causative agent. Available data suggest that the pathogenesis of SSPE as a persistent infection of the CNS with measles virus is secondary to an abnormal host response to the initial measles infection and the generation of viral mutants during the acute infection that can establish persistence. The mean age at presentation with symptoms was around 6 years before vaccination programs. The child presents with psycho-intellectual disturbances (emotional lability, a decrease in school performance, and hyperactivity). Within 6 months, a variety of motor or convulsive findings become manifest, sometimes with severe myoclonic jerks. Spasticity may evolve during this stage.[70] The illness progresses to frequent and severe myoclonic jerks, rigidity, and decerebrate or decorticate posturing. Hypothalamic dysfunction is expected, with spells of diaphoresis, hyerpyrexia, and flushing. Death is usually secondary to a complication of living in a vegetative state.

## ■ Conclusion

CNS viral infections have a broad spectrum of severity, depending on the nature of the infecting virus and on host factors such as age and immune status. A clinical diagnosis of CNS viral infection requires a detailed history and physical examination to uncover clues to the most likely etiologic agent. Advances in molecular viral diagnostic testing have facilitated the identification of infecting agents and enabled further understanding of the pathogenesis and spectrum of disease. Treatment is largely supportive; however, some viral infections of the CNS require the prompt initiation of antiviral agents, and other infections may benefit from emerging therapies whose benefit is yet to be proven.

### References

1. Tsai TF. New initiatives for the control of Japanese encephalitis by vaccination: minutes of a WHO/CVI meeting, Bangkok, Thailand, 13-15 October 1998. Vaccine 2000;18(Suppl 2):1–25
2. Centers for Disease Control and Prevention. West Nile virus activity—United States Jan 1-Dec 2005. Morb Mortal Wkly Rep 2005;54:1253–1256
3. Hayes EB, O'Leary DR. West Nile virus infection: a pediatric perspective. Pediatrics 2004;113(5):1375–1381
4. Dayan GH, Quinlisk MP, Parker AA, et al. Recent resurgence of mumps in the United States. N Engl J Med 2008;358(15):1580–1589
5. Centers for Disease Control. Encephalitis surveillance: annual summary 1977. Issued December 1979
6. Bellini WJ, Harcourt BH, Bowden N, Rota PA. Nipah virus: an emergent paramyxovirus causing severe encephalitis in humans. J Neurovirol 2005;11(5):481–487
7. World Health Organization. WHO expert consultation on rabies. WHO Technical Report Series 2005;931:1–121
8. Whitley RJ, Kimberlin DW. Herpes simplex encephalitis: children and adolescents. Semin Pediatr Infect Dis 2005;16(1):17–23
9. Rantala H, Uhari M. Occurrence of childhood encephalitis: a population-based study. Pediatr Infect Dis J 1989;8(7):426–430
10. Whitley RJ. Herpes simplex encephalitis: adolescents and adults. Antiviral Res 2006;71(2-3):141–148
11. Nahmias AJ, Whitley RJ, Visintine AN, Takei Y, Alford CA Jr. Herpes simplex virus encephalitis: laboratory evaluations and their diagnostic significance. J Infect Dis 1982;145(6):829–836
12. Koskiniemi M, Vaheri A, Taskinen E. Cerebrospinal fluid alterations in herpes simplex virus encephalitis. Rev Infect Dis 1984;6(5):608–618
13. Lakeman FD, Whitley RJ; National Institute of Allergy and Infectious Diseases Collaborative Antiviral Study Group. Diagnosis of herpes simplex encephalitis: application of polymerase chain reaction to cerebrospinal fluid from brain-biopsied patients and correlation with disease. J Infect Dis 1995;171(4):857–863
14. Schroth G, Gawehn J, Thron A, Vallbracht A, Voigt K. Early diagnosis of herpes simplex encephalitis by MRI. Neurology 1987;37(2):179–183
15. Morawetz RB, Whitley RJ, Murphy DM. Experience with brain biopsy for suspected herpes en-

cephalitis: a review of forty consecutive cases. Neurosurgery 1983;12(6):654–657

16. Domachowske JB, Cunningham CK, Cummings DL, Crosley CJ, Hannan WP, Weiner LB. Acute manifestations and neurologic sequelae of Epstein-Barr virus encephalitis in children. Pediatr Infect Dis J 1996;15(10):871–875

17. Connelly KP, DeWitt LD. Neurologic complications of infectious mononucleosis. Pediatr Neurol 1994;10(3):181–184

18. North K, de Silva L, Procopis P. Brain-stem encephalitis caused by Epstein-Barr virus. J Child Neurol 1993;8(1):40–42

19. Bale JF Jr. Human cytomegalovirus infection and disorders of the nervous system. Arch Neurol 1984;41(3):310–320

20. Rafailidis PI, Mourtzoukou EG, Varbotis IC, Falagas ME. Severe cytomegalovirus infection in apparently immunocompetent patients: a systematic review. Virol J 2008;5:47–51

21. Nielsen SL, Petito CK, Urmacher CD, Posner JB. Subacute encephalitis in acquired immune deficiency syndrome: a postmortem study. Am J Clin Pathol 1984;82(6):678–682

22. Johnson R, Milbourn PE. Central nervous system manifestations of chickenpox. Can Med Assoc J 1970;102(8):831–834

23. Cohen JI, Davenport DS, Stewart JA, Deitchman S, Hilliard JK, Chapman LE; B Virus Working Group. Recommendations for prevention of and therapy for exposure to B virus (cercopithecine herpesvirus 1). Clin Infect Dis 2002;35(10):1191–1203

24. Wang SM, Liu CC, Tseng HW, et al. Clinical spectrum of enterovirus 71 infection in children in southern Taiwan, with an emphasis on neurological complications. Clin Infect Dis 1999;29(1):184–190

25. Hayward JC, Gillespie SM, Kaplan KM, et al. Outbreak of poliomyelitis-like paralysis associated with enterovirus 71. Pediatr Infect Dis J 1989;8(9):611–616

26. Grist NR, Bell EJ. Enteroviral etiology of the paralytic poliomyelitis syndrome. Arch Environ Health 1970;21(3):382–387

27. Kelsey DS. Adenovirus meningoencephalitis. Pediatrics 1978;61(2):291–293

28. Reeves WC. The discovery decade of arbovirus research in western North America, 1940-1949. Am J Trop Med Hyg 1987;37(3, Suppl):94S–100S

29. Weaver SC, Salas R, Rico-Hesse R, et al; VEE Study Group. Re-emergence of epidemic Venezuelan equine encephalomyelitis in South America. Lancet 1996;348(9025):436–440

30. Centers for Disease Control and Prevention. West Nile virus disease and other arboviral diseases—United States 2010. Morb Mortal Wkly Rep 2011;60:1009–1013

31. Spruance SL, Bailey A. Colorado tick fever. A review of 115 laboratory confirmed cases. Arch Intern Med 1973;131:288–293

32. Warrell DA. The clinical picture of rabies in man. Trans R Soc Trop Med Hyg 1976;70(3):188–195

33. Hemachudha T, Wacharapluesadee S, Mitrabhakdi E, Wilde H, Morimoto K, Lewis RA. Pathophysiology of human paralytic rabies. J Neurovirol 2005;11(1):93–100

34. Koch FJ, Sagartz JW, Davidson DE, Lawhaswasdi K. Diagnosis of human rabies by the cornea test. Am J Clin Pathol 1975;63(4):509–515

35. Porras C, Barboza JJ, Fuenzalida E, Adaros HL, Oviedo AM, Furst J. Recovery from rabies in man. Ann Intern Med 1976;85(1):44–48

36. Willoughby RE Jr, Tieves KS, Hoffman GM, et al. Survival after treatment of rabies with induction of coma. N Engl J Med 2005;352(24):2508–2514

37. Jackson AC. Therapy of human rabies. Adv Virus Res 2011;79:365–375

38. Barton LL, Hyndman NJ. Lymphocytic choriomeningitis virus: reemerging central nervous system pathogen. Pediatrics 2000;105(3):E35

39. Berger JR, Levy RM. The neurologic complications of human immunodeficiency virus infection. Med Clin North Am 1993;77(1):1–23

40. Berger JR, Pall L, Lanska D, Whiteman M. Progressive multifocal leukoencephalopathy in patients with HIV infection. J Neurovirol 1998;4(1):59–68

41. Telenti A, Aksamit AJJ Jr, Proper J, Smith TF. Detection of JC virus DNA by polymerase chain reaction in patients with progressive multifocal leukoencephalopathy. J Infect Dis 1990;162(4):858–861

42. de Luca A, Cingolani A, Linzalone A, et al. Improved detection of JC virus DNA in cerebrospinal fluid for diagnosis of AIDS-related progressive multifocal leukoencephalopathy. J Clin Microbiol 1996;34(5):1343–1346

43. Vazeux R, Cumont M, Girard PM, et al. Severe encephalitis resulting from coinfections with HIV and JC virus. Neurology 1990;40(6):944–948

44. World Health Organization. Report of the Scientific Group on HTLV-1 and Associated Diseases, Kogoshima, Japan, December 1988: Viral Diseases. Wkly Epidemiol Rec 1989;49:382–383

45. Maloney EM, Cleghorn FR, Morgan OS, et al. Incidence of HTLV-I-associated myelopathy/tropical spastic paraparesis (HAM/TSP) in Jamaica and Trinidad. J Acquir Immune Defic Syndr Hum Retrovirol 1998;17(2):167–170

46. Gout O, Gessain A, Iba-Zizen M, et al. The effect of zidovudine on chronic myelopathy associated with HTLV-1. J Neurol 1991;238(2):108–109

47. Murphy EL, Engstrom JW, Miller K, Sacher RA, Busch MP, Hollingsworth CG; REDS Investigators. HTLV-II associated myelopathy in 43-year-old woman. Lancet 1993;341(8847):757–758

48. Hadlow WJ. Scrapie and kuru. Lancet 1959;2:289–290

49. Brown P, Will RG, Bradley R, Asher DM, Detwiler L. Bovine spongiform encephalopathy and variant Creutzfeldt-Jakob disease: background, evolution, and current concerns. Emerg Infect Dis 2001;7(1):6–16

50. Brown P, Cathala F, Raubertas RF, Gajdusek DC, Castaigne P. The epidemiology of Creutzfeldt-Jakob disease: conclusion of a 15-year investigation in France and review of the world literature. Neurology 1987;37(6):895–904

51. Brown P, Preece M, Brandel JP, et al. Iatrogenic Creutzfeldt-Jakob disease at the millennium. Neurology 2000;55(8):1075–1081

52. Richt JA, Kunkle RA, Alt D, et al. Identification and characterization of two bovine spongiform encephalopathy cases diagnosed in the United States. J Vet Diagn Invest 2007;19(2):142–154

53. Brown P, Cathala F, Castaigne P, Gajdusek DC. Creutzfeldt-Jakob disease: clinical analysis of a consecutive series of 230 neuropathologically verified cases. Ann Neurol 1986;20(5):597–602

54. Finkenstaedt M, Szudra A, Zerr I, et al. MR imaging of Creutzfeldt-Jakob disease. Radiology 1996;199(3):793–798

55. Budka H, Aguzzi A, Brown P, et al. Neuropathological diagnostic criteria for Creutzfeldt-Jakob disease (CJD) and other human spongiform encephalopathies (prion diseases). Brain Pathol 1995; 5(4):459–466

56. WHO infection control guidelines for transmissible spongiform encephalopathies. Report of a WHO consultation, Geneva, Switzerland, 23–26 March, 1999

57. Cunningham CK, Bonville CA, Ochs HD, et al. Enteroviral meningoencephalitis as a complication of X-linked hyper IgM syndrome. J Pediatr 1999;134(5):584–588

58. Winkelstein JA, Marino MC, Lederman HM, et al. X-linked agammaglobulinemia: report on a United States registry of 201 patients. Medicine (Baltimore) 2006;85(4):193–202

59. Dropulic LK, Cohen JI. Severe viral infections and primary immunodeficiencies. Clin Infect Dis 2011;53(9):897–909

60. Cinbis M, Aysun S. Alice in Wonderland syndrome as an initial manifestation of Epstein-Barr virus infection. Br J Ophthalmol 1992;76(5):316–318

61. Cassady KA, Whitley RJ. Pathogenesis and pathophysiology of viral central nervous system infections. In: Scheld WM, Whitley RJ, Durack DT, eds. Infections of the Central Nervous System. 2nd ed. Philadelphia, PA: Lippincott–Raven Publishers; 1997:7–22

62. Bale JF Jr. Viral encephalitis. Med Clin North Am 1993;77(1):25–42

63. Centers for Disease Control and Prevention. Expanded program on immunization: certification of poliomyelitis eradication—the Americas. Morb Mortal Wkly Rep 1994;43:720–722

64. Rosen L. The natural history of Japanese encephalitis virus. Annu Rev Microbiol 1986;40:395–414

65. Yan HJ. Herpes simplex encephalitis: the role of surgical decompression. Surg Neurol 2002; 57(1):20–24

66. Ho DD, Hirsch MS. Acute viral encephalitis. Med Clin North Am 1985;69(2):415–429

67. Misra UK, Tan CT, Kalita J. Viral encephalitis and epilepsy. Epilepsia 2008;49(Suppl 6):13–18

68. Yohannan MD, Ramia S, al Frayh ARS. Acute paralytic poliomyelitis presenting as Guillain-Barré syndrome. J Infect 1991;22(2):129–133

69. Detels R, Brody JA, McNew J, Edgar AH. Further epidemiological studies of subacute sclerosing panencephalitis. Lancet 1973;2(7819):11–14

70. Risk WS, Haddad FS. The variable natural history of subacute sclerosing panencephalitis: a study of 118 cases from the Middle East. Arch Neurol 1979;36(10):610–614

# 6

# Fungal Infections of the Central Nervous System

Walter A. Hall and Peter D. Kim

Fungal infections that affect the central nervous system (CNS) usually cause chronic meningitis or brain abscess. Most clinically significant fungal infections involve patients with altered immune function, although immunocompetent hosts can also become infected. Fungal infections are often overlooked as a cause of CNS disease, and delays in diagnosis from 2 months to 11 years have been reported.[1] No consistent guidelines regarding the neurosurgical management of these infections have been established because of their infrequent occurrence. This chapter focuses on the medical and surgical management of these uncommon entities.

## ■ Incidence and Demographics

The incidence of fungal infections involving the CNS has increased in recent years because of the growing number of patients with compromised immune systems. This is in large part due to the increased use of immunosuppressive agents, which are commonly given to treat inflammatory conditions, malignancies, and acquired immunodeficiency syndrome (AIDS). They are also given to transplant recipients.

The most common causes of fungal meningitis are *Cryptococcus neoformans* and *Cryptococcus gattii. C. neoformans* is found throughout the world in soil contaminated by bird feces and in fruits, vegetables, and dairy products.[2] In contrast,

*C. gattii* is endemic in Australia and can be isolated from eucalyptus trees.

The incidence of fungal brain abscess has increased because of the administration of corticosteroids, immunosuppressive agents, and broad-spectrum antibiotics.[3] Many cases of fungal brain abscess remain undiagnosed until autopsy. Fungal brain abscess is due to *Aspergillus* species in 18 to 28% of patients.[4] *Aspergillus* meningitis rarely occurs because of the large size of the hyphae (**Fig. 6.1**) at body temperature, which are unable to infiltrate the microvasculature of the meninges.[4]

Some fungal infections are associated with specific geographic locations. Coccidioidomycosis is found in the southwestern United States, particularly in Arizona and California's San Joaquin Valley. Histoplasmosis is found throughout the United

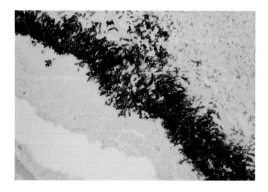

**Fig. 6.1** Gomori methenamine silver stain showing the large fugal hyphae of *Aspergillus* species (magnification x 64).

States except for the Rocky Mountain states and the Pacific Northwest and is endemic in the valleys of the Ohio, Mississippi, St. Lawrence, and Rio Grande Rivers. *Histoplasma capsulatum* is the most common fungus causing pulmonary infections.[4] *Blastomyces dermatitidis* is found throughout the southern and central United States, and young men are most often infected because of greater environmental exposure to the fungus.[5]

## ■ Etiology and Pathogenesis

*Candida* species are normal flora for the mucosa of the genital and gastrointestinal tracts.[5] Common clinical manifestations of infection due to *Candida* species are thrush and vulvovaginitis. Of all the *Candida* species identified, only 10 have been found to cause human disease, with *Candida albicans, Candida krusei*, and *Torulopsis glabrata* the most frequently identified agents.[4] These thin-walled oval organisms reproduce in the yeast form, and true hyphae are usually found only in active infection.[4] Systemic candidiasis results when organisms enter the bloodstream after penetrating the mucosal surface following surgery, with intravenous drug use, or in the presence of an indwelling intravenous catheter. Nearly half of patients with systemic disease develop CNS involvement, although the incidence reaches nearly 80% in the presence of endocarditis.[4] CNS infection with *Candida* species is nosocomial in 95% of patients, but infection after neurosurgery is rare.[1]

The most common etiologic agents for fungal brain abscess at autopsy are *Candida* species, which can cause microabscesses, macroabscesses, noncaseating granulomas, and glial nodules located at the gray–white junction.[3] Other infectious CNS manifestations associated with *Candida* species are mycotic aneurysms, vasculitis leading to vessel thrombosis and infarction, and intraventricular fungal balls.[1] Patients at risk for *Candida* species brain abscess are premature infants with a low birth weight and those who have cancer, neutropenia,

diabetes mellitus, chronic granulomatous disease, or thermal injuries. Also at risk are patients who have a central venous catheter or who have received chemotherapy, antimicrobial therapy, corticosteroids, or immunosuppressive therapy following a bone marrow or solid-organ transplant.[3,4]

The fungal species *C. neoformans* forms the only known encapsulated yeast that is pathogenic to humans.[4-6] The polysaccharide capsule is responsible for the virulence of the organism because it inhibits phagocytosis and antigen presentation.[4,5] This organism reproduces by budding. The primary site of entry of *C. neoformans* into the host is through the lungs by the inhalation of infected soil or dust. Hematogenous dissemination of the organism to the CNS occurs most often in immunocompromised patients or in the face of overwhelming exposure in immunocompetent individuals. CNS involvement is in the form of meningoencephalitis (**Fig. 6.2**) in 90% of patients with disseminated disease.[4] Defective T-lymphocyte function is the primary pre-

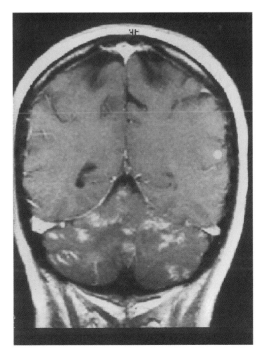

**Fig. 6.2** Coronal T1-weighted contrast-enhanced magnetic resonance image demonstrating cryptococcal meningoencephalitis of the cerebellum.

disposing factor for cryptococcosis and is associated with AIDS, hematologic malignancies, collagen vascular diseases, immunosuppression following organ transplant, and corticosteroid use.[4,5] Early in the AIDS epidemic, 6 to 8% of patients developed cryptococcal meningoencephalitis.[7] Because of the presence of global immune dysfunction, AIDS patients do not develop a significant inflammatory response, necrotizing granulomas do not form, and lymphocyte-mediated activation of macrophages is impaired.[8] The widespread CNS involvement that is seen in AIDS patients with cryptococcal meningoencephalitis is due to the inability of the microglia and astrocytes within the brain to contain the infection. *C. neoformans* can replicate and survive within human microglia.[1]

*Coccidioides immitis* forms nonseptate hyphae that become airborne and are inhaled as arthroconidia in infected dust. Disease due to *C. immitis* is usually restricted to the lungs and causes flulike symptoms, although dissemination can occur through lymphatic and hematogenous routes, leading to caseous granulomas. One-third to one-half of patients with disseminated coccidioidomycosis develop CNS involvement, usually 4 to 12 weeks after the pulmonary infection.[4] Basilar leptomeningitis with cerebrospinal fluid (CSF) obstruction leading to hydrocephalus is the most common form of CNS involvement in coccidioidomycosis. Other CNS infectious processes due to *C. immitis* are encephalitis, multiple miliary granulomas, and solitary brain abscess. Vasculitis of the small and medium-size arteries due to *C. immitis* can result in cerebral ischemia and infarction of the deep white matter and basal ganglia or the formation of mycotic aneurysms. The spinal meninges can also be involved, resulting in paraplegia from occlusion of the anterior spinal artery or necrotizing meningomyelitis.[4]

*H. capsulatum* is found in soil contaminated by bird feces. This fungus is present in the mycelial form in the wild but converts to a budding yeast form at human body temperature.[4] Infection with *H. capsulatum* is contracted by inhaling con-taminated dust and is usually limited to the lungs. Acute disease manifests as fever, hypoxia, and pulmonary infiltrates, with severity dependent on the size of the infectious inoculum. The normal immune response in an immunocompetent individual is the formation of caseating granulomas, which calcify and restrict disease to the lungs. Disseminated disease is uncommon in immunocompetent individuals and is usually associated with immunosuppression following organ transplant or AIDS. Systemic disease is characterized by anemia, splenomegaly, leukopenia, cachexia, and fever.[5] Involvement of the CNS occurs in 10 to 20% of disseminated cases through hematogenous spread.[4] The two primary modes of CNS involvement are (1) basilar leptomeningitis with multiple cranial neuropathies, hydrocephalus, and seizures and (2) intraparenchymal mass lesions ranging from multiple miliary granulomas to large histoplasmomas, with symptomatology referable to their location in the brain. Spinal histoplasmomas can cause myelopathy but the infection is usually clinically silent.[1]

*B. dermatitidis* is found in soil and decaying wood in its hyphal form; however, in infected tissue it forms spherical yeasts.[4] Conidia are initially inhaled in the lungs in most cases of blastomycosis, although the disease can be contracted via exposed areas of the skin that will develop subcutaneous nodules and can ulcerate.[5] The genitourinary tract and the skull can become infected with *B. dermatitidis*. The CNS is infected in fewer than 5% of cases of disseminated disease by hematogenous spread or through direct extension of cranial or vertebral osteomyelitis.[4,6] Intracerebral blastomycomas and chronic meningitis are the most common forms of CNS involvement.

Fungal infection can involve the brain in 10 to 50% of patients with invasive aspergillosis. The primary site of infection is usually the lungs.[4] In immunocompetent individuals, a local immediate hypersensitivity reaction in the lungs leads to the formation of granulomas that contain the organism.[4] Dissemination to the brain is either through the bloodstream or by direct extension from the paranasal sinuses.[1] Risk factors for *Aspergillus* species infection of the brain include neutropenia from a hematologic malignancy, hepatic disease, Cushing syndrome, AIDS, diabetes mellitus, chronic granulomatous disease, intravenous drug use, organ transplant, bone marrow and stem cell transplant, chronic corticosteroid use, malnutrition, chronic pulmonary disease, and prior craniotomy.[3,4,9] Of the 350 different *Aspergillus* species, *Aspergillus fumigatus* and *Aspergillus flavus*, acting as opportunistic pathogens, cause most infections in humans.[4]

*Aspergillus* species have a predilection for invading blood vessel walls (**Fig. 6.3**) in medium-size to large arteries, where they destroy the internal elastic layer, causing thrombosis, vascular occlusion, and subsequent cerebral infarction in the distribution of the artery. The resulting necrotic brain parenchyma serves as an ideal environment for fungal proliferation, leading to the formation of a brain abscess that can reach several centimeters in diameter. In addition to causing brain abscesses, *Aspergillus* species can cause mycotic aneurysms (**Fig. 6.4**) to form through their effect on the wall of the blood vessel, which is usually an anterior or middle cerebral artery. Rupture of these intracranial aneurysms can result in intracerebral hematomas (**Fig. 6.5**) or subarachnoid hemorrhage.[4] Direct extension of *Aspergillus* species from the paranasal sinuses (**Fig. 6.6**) or orbits can lead to a solitary frontal lobe brain abscess adjacent to the site of intracranial entry.

Organisms of the genera *Rhizopus*, *Absidia*, and *Mucor* (family Mucoraceae) cause mucormycosis. The *Mucor* mold is found worldwide in rotting organic matter. The nonseptate hyphae branch at right angles. The fungal spores become airborne as infected dust and can be cultured from the nose and throat of healthy individuals. This fungal infection enters the skin after trauma or a burn.[4] Like *Aspergillus* species, this fungus frequently involves medium-size and large blood vessels, resulting in thrombosis and widespread necrosis of the mucosa and skull base, which creates an ideal environment for growth and dissemination.

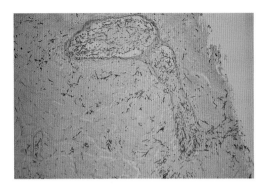

**Fig. 6.3** Gomori methenamine silver stain revealing *Aspergillus fumigatus* hyphae in the wall of a fungal mycotic aneurysm (magnification unknown). This fungus has a propensity to invade blood vessel walls, leading to thrombosis, occlusion, and infarction.

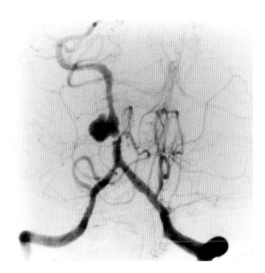

**Fig. 6.4** This posterior circulation cerebral angiogram shows a large *Aspergillus* species fungal mycotic aneurysm arising from the trunk of the basilar artery.

Mucormycosis is an aggressive fungal infection that can involve the brain through hematogenous spread or after head trauma, but it typically results from direct extension of an infection involving the face or nasopharynx (**Fig. 6.7**). Predisposing conditions for mucormycosis are the following: diabetes mellitus (70% of patients, usually with ketoacidosis); acidemia from sepsis, dehydration, diarrhea, or renal failure; intravenous drug abuse;

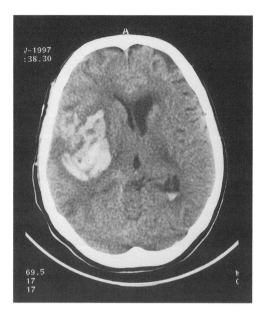

**Fig. 6.5** Computed tomographic scan of the brain showing a large intracerebral hematoma in a patient known to have a systemic *Aspergillus* species infection that was presumed to be due to the rupture of a fungal mycotic aneurysm.

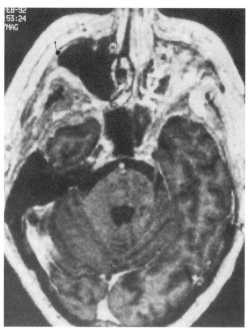

**Fig. 6.6** Axial T1-weighted contrast-enhanced magnetic resonance image of the brain demonstrates an *Aspergillus* species infection in the left maxillary sinus. A frontal brain abscess eventually developed through direct extension in this patient with a bone marrow transplant.

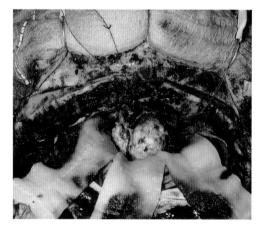

**Fig. 6.7** Intraoperative photograph shows a bifrontal *Mucor* species brain abscess that invaded the brain from the paranasal sinuses by direct extension. The patient had poorly controlled juvenile diabetes mellitus.

hematologic malignancy; renal transplant; and the use of deferoxamine for iron overload.[3,10] Intravenous drug abusers are at risk for cerebral mucormycosis via direct inoculation of the blood stream with fungus from contaminated needles. Normal hosts account for fewer than 5% of cases of CNS mucormycosis. *Rhizopus arrhizus* is one of the most common of the *Mucor* species causing brain abscess and belongs to the order Mucorales. *R. arrhizus* and *Rhizopus oryzae* are responsible for 95% of infections in humans.[5]

*Scedosporium apiospermum* is the asexual form of *Pseudallescheria boydii.* It can enter the CNS by direct extension from trauma or infected sinuses, by hematogenous dissemination from a pulmonary focus, or by an intravenous catheter. Normal hosts or immunocompromised individuals with neutropenia or cellular immunodeficiency can develop CNS infection from *Scedosporium* species.[11] Brain abscess is the most common CNS manifestation of *Scedosporium* species infection, although meningitis and ventriculitis can occur.

Other fungi that have been reported to cause brain abscess include *Cladophia-*

*lophora bantiana, Bipolaris hawaiiensis, Bipolaris spicifera, Exophiala (Wangiella) dermatitidis, Ochroconis gallopava (Dactylaria constricta* var. *gallopava), Ramichloridium mackenziei, Curvularia pallescens,* and *Acrophialophora fusispora.*[3]

## ■ Presentation

### Clinical Features

Chronic meningitis usually presents with the onset of indolent symptoms of at least 4 weeks' duration.[12] It is necessary to distinguish this entity from recurrent aseptic meningitis and persistent encephalitis. Determining the date of the onset of symptoms and the timing of symptom development can be important in confirming the diagnosis of chronic meningitis. Symptoms associated with chronic meningitis can wax and wane for weeks to months. Early symptoms may include headache, nausea, decreased memory and comprehension, decreased vision, double vision, vomiting, confusion, unsteady gait, and cranial nerve palsies. A dementia-like picture can be present in the face of hydrocephalus. With worsening cerebral edema, papilledema and brainstem compression with upper motor neuron signs, increased deep tendon reflexes, and Cheyne-Stokes respiration can develop.

A normal neurologic examination and an absence of fever may be seen in patients with chronic meningitis. Skin lesions may require a biopsy for the diagnosis of cryptococcosis, coccidioidomycosis, blastomycosis, or sporotrichosis. Skin lesions will precede meningeal symptoms in 10% of patients with cryptococcosis.[13] Lymphadenopathy may be present with histoplasmosis. Retinal lesions are sometimes present in patients with cryptococcosis or coccidioidomycosis.

*Candida* meningitis is rare except in patients who are immunosuppressed, have had prior neurosurgery, or have a hematologic malignancy, and in very low birth weight newborns.[14] Newborns with *Candida* meningitis have typically had long intensive care unit stays and have for pro-

longed periods required indwelling intravenous catheters through which the fungus has access to the bloodstream. Congenital malformations of the intestine or urinary tract that have required surgical repair can also act as a portal for *Candida* entry into the blood. Hydrocephalus can already be present when *Candida* meningitis is diagnosed, and CSF shunts that become infected with *Candida* are at risk for partial or complete obstruction, usually requiring multiple surgical revisions. One retrospective review of pediatric shunt infections found that 17% were *Candida*-related.[15] The etiology of shunt infection due to *Candida* species was either contamination at the time of placement or hematogenous dissemination from a remote source.[4]

Patients with cryptococcal meningoencephalitis often have an insidious clinical presentation, leading to a delay in diagnosis. Underlying disease entities that predispose to cryptococcal meningitis are corticosteroid therapy and AIDS. Symptoms associated with raised intracranial pressure due to hydrocephalus, such as headaches, nausea, and vomiting, may be the only complaints.[4] Psychosis and confusion can be presenting symptoms. Visual symptoms such as decreased acuity due to papilledema or rapid visual deterioration from neuritis of the optic nerves or chiasm can occur.[1]

Exposure to *Coccidioides* species is necessary for infection, which usually begins as a pulmonary process 2 to 4 weeks after exposure. In immunosuppressed patients, coccidioidal meningitis presents as a systemic illness with fever, malaise, headache, cranial nerve findings, and skin lesions. *Histoplasma* meningitis can occur in immunosuppressed patients who have AIDS, are organ transplant recipients, or are taking corticosteroids or tumor necrosis factor-α inhibitors.[16]

Fungal abscesses can develop in any part of the brain, and the clinical presentation depends on their location. Headache, seizures, altered level of consciousness, encephalopathy, focal neurologic deficits, meningismus, personality changes, and aphasia can be seen with fungal brain abscess. Nearly a third of bone marrow transplant recipients who have *Candida* species brain abscesses may have no clinical findings.[3] Blastomycomas will be either asymptomatic or cause symptoms related to their location in the brain. Chronic meningitis can also result from *B. dermatitidis* infection, which presents similarly to tuberculous meningitis and often results in the development of hydrocephalus. The presentation of cranial and spinal epidural blastomyccocal abscesses can be due to the underlying mass effect on the brain or spinal cord. Histoplasmomas can occur throughout the brain and cause symptoms that reflect their location.

*Aspergillus* species brain abscess can present with a strokelike syndrome due either to vascular occlusion or to hemorrhage that is referable to the area of the brain that is involved. Severely immunocompromised patients can present with relatively nonspecific clinical findings, such as altered consciousness or seizure activity, whereas immunocompetent individuals may have headache or focal neurologic findings.[3] Rhinocerebral mucormycosis will usually present with findings referable to the eyes or the sinuses, such as headache, facial pain or edema, nasal congestion, and epistaxis.[10] Fever and abnormalities involving cranial nerves II through VII are common, and blindness, diplopia, chemosis, proptosis, and ophthalmoplegia can also result from invasion of the orbit, cavernous sinus, and ophthalmic artery. Invasion of the carotid artery with thrombosis and hemiparesis is possible because of the potential for this mold to invade blood vessels. As the infection spreads to adjacent structures, necrotic lesions can involve the nares, turbinates, hard palate, sphenoid sinus, sella turcica, and cribriform plate. Findings in advanced mucormycosis include blindness, diabetes insipidus, carotid artery occlusion, cavernous sinus thrombosis, and bifrontal brain abscess (**Fig. 6.8**).[4,17] Hematogenous dissemination of *Mucor* species to the basal ganglia in intravenous drug abusers can lead to brain abscess that presents with fever, headache, and a neurologic deficit such as a hemiparesis.[3] *Scedosporium apiospermum* can cause brain abscess in

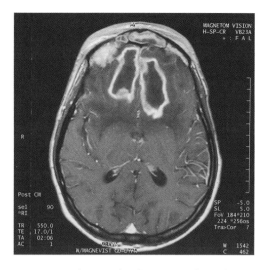

**Fig. 6.8** Axial T1-weighted contrast-enhanced magnetic resonance image of the brain shows the bifrontal *Mucor* species brain abscess that is visible in the intraoperative photograph of **Fig. 6.7**.

immunocompromised patients or in immunocompetent patients 15 to 30 days after near-drowning.[3]

## Microbiology

The CSF will show signs of inflammation in chronic meningitis.[12] To recover fungi from the CSF, it is important to obtain an adequate CSF volume of 3 to 5 mL for culture.[13] In the presence of *Candida* species meningitis, microscopic analysis of the CSF will often reveal the organism, which can be cultured, and a polymorphonuclear pleocytosis.[6] In patients with AIDS, CSF cultures for cryptococcal meningitis can become positive within a few days; however, a longer incubation period is necessary in immunocompetent patients. In immunocompromised individuals, *C. neoformans* can occasionally be isolated from the blood or urine.[4,18] An India ink preparation can occasionally demonstrate the organism in the CSF.[5] CNS blastomycosis can be difficult to diagnose in the absence of chronic pulmonary blastomycosis; however, with chronic meningeal involvement, the organisms can occasionally be identified microscopically or by culture.

## ■ Diagnosis

### Laboratory

When the CSF is sampled, the opening pressure is usually elevated and the glucose concentration is below 40 mg/dL in fungal meningitis.[13] A *Candida*-specific mannan antigen titer and a polymerase chain reaction (PCR)–based test for the detection of *C. albicans* in the CSF are available.[4] There is no reliable serologic test for CNS candidiasis.[1,6]

Other tests that may identify fungal infection in the CSF are cryptococcal antigen, complement fixation antibody to *Coccidioides* species, *Histoplasma* antigen, and *Aspergillus* galactomannan.[13] Rapid latex agglutination and enzyme immunoassays can detect the cryptococcal capsular polysaccharide antigen in the blood and CSF.[1] Serum serology can be useful in diagnosing coccidioidomycosis. Serum antigen tests for *Cryptococcus* species and serum or urine antigen tests for *Histoplasma* can be useful for establishing a diagnosis, particularly in the presence of disseminated disease. Eosinophilia in the blood or CSF can be a sign of coccidioidal meningitis, although the single best test for diagnosis is a positive complement fixation test of CSF. This test is sensitive and specific, unlike an immunodiffusion test, which is less specific, or enzyme-linked immunosorbent assays (ELISAs), which lack both sensitivity and specificity.[13]

In a patient with a ring-enhancing intracranial mass consistent with a brain abscess surrounded by cerebral edema, a lumbar puncture is usually contraindicated because of the risk for cerebral herniation. Furthermore, when CSF is obtained from a patient with an *Aspergillus* species brain abscess, the findings are usually nonspecific and nondiagnostic. There is no reliable serologic test for aspergillosis, but diagnostic tests such as PCR and Western blot analysis are under development.[1] Diagnosing cerebral mucormycosis can be difficult because the CSF findings are nonspecific and the serologic testing is unreliable.[4]

### Imaging

*Candida* species can cause multiple brain abscesses in patients with disseminated disease. These microabscesses are often less than 1 mm in size, can be difficult to detect on imaging, and may or may not enhance with contrast.[4] Foci of high signal on T2-weighted and proton density–weighted magnetic resonance (MR) imaging can be indicative of *Candida* species infection in the CNS.[1] In the early stages of CNS cryptococcal infection, the perivascular subarachnoid spaces can appear dilated with hypodense lesions on computed tomographic (CT) scans because of the formation of gelatinous pseudocysts.[4] These lesions are usually hyperintense on T2-weighted imaging and hypointense on T1-weighted imaging, and they do not enhance with contrast administration on either CT scans or MR images. In contrast to these pseudocysts, cryptococcomas enhance after contrast administration on CT scans or MR images and display varying degrees of vasogenic edema. A contrast-enhanced MR image can demonstrate hydrocephalus or intracranial mass lesions such as granulomas due to cryptococcosis or histoplasmosis. Increased intracranial pressure may be inferred if there is flattening of the cerebral gyri over the convexities of the hemispheres.

Blastomycosis can result in chronic meningitis or brain abscess formation. Blastomycomas enhance homogeneously or in a ringlike manner on CT scans and MR images with contrast administration when surrounded by vasogenic edema.[4] Histoplasmomas can be ring-enhancing on contrast CT and MR imaging and demonstrate varying degrees of surrounding cerebral edema.

*Aspergillus* species brain abscesses typically are ring-enhancing lesions with surrounding edema on contrast CT or MR imaging (**Fig. 6.9**). However, there may be little (**Fig. 6.10**) or no enhancement on MR imaging in immunosuppressed patients with CNS aspergillosis.[19] An MR image of the paranasal sinuses can demonstrate an infection due to mold. Radiographic findings of rhinocerebral mucormycosis can include sinus opacification, bone erosion,

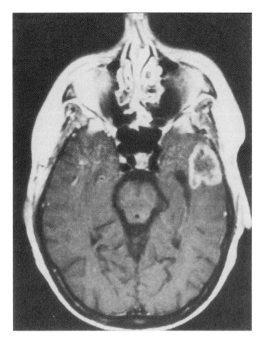

**Fig. 6.9** *Aspergillus* species brain abscess of the left temporal lobe as seen on a contrast-enhanced T1-weighted axial magnetic resonance image in a patient with a history of chronic pulmonary disease.

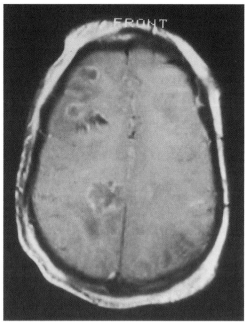

**Fig. 6.10** Weak, patchy enhancement can be seen in the anterior and posterior right frontal regions on a contrast-enhanced T1-weighted axial magnetic resonance image in this recipient of a hepatic transplant.

frontal lobe infiltration, and cavernous sinus involvement. CT may demonstrate bony destruction of the facial bones and skull base with air–fluid levels in the paranasal sinuses.[4] The infected mucosa of the paranasal sinuses and nasopharynx demonstrates a low signal intensity on T1-weighted, T2-weighted, and proton density–weighted MR images.[1] This appearance on MR imaging is thought to be due to the paramagnetic metals associated with the fungal infection and can help distinguish infection from benign mucosal swelling.[1] *Mucor* species brain abscess can demonstrate ring enhancement on CT and MR imaging and hemorrhage within the infectious collection. Contrast enhancement of the infected mucosa (**Fig. 6.11**), orbital structures, and dura mater can be seen on MR imaging. Absence of contrast enhancement in mucormycosis carries a poor prognosis because it suggests that the host defenses can no longer encapsulate the or-

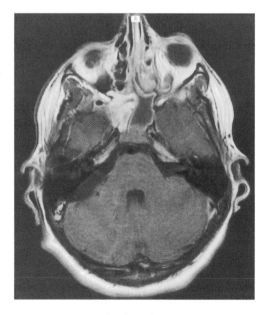

**Fig. 6.11** T1-weighted axial magnetic resonance image of the brain in a patient with diabetes mellitus shows contrast enhancement of infected mucosa in the sphenoid sinus that is due to *Mucor* species.

ganism.[3] Vascular imaging is useful for detecting thrombosis of the internal carotid arteries or cavernous sinus.

## Histology

On histologic examination of tissue specimens, *Aspergillus* species have septate hyphae with acute-angle, dichotomous branching at regular intervals. Irregular hyphae with right-angle branching and absence of septa are seen with mucormycosis. The diagnosis of mucormycosis will often require the histopathologic examination of biopsied or debrided necrotic tissue to show these findings. *Scedosporium apiospermum*, *Scedosporium prolificans*, and *Fusarium* hyphae cannot be distinguished histologically from *Aspergillus* species.[20]

## Treatment

### Surgical Approaches

The initial evaluation of the patient suspected to have a brain abscess should include contrast-enhanced CT or MR imaging of the brain. If one or more ring-enhancing brain lesions measuring greater than 2.5 cm in diameter are found, the patient should be taken to the operating room for either surgical excision or aspiration. The surgical specimens should be sent for pathologic examination and culture and sensitivity. If the lesions are smaller than 2.5 cm or in the cerebritis stage, the largest lesion should be biopsied or aspirated for diagnosis and identification of the organism.[3] An open or stereotactic biopsy is often the only way to confirm the presence of a histoplasmoma or blastomycoma. Excisional surgery or drainage is a key factor for success in treating CNS aspergillosis.[21] Repeat surgical debridement of the *Aspergillus* species abscess or a hemorrhagic infarct may be necessary, even at multiple intracranial sites, in the face of progressive disease despite appropriate antimicrobial therapy.

The role of surgery in the treatment of cerebral mucormycosis cannot be overlooked. The propensity of *Mucor* species to invade blood vessels, leading to cerebral infarction, can result in the decreased delivery of antifungal agents to the location of the infection. Radical surgical removal of necrotic, infected tissue is often the only effective way to reduce the number of invading fungal elements and to prevent them from spreading locally within the intracranial compartment. Once intracranial extension is established, surgical resection of the abscess capsule is required for prolonged survival.[16] As with other CNS fungal infections, surgical drainage is the cornerstone of effective treatment for *Scedosporium* brain abscess.[20]

*C. albicans* shunt infections should be treated with removal of the entire shunt system and placement of an external ventricular drain, in combination with the administration of intravenous amphotericin B. The *Candida*-specific mannan antigen levels can be followed during treatment with amphotericin B and should be normal for 1 week before replacement of a previously *Candida*-infected shunt.[22] CNS cryptococcomas rarely need to be surgically removed, but months of antimicrobial treatment may be required before they decrease in size on CT scans or MR images.[23] In the presence of symptomatic hydrocephalus and the absence of an intracranial mass lesion, external CSF drainage via repeat lumbar punctures or placement of an external ventricular or lumbar drain is indicated. Persistent hydrocephalus may require permanent CSF diversion by placement of a shunt, which can be performed successfully in an ongoing infection as long as the foreign body is placed after the initiation of antifungal therapy for cryptococcosis.[23] Permanent CSF diversion can be necessary to treat hydrocephalus resulting from basilar meningitis due to *H. capsulatum*.

### Medical Approaches

### Antimicrobial Agents

Once the offending organism has been identified, antimicrobial agents can be adjusted for optimal treatment. In immunocompromised patients, the mortality rate remains high, even with appropriate treatment. However, these infections can be effectively treated if the white blood cell counts return to normal or the immunosuppressive drug dose is lowered or discontinued.

Amphotericin B is the primary treatment for cryptococcal meningitis at a dose of 0.7 mg/kg per day for 6 weeks. Liposomal amphotericin B and the lipid complex at doses of 3 to 6 mg/kg per day have provided successful treatment for cryptococcal meningitis with reduced renal toxicity.[23] Because of the development of resistance, flucytosine cannot be used as a single agent against *Cryptococcus* species and is generally combined with amphotericin B at a dose of 100 mg/kg per day.[23] Fluconazole and itraconazole have been used successfully to treat cryptococcal meningitis. Maintenance therapy with fluconazole appears to be more effective than itraconazole, but the latter agent should be used when the former is not tolerated.[1] Criteria for the discontinuation of antifungal therapy are not well defined but have included the resolution of symptoms, two negative CSF cultures, and a normal CSF glucose level.[23] The return of new clinical signs or symptoms and repeat positive CSF cultures are the two clearest signs of relapse necessitating a change in treatment.[23]

For candidal meningitis and brain abscess, the treatment of choice is amphotericin B deoxycholate, liposomal amphotericin B, or amphotericin B lipid complex with 5-flucytosine. Fluconazole is a second-line agent that has not been formally evaluated. The dosages for *C. albicans* brain abscess are 0.6 to 1.0 mg/kg every 24 hours for amphotericin B deoxycholate and 5 mg/kg every 24 hours for amphotericin B lipid complex. The dose of 5-flucytosine is 100 mg/kg orally every 6 hours, and the dose of fluconazole is 400 to 800 mg ever 24 hours. Liposomal amphotericin B (3 to 5 mg/kg per day for 4 to 6 weeks) remains the treatment of choice for CNS histoplasmosis, followed by itraconazole (200 mg two to three times daily for at least 1 year).[24] Azole agents are not recommended for patients with life-threatening CNS histoplasmosis. CNS blastomycosis should be treated with amphotericin B because azole agents poorly cross the blood–brain barrier. However, in the absence of CNS involvement, systemic blastomycosis has been successfully treated with itraconazole or ketoconazole.[1]

Previously, the treatment for *Aspergillus* brain abscess was amphotericin B deoxycholate (0.8 to 1.25 mg/kg per day up to 1.5 mg/kg per day depending on the therapeutic response); however, few instances of survival have been reported.[25] Eradication of CNS *Aspergillus* has required more than a total of 3 g of amphotericin B. Even though high-dose itraconazole has resulted in the successful eradication of CNS *Aspergillus* in a few case reports, because of limited experience and unreliable absorption, this agent and posaconazole are better for salvage therapy than as a primary treatment.[3] Amphotericin B has been placed in an *Aspergillus* abscess cavity even though it is neurotoxic to the brain.[26] Voriconazole is now considered the drug of choice for treating CNS aspergillosis.[21] The response rate to voriconazole in patients with invasive aspergillosis in studies has been approximately 35%.[21] The total duration of treatment with antifungal agents remains unclear, although patients receiving cumulative doses of intravenous amphotericin B of 9.5 g and 11.45 g followed by 3 to 6 months of high-dose oral itraconazole have responded to treatment.[1]

Mucormycosis should be treated with amphotericin B deoxycholate, liposomal amphotericin B, or amphotericin B lipid complex; aggressive surgical debridement; and the correction of any underlying metabolic abnormalities.[3,27] Amphotericin B has been applied topically in the orbital cavities to treat mucormycosis, but this practice is of unknown benefit.[27] In addition to the intravenous administration of amphotericin B for mucormycosis, some have advocated its administration into the CSF and the abscess cavity.[28] Posaconazole (800 mg/day given every 6 or 12 hours) is considered an effective salvage therapy for patients with mucormycosis who have either not responded to or become unable to tolerate amphotericin B, provided that they can tolerate oral administration.[29] Hyperbaric oxygen has been used as an adjunctive treatment for mucormycosis.[3] Correction of any underlying metabolic abnormality is an essential aspect to treating the patient with mucormycosis.

Voraconazole (8 mg/kg per day given every 12 hours after a loading dose of 6 mg/kg given twice intravenously 12 hours apart) has emerged as the antifungal treatment of choice for *Scedosporium* brain abscess based on clinical experience, a lack of effective alternative treatments, and the in vitro resistance of this organism to amphotericin B.[3,20] In one report of 21 patients with CNS scedosporiosis, a 43% therapeutic response rate to voriconazole was observed.[30]

### Anticonvulsants

Anticonvulsants should be used in the early stages of treatment of CNS fungal infections to prevent seizures.

### Steroids

Corticosteroids can be initiated in patients with significant surrounding cerebral edema causing increased intracranial pressure or in patients with evidence of transtentorial herniation. However, they should be used sparingly, particularly in patients who are already immunocompromised, to avoid the detrimental effects of immune suppression.

### Sequelae

Despite favorable survival rates in patients treated for *Candida* meningitis, neurologic sequelae are common, with 56% of neonates having psychomotor retardation and 50% developing hydrocephalus.[6]

### Prognosis

The cure rates for *Candida* meningitis treated with amphotericin B are 71 to 100% in neonates and 67 to 89% in adults.[6] Cryptococcal meningitis is difficult to eradicate despite aggressive treatment and carries a mortality rate of 6%.[4] Prognostic factors that have been associated with a poor outcome in cryptococcal meningitis include lethargy or obtundation, a high CSF cryptococcal antigen titer, a low CSF leukocyte count at presentation, and infection with *C. neoformans*.[4,18]

The prognosis for patients with cerebral aspergillosis is poor, with a survival rate of less than 5%. Death often occurs within a matter of days following the onset of neurologic symptoms in CNS aspergillosis. A delay in diagnosis is often responsible for the poor outcome. A high degree of suspicion is often necessary to diagnose CNS aspergillosis early in the course of the disease.

The combination of antifungal therapy with radical surgical debridement has improved the prognosis of paranasal sinus mucormycosis, with reported survival rates of greater than 80%.[31] Cerebral involvement by *Mucor* species is associated with a much worse prognosis than paranasal involvement, particularly if the basal ganglia are involved, which removes surgical debridement as a reasonable option.[32] As with aspergillosis, the strongest predictive factor for a poor outcome in mucormycosis is a delay in diagnosis and initiation of treatment.[4] The correction of any underlying systemic metabolic disorders such as diabetic ketoacidosis is essential for any possibility of recovery.

### ■ Conclusion

The prognosis for most fungal infections of the CNS remains poor. Most patients who develop these infections have a compromised immune system, and discontinuation of the immunosuppression when possible can help aid in recovery. Infections are in the form of either a chronic meningoencephalitis or a brain abscess. Amphotericin B or the newer lipid formulations remain the primary medical treatments for CNS fungal infections. In the face of a brain abscess due to *Aspergillus* species or *Mucor* species in an immunocompromised patient, aggressive surgical debridement combined with amphotericin B may be the only possible treatment with any potential for a good clinical outcome. The rapid identification of a CNS fungal infection and the prompt initiation of treatment offer the best chance for a positive therapeutic response. The clinical condition of the patient at the time of diagnosis is the strongest predictor of clinical outcome.

## References

1. Hall WA, Anker L. Fungal infections in the brain. In: Batjer HH, Loftus CM, eds. Textbook of Neurological Surgery. Principles and Practice. Vol 4. Philadelphia, PA: Lippincott Williams & Wilkins; 2003:3157–3165
2. Levitz SM. The ecology of *Cryptococcus neoformans* and the epidemiology of cryptococcosis. Rev Infect Dis 1991;13(6):1163–1169
3. Tunkel AR. Brain abscess. In: Mandell GL, Bennett JE, Dolin R, eds. Mandell, Douglas, and Bennett's Principles and Practice of Infectious Diseases. Philadelphia, PA: Churchill Livingstone Elsevier; 2010:1265–1278
4. Anker L, Hall WA. Fungal infections. In: Hall WA, McCutcheon IA, eds. Infections in Neurosurgery. Park Ridge, IL: American Association of Neurological Surgeons Publications; 2000: 219–235
5. Chimelli L, Mahler-Araujo MB. Fungal infections. Brain Pathol 1997;7(1):613–627
6. Slavoski LA, Tunkel AR. Therapy of fungal meningitis. Clin Neuropharmacol 1995;18(2):95–112
7. Currie BP, Casadevall A. Estimation of the prevalence of cryptococcal infection among patients infected with the human immunodeficiency virus in New York City. Clin Infect Dis 1994;19(6): 1029–1033
8. Lee SC, Dickson DW, Casadevall A. Pathology of cryptococcal meningoencephalitis: analysis of 27 patients with pathogenetic implications. Hum Pathol 1996;27(8):839–847
9. Denning DW. Invasive aspergillosis. Clin Infect Dis 1998;26(4):781–803, quiz 804–805
10. Sugar AM. Mucormycosis. Clin Infect Dis 1992; 14(Suppl 1):S126–S129
11. Lamaris GA, Chamilos G, Lewis RE, Safdar A, Raad II, Kontoyiannis DP. *Scedosporium* infection in a tertiary care cancer center: a review of 25 cases from 1989-2006. Clin Infect Dis 2006;43(12): 1580–1584
12. Helbok R, Broessner G, Pfausler B, Schmutzhard E. Chronic meningitis. J Neurol 2009;256(2): 168–175
13. Bennett JE. Chronic meningitis. In: Mandell GL, Bennett JE, Dolin R, eds. Mandell, Douglas, and Bennett's Principles and Practice of Infectious Diseases. Philadelphia, PA: Churchill Livingstone Elsevier; 2010:1237–1241
14. Nguyen MH, Yu VL. Meningitis caused by *Candida* species: an emerging problem in neurosurgical patients. Clin Infect Dis 1995;21(2):323–327
15. Chiou CC, Wong TT, Lin HH, et al. Fungal infection of ventriculoperitoneal shunts in children. Clin Infect Dis 1994;19(6):1049–1053
16. Wheat LJ, Musial CE, Jenny-Avital E. Diagnosis and management of central nervous system histoplasmosis. Clin Infect Dis 2005;40(6):844–852
17. Weprin BE, Hall WA, Goodman J, Adams GL. Long-term survival in rhinocerebral mucormycosis. Case report. J Neurosurg 1998;88(3):570–575
18. Speed B, Dunt D. Clinical and host differences between infections with the two varieties of *Cryptococcus neoformans*. Clin Infect Dis 1995; 21(1):28–34, discussion 35–36
19. Ruhnke M, Kofla G, Otto K, Schwartz S. CNS aspergillosis: recognition, diagnosis and management. CNS Drugs 2007;21(8):659–676
20. Berenguer J, Diaz-Mediavilla J, Urra D, Muñoz P. Central nervous system infection caused by *Pseudallescheria boydii*: case report and review. Rev Infect Dis 1989;11(6):890–896
21. Walsh TJ, Anaissie EJ, Denning DW, et al; Infectious Diseases Society of America. Treatment of aspergillosis: clinical practice guidelines of the Infectious Diseases Society of America. Clin Infect Dis 2008;46(3):327–360
22. Ikeda K, Yamashita J, Fujisawa H, Fujita S. Cerebral granuloma and meningitis caused by *Candida albicans*: useful monitoring of mannan antigen in cerebrospinal fluid. Neurosurgery 1990;26(5):860–863
23. Perfect JR. *Cryptococcus neoformans*. In: Mandell GL, Bennett JE, Dolin R, eds. Mandell, Douglas, and Bennett's Principles and Practice of Infectious Diseases. Philadelphia, PA: Churchill Livingstone Elsevier; 2010:3287–3303
24. Deepe GS Jr. *Histoplasma capsulatum*. In: Mandell GL, Bennett JE, Dolin R, eds. Mandell, Douglas, and Bennett's Principles and Practice of Infectious Diseases. Philadelphia, PA: Churchill Livingstone Elsevier; 2010:3305–3318
25. Denning DW, Stevens DA. Antifungal and surgical treatment of invasive aspergillosis: review of 2,121 published cases. Rev Infect Dis 1990; 12(6):1147–1201
26. Erdogan E, Beyzadeoglu M, Arpaci F, Celasun B. Cerebellar aspergillosis: case report and literature review. Neurosurgery 2002;50(4):874–876, discussion 876–877
27. Talmi YP, Goldschmied-Reouven A, Bakon M, et al. Rhino-orbital and rhino-orbito-cerebral mucormycosis. Otolaryngol Head Neck Surg 2002; 127(1):22–31
28. Adler DE, Milhorat TH, Miller JI. Treatment of rhinocerebral mucormycosis with intravenous, interstitial, and cerebrospinal fluid administration of amphotericin B: case report. Neurosurgery 1998;42(3):644–648, discussion 648–649
29. van Burik JA, Hare RS, Solomon HF, Corrado ML, Kontoyiannis DP. Posaconazole is effective as salvage therapy in zygomycosis: a retrospective summary of 91 cases. Clin Infect Dis 2006; 42(7):e61–e65
30. Troke P, Aguirrebengoa K, Arteaga C, et al; Global *Scedosporium* Study Group. Treatment of scedosporiosis with voriconazole: clinical experience with 107 patients. Antimicrob Agents Chemother 2008;52(5):1743–1750
31. Blitzer A, Lawson W, Meyers BR, Biller HF. Patient survival factors in paranasal sinus mucormycosis. Laryngoscope 1980;90(4):635–648
32. Nussbaum ES, Hall WA. Rhinocerebral mucormycosis: changing patterns of disease. Surg Neurol 1994;41(2):152–156

# 7

# Parasitic Infections of the Central Nervous System

Ali Akhaddar and Mohamed Boucetta

> Man can see only what he knows.
> —*Johann Wolfgang von Goethe (1749–1832)*

Parasitic infections of the central nervous system (CNS) were once considered unusual, if not rare. However, because of the increase in international travel to areas where parasitic infections are endemic and the migration of individuals infected with the disease, neuroparasitosis is becoming more common worldwide. Despite this occurrence, parasitic infection is often overlooked in the differential diagnosis of CNS disease. Improvements in neuroimaging and serologic assessment, as well as better understanding of the natural progression of the disease and the response to antiparasitic drugs, have resulted in better treatment paradigms. This chapter focuses on the most pertinent CNS parasitic diseases encountered in neurosurgical practice, especially in immunocompetent hosts (**Table 7.1**).

## ▪ Cysticercosis

Cysticercosis is the most common parasitic disease of the CNS and is secondary to infection by the larval form of the pork tapeworm *Taenia solium*. Within the CNS, the brain parenchyma is the most commonly affected site. CNS infection with *T. solium* is a major cause of acquired epilepsy.[1,2]

### Incidence and Demographics

Neurocysticercosis is an infection with worldwide prevalence and has endemic sta-

**Table 7.1** Parasitic infections that potentially involve the central nervous system in humans

| Parasitic Groups | Parasitic Infections |
|---|---|
| Helminth tapeworms | **Cysticercosis**[a]<br>**Echinococcosis**[a]<br>Coenurosis<br>Fascioliasis<br>Sparganosis |
| Helminth flukes | **Schistosomiasis**[a]<br>Paragonimiasis |
| Helminth roundworms | Baylisascariasis<br>Filariasis<br>Gnathostomiasis<br>Angiostrongyliasis<br>Strongyloidiasis<br>Toxocariasis<br>Trichinosis |
| Protozoa | **Amebiasis**[a]<br>Malaria<br>Toxoplasmosis<br>Trypanosomiasis |

[a] May be encountered in neurosurgical practice, especially in immunocompetent individuals.

tus in parts of Latin America, India, Africa, East Asia, and China.[3–6] This infection is rare in Islamic countries because of the prohibition of pork consumption. Neurocysticercosis is becoming increasingly prevalent in developed countries.[5,7,8] CNS cysticercosis occurs often in young and middle-aged adults. Over 50 million people worldwide were affected, with approximately 50,000 deaths per year.[4,9] Spinal forms are rare; fewer than 200 cases have been previously reported.[10,11]

## Etiology and Pathogenesis

The life cycle of *T. solium* is well known, in which pigs are the intermediate host and humans are the definitive host. Additionally, humans may accidentally ingest the eggs and become the intermediate host. The ova penetrate the intestinal wall and enter the bloodstream. They are then dispersed to the skin, skeletal muscles, heart, eyes, and most importantly, the brain.[3] Involvement of the CNS occurs in 60 to 90% of infected patients. The most commonly involved locations are brain parenchyma (60%) and the subarachnoid space (40%).[4,5,12] The spinal cord is more rarely involved (fewer than 6% of cases).[8,10,11] After entering the CNS, cysticerci elicit a scarce inflammatory reaction in the surrounding tissues. During this stage, parasites have a clear vesicular fluid and a normal scolex (vesicular stage). Cysticerci may remain viable or enter into a process of degeneration.

The first stage of involution is the colloidal stage, in which the vesicular fluid becomes turbid and the scolex shows signs of degeneration. Colloidal cysticerci are surrounded by a thick collagen capsule, with associated astrocytic gliosis and diffuse cerebral edema. Thereafter, the wall of the cyst thickens, and the scolex is transformed into coarse, mineralized granules (nodular–granular stage). Finally, in the calcified stage, the parasite remnants appear as a mineralized nodule. In the last two stages, the edema subsides but the astrocytic changes become more intense. Seizures are thought to occur either from parenchymal irritation or gliosis or because of active inflammation.[13]

## Presentation

When the lesions diffusely infect the brain parenchyma, they produce encephalitis, raised intracranial pressure, and seizures (50 to 80% of patients).[4] In the meninges, they produce basal meningitis and arterial thrombosis. The lesions may occur in the ventricles, causing hydrocephalus by obstruction of the aqueduct of Sylvius or even the fourth ventricle. Cerebral infarction is another serious complication that results from vasculitis of small perforating arteries.[12] Spinal cord involvement may cause arachnoiditis, meningitis, myelitis, or cord compression.[10,11] Most patients with intramedullary cysts present with thoracic spastic paraparesis and bladder dysfunction.[10]

## Diagnosis

The peripheral white blood cell count, eosinophil count, and erythrocyte sedimentation rate are usually normal. Stool examination for *T. solium* eggs is positive in only 5 to 10% of patients. The cerebrospinal fluid (CSF) is also usually unremarkable except in cases with meningeal involvement (low glucose level with eosinophilia).[14] Enzyme-linked immunosorbent assay (ELISA) of the blood or CSF should be interpreted with caution. In serum, it has 50% sensitivity and 65% specificity.[15] Sensitivity and specificity are higher in CSF (85 and 100%, respectively). Enzyme-linked immunoelectrotransfer blot (EITB) has been the gold standard serodiagnostic assay. This test is reported to have a sensitivity of 98% and a specificity of 100% but has only 30% sensitivity in the patient with a single brain lesion.[16,17] Biopsy of brain (stereotactic), skin, or muscle can provide a definitive diagnosis in an otherwise ambiguous clinical situation.[18] At the vesicular stage, magnetic resonance (MR) imaging demonstrates a cystic lesion isointense to the CSF. The lesion contains an eccentric scolex hyperintense to the CSF with no surrounding edema and little or no rim enhancement after intravenous gadolinium (Gd) administration. At the colloidal stage, MR imaging shows the cyst with hyperintense content relative to the CSF and mild or marked surrounding edema. After Gd administration, the cyst wall enhances as well as the eccentric scolex. At the nodular–granular stage, MR imaging shows a retracted, thickened cyst with mild surrounding edema and homogeneous Gd enhancement. At the calcified stage, computed tomography (CT) demonstrates multiple small calcified nodules with no surrounding edema. MR imaging shows a small calcified lesion, better identified on T2* gradient echo sequences. Cysticercosis in an intraventricular location usually presents as a single cyst, but on MR imaging, the cyst wall and content may be difficult to identify. Gd-enhanced T1-weighted MR imaging shows enhancement of the cyst wall and scolex. In the subarachnoid spaces, the content of the cysts appears isointense to the CSF.[1,6,19] Spinal cysticercosis usually involves the subarachnoid space, with the formation of intradural cysts or arachnoiditis. The intradural and intramedullary cysts are identified on MR imaging by the same findings as those of cerebral subarachnoid and intraparenchymal cysts, respectively.[10,11]

### Treatment

Ventricular CSF shunting is the most common surgical indication for neurocysticercosis to resolve hydrocephalus. Neuroendoscopy may be used for resection of some intraventricular cysts.[20] Other surgical indications include brain biopsy and resection of mass lesions.[12,18] In cases of spinal cord involvement, surgery is always mandatory in the presence of medullary compression. The two widely accepted anticysticercal drugs are albendazole and praziquantel; however, albendazole is superior in terms of cyst eradication, seizure control, and tolerability.[21] Anticysticercal drugs must be used with caution in patients with increased intracranial pressure and encephalitis.[6,15] Corticosteroids are the primary form of therapy for cysticercotic encephalitis, angiitis, and arachnoiditis.[22] In patients with giant subarachnoid cysticerci, ventricular cysts, spinal cysts, and multiple parenchymal brain cysts, corticosteroids must be administered before, during, and even after the course of cysticidal drugs to avoid cerebral infarction, acute hydrocephalus, spinal cord swelling, and massive brain edema.[8,22] Antiepileptic therapy must be administered early.[13,23]

### Outcome

A large number of patients treated with ventriculoperitoneal shunts require repeat intervention to release obstruction.[24] The prognosis is better for intraparenchymal lesions. The mortality rate is lower than 10%.[14] Worse outcome is observed for extraparenchymal lesions as well as cases complicated by basilar arachnoiditis and vasculitis with subsequent cerebral ischemia.[5,18] The most common sequelae are seizures.[13,23] True disease control is achieved only by avoiding transmission, with proper sanitary measures (public health education and pig vaccination).

### Conclusion

Neurocysticercosis remains a significant cause of morbidity and mortality throughout the world. This disease has multiple forms of neurologic presentation. Patients with intraparenchymal lesions have a favorable course and respond well to clinical treatment. Those with subarachnoid and intraventricular cysts have a greater morbidity and mortality. The vast majority of patients require anticonvulsive therapy. Control and eradication programs are urgently needed in areas where the disease is endemic.

## ■ Echinococcosis

Echinococcosis is a parasitic infection caused by larvae (metacestodes) of the tapeworm *Echinococcus*. Three forms that occur in humans: cystic (*Echinococcus granulosus*), alveolar (*Echinococcus multilocularis*), and polycystic (*Echinococcus vogeli* and *Echinococcus oligarthrus*), which is rare.[25] The cystic strain (cystic hydatidosis) is the most common form to occur in humans.[26,27] Both cerebral and spinal structures may be involved. This chapter focuses on cystic hydatidosis because it is the most frequent and most important CNS echinococcosis.

### Incidence and Demographics

Although rare in western Europe and North America, hydatidosis is a significant cause of morbidity and mortality in large geographic regions like the Middle East,

Mediterranean area, South America, Australia, and northwestern China. This infection is currently considered an emerging or reemerging disease.[26-30] Annual incidence rates of diagnosed human cases vary widely, from 1 to 200 cases per 100,000 inhabitants.[29] Approximately 2 to 3% of all reported hydatid cysts are found in the CNS. The brain is affected in approximately 2% and the spine in fewer than 1% of all patients.[30-33] Individuals of all ages may be affected, although children and young adults are particularly vulnerable.[15,34,35]

### Etiology and Pathogenesis

The adult parasites live in the intestines of dogs and wild canids. Infective eggs, passed in the feces, are ingested by intermediate hosts, including sheep, cattle, and humans. The life cycle is maintained when dogs ingest the carcasses of infected intermediate hosts. In humans, echinococcal infestation occurs through the fecal–oral route.[3] Unilocular cysts most commonly develop in the liver (75% of cases), lungs (15% of cases), and other organs, including the brain and spine.[25,28] The host reacts to the presence of this lesion by enveloping it in a fibroblastic capsule (adventitial membrane), but this occurs to a much lesser degree in the brain. Occasionally, hydatid cysts degenerate and die.[25,26] When an embryo of *E. granulosus* is lodged in the brain, a solitary cyst develops.

Multiple cysts are rare (5%).[31,36] The brain cysts are usually spherical, with a wall that is white, smooth, soft, and elastic. The location of primary hydatid cysts of the brain is supratentorial in 90% of cases and subcortical. Intraventricular and infratentorial infections are unusual.[31,37] A hydatid cyst is a slow-growing lesion (1 to 5 cm annually) that does not invade the brain.[36] In the spine, the vertebral body is affected through invasion of the venous portovertebral shunts. Spinal lesions are microvesicular, multiple, and invasive. The parasite grows along the bony intratrabecular space, then infiltrates and destroys the bone; thereafter, it extends into the extradural space or paraspinal tissues. During this extraosseous stage, the cyst may impinge on nerve roots and the spinal cord, causing neurologic symptoms.[32,38] Spinal hydatid cysts are classified in five categories: (1) intramedullary, (2) intradural extramedullary, (3) extradural, (4) vertebral, and (5) paravertebral lesions.[39] The first three categories are rare.[40] The most common sites involved are the lower dorsal and lumbar regions, in about two-thirds of cases.[31,35]

### Presentation

Symptoms depend on the involvement of intracranial structures and may vary from simple headache to uncal herniation. Headache is the most common presenting symptom in 70 to 75% of cases, followed by weakness of the extremities in 40%. Other symptoms that occur are epilepsy, mental changes, skull deformities, change in school or job performance, and psychotic syndromes.

Papilledema may lead to optic atrophy with unilateral or bilateral blindness.[31,36,41] During the intraosseous phase of spinal hydatidosis, no symptoms are typically present. Thereafter, the initial symptoms are either radicular pain in 75% of patients or muscle weakness in 20%.[35,42] Trauma may produce a pathologic fracture with acute neurologic signs.[32] Other symptoms of systemic involvement may be associated that are most often referable to involvement of the liver and lungs.

### Diagnosis

Eosinophilic pleocytosis, elevated sedimentation rate, and Casoni reaction are supportive evidence of infection but not specific. The sensitivity of indirect agglutination and indirect hemagglutination is high (60 to 100%); however, they have limited specificity.[43] Currently, the gold standard for diagnosis is serologic and is based on the detection of immunoglobulin G antibodies to hydatid cyst fluid–derived native or recombinant antigen B subunits, either in ELISA or in immunoblot formats.[25,43] On CT, the brain lesion presents as a spherical, well-defined, homogeneous, smooth, thin-walled, cystic lesion isodense to the CSF without surrounding cerebral edema. The cyst wall is iso- or hyperdense relative to the brain parenchyma. Wall calcifications are rare.[33,36] After contrast administration, there is typically no enhancement (**Fig. 7.1a**). On MR imaging, the cyst is isointense to CSF on T1- and T2-weighted images and has a hypointense rim on T1- and T2-weighted images without perilesional edema (**Fig. 7.1b,c**). On FLAIR (fluid-attenuated inversion recovery) images, the fluid in the hydatid cyst is hyperintense. The Gd-enhanced T1-weighted MR image classically shows no enhancement.[14,44,45] In spinal hydatidosis, CT reveals irregular bony erosions of the vertebral body, neural arch, and head of the ribs. In the paraspinal soft tissues, the occurrence of spherical formations with multiple daughter cysts is common. Enhancement is rare and is often related to concomitant bacterial infection.[35,42] On MR imaging, the cyst appears as a multiloculate, hypointense mass on T1-weighted images but is brightly hyperintense on T2-weighted images (**Fig. 7.2**). The alteration in signal intensity can be used to demonstrate cyst viability.

## Treatment

In the brain, the Dowling method is frequently used and consists of the spontaneous delivery of the intact brain hydatid cyst through a large cranial flap and corticectomy (**Fig. 7.3**). The cyst is delivered by using saline irrigation between the cyst wall and the surrounding brain with soft-tipped catheters (hydrodissection).[33,37,46] If the cyst ruptures during surgery, which occurs in approximately 20 to 25% of cases,[31,36,44] local parasiticidal solution (hypertonic saline or oxygenic water) should be used to prevent recurrence. Anaphylactic shock can be observed when intraoperative spillage occurs. In the spine, different approaches have been used to eradicate the vesicular lesions, including posterior (**Fig. 7.4**) or anterior approaches. Spinal instability and deformity are treated when necessary to prevent possible neurologic complications. At the completion of surgery for extradural lesions, the area should be irrigated with a parasiticidal solution. Surgery is the mainstay of treatment for neurohydatidosis; however, anthelmintic treatment may be used before and/or after the operation to prevent recurrence.[32,35,36] Although their effectiveness in neurohydatidosis is not well established, albendazole and mebendazole are the most frequently used anthelmintic agents. Albendazole is a broad-spectrum anthelmintic agent with good oral absorption but may be hepatotoxic.[47] Preoperative seizures require long-term antiepileptic therapy. Adequate rehabilitation is crucial for a successful outcome.[41]

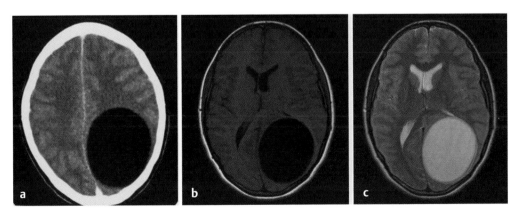

**Fig. 7.1a–c** **(a)** Axial computed tomographic scan with contrast injection, **(b)** axial T1-weighted magnetic resonance (MR) image, and **(c)** T2-weighted MR image showing a large cerebral hydatid cyst located in the left parieto-occipital area compressing the lateral ventricle and causing shift of the midline structures.

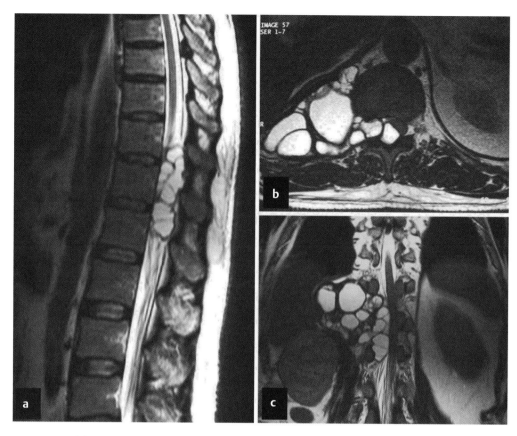

**Fig. 7.2a–c** **(a)** Sagittal, **(b)** axial, and **(c)** coronal T2-weighed magnetic resonance images revealing hyperintense, multiloculate, low-thoracic intraspinal lesions extending into the right foramina and compressing the spinal cord.

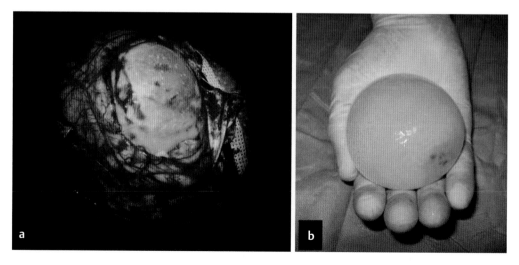

**Fig. 7.3a,b** **(a)** Operative view of the brain cyst before warm saline was injected between the cyst wall and the surrounding brain to remove the cyst (Dowling technique) . **(b)** The hydatid cyst was extracted without rupture.

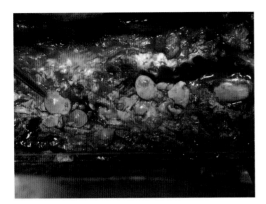

**Fig. 7.4** Operative view after thoracic laminectomy showing multivesicular hydatid cysts in the epidural space.

## Outcome

Rapid recovery from neurologic deficits occurs in most patients operated on for brain hydatidosis. The postoperative course may be complicated by subdural effusion, extradural hematoma, and infection. The death rate is less than 10%.[31,36] Recurrence in the brain occurs in 10 to 20% of cases and is often due to spillage of the cyst contents at the time of its removal.[31,33,41,44] When the spine is affected, no improvement can be expected in patients with complete paraplegia. Because its eradication is nearly impossible, even after repeated surgical intervention and chemotherapy, spinal hydatidosis has a high rate of recurrence (40 to 100% of cases).[31,35,37,38] The death rate is approximately 4%.[31,38] Hydatidosis is potentially an eradicable parasitic disease, and efforts must focus on the numerous human factors that are involved in maintenance of the parasitic cycle.[26,27]

## Conclusion

In hydatid cyst of the brain, every attempt should be made to deliver the cyst unruptured. Spinal hydatidosis is highly likely to recur, leading to progressive destruction of the vertebral column and neurologic deterioration. Anthelmintic treatment must also be considered to control the disease locally, avoid systemic spread, and prevent recurrence. Preventive programs must focus on breaking the parasite's life cycle and on educating people in areas of endemicity.

## ■ Schistosomiasis

Schistosomiasis (bilharziasis) is a snail-transmitted parasitic infection caused by the trematode platyhelminth of the genus *Schistosoma*. Five species of *Schistosoma* infect humans: *Schistosoma mansoni*, *Schistosoma haematobium*, *Schistosoma japonicum*, *Schistosoma mekongi*, and *Schistosoma intercalatum*.[48] CNS complications usually occur in chronically infected individuals. Both the brain and spinal cord may be involved.[49]

### Incidence and Demographics

Only the first three species of *Schistosoma* cause significant disease in humans and are endemic in certain parts of the world: *S. mansoni* in Africa, Latin America, and some Caribbean islands; *S. japonicum* in China, Indonesia, Thailand, and the Philippines; and *S. haematobium* in Africa and the Middle East.[48,49] Worldwide, 20,000 deaths per year are associated with the severe consequences of this parasitic infection. An estimated 600 million people are at risk for infection in 79 countries where it is endemic.[48,50] The incidence of neuroschistosomiasis was estimated at approximately 2 to 4% of persons infected systemically.[51]

### Etiology and Pathogenesis

Schistosomes use humans and other mammals as definitive hosts and aquatic snails as intermediate hosts. Infection is acquired via direct contact with water contaminated by the larval form of the parasite. These larvae penetrate the human skin and reach the vascular system, where they mature. Adult parasites localize in the venous system, draining the colon (*S. mansoni* and *S. japonicum*) or the urinary tract (*S. haematobium*). Other organs, such as the lungs, liver, and CNS, may be involved.[48,49,52] After the eggs die, circumscribed granulomas form around the degenerating eggs.

Ultimately, the only residue of disease is fibrosis surrounding a zone of necrosis.[53] The eggs of *S. japonicum* have a tendency to calcify. CNS involvement is uncommon; cerebral lesions most frequently occur in cases of *S. japonicum* infection, whereas *S. mansoni* and *S. haematobium* infections may involve the spinal cord.[49] A tumorlike presentation can develop as a result of slowly expanding intracranial lesions.[54] The granulomas are rimmed by a zone of reactive astrocytosis. The adult worm may be present within blood vessels in the brain, inducing vasculitis with rupture of blood vessels and secondary hemorrhage.[54] Schistosome-induced myelopathy results from the inflammatory reaction accompanying the deposition of ova in the venules located in and around the lower part of the spinal cord. The ova, which normally are deposited in the inferior mesenteric vein of the portal system, reach the spinal veins via the Batson plexus.[55–58]

## Presentation

*S. japonicum* infection is almost always associated with cerebral manifestations, and *S. mansoni* and *S. haematobium* infection with a myeloradicular syndrome. Symptoms of cutaneous allergic response, fever, hematuria, hepatosplenomegaly, and peripheral eosinophilia may be present before the neurologic symptoms appear.[57] Young men, teenagers, and children are mostly affected.

Cerebral lesions may be unique or multiple and have presented with headache, seizures, and focal neurologic deficits, whereas nausea, vomiting, ataxia, and brain herniation are more common in posterior fossa schistosomiasis.[57,58] The seizure semiology consists mainly of motor seizures.[57,59] Acute cerebral schistosomiasis can provoke encephalitis and strokelike symptoms due to cerebral vasculitis. Spinal cord schistosomiasis has a spectrum of severity ranging from asymptomatic egg deposits to severe acute transverse myelitis. Patients present with back pain as the first symptom in 79 to 100% of cases.[60–62] Classically, there are three clinical forms: medullary (27% of cases), my-

eloradicular (55%), and conus–cauda equina syndrome (18%).[63] Because of the location of parasitic infestation, sensory disturbances rarely ascend higher than the T9 level.[61]

## Diagnosis

Laboratory changes, such as eosinophilia, and evidence of eggs in the urine or feces may or may not be present. Rectal biopsy has an important sensitivity, allowing identification of the eggs in 95 to 100% of cases.[64] CSF examination generally shows an inflammatory pattern. Antibody detection (indirect hemagglutination, indirect immunofluorescence tests, or ELISA) in samples of blood or CSF is useful in only a few specific circumstances. The existence of other forms of visceral involvement is important.[48,57,65] Definitive diagnosis requires the pathologic demonstration of parasitic eggs in brain, spinal cord, or spinal nerve root tissue obtained at biopsy.[66] On MR imaging, the tumorlike lesion is heterogeneous, isointense to the gray matter on T1-weighted, and hyperintense on T2-weighted imaging. It is most commonly located in the cerebellum, less often in the thalamus and hemispheres. After Gd administration, MR imaging may reveal either homogeneous nodular enhancement of the mass or a punctate pattern of enhancement with multiple enhancing nodules distributed throughout the mass.[19,58,66–68] In the spinal cord, the most frequent findings are medullary enlargement (particularly the lower spinal cord) and thickening of the spinal roots (especially the cauda equina) on T1-weighted imaging, signal hyperintensity on T2-weighted imaging, and a heterogeneous pattern of Gd enhancement.[56,62]

## Treatment

Surgical treatment should be considered for brain involvement when the lesion causes a mass effect, the neurologic signs and symptoms progress despite clinical treatment, or the diagnosis is uncertain. Decompression for the posterior fossa lesions is often necessary to prevent the development of hydrocephalus.[51,58] Praziquantel and oxamniquine are the antischistosomal agents recommended for treatment.[59,64] These agents destroy the adult worms and thereby prevent further oviposition.[64] Corticosteroids are utilized to diminish granulomatous inflammation and edema. In addition, there is some evidence that corticosteroids reduce ova deposition by adult worms.[63,69] The therapeutic decision for patients with the new onset of seizures should be made based on the type of seizures.[57,59] In spinal cord involvement, Nobre et al reported that 22% of their patients exhibited a full response to medical treatment, 57% had a partial response without functional limitations, and 17% had partial improvement with limitations or no response to treatment.[62] With intracranial lesions, if there is no clinical improvement after the institution of antischistosomal medications or if neurologic deterioration occurs, surgical decompression and biopsy sampling should be considered.

### Outcome

Outcome is largely dependent on early treatment, particularly with spinal cord involvement, and is better for cerebral schistosomiasis. Improvement is usually progressive and more rapid at the onset of corticosteroid and antischistosomal drug treatment.[69] For some authors, microsurgery is effective for the total resection of lesions and can assist in protection of the brain, increasing the cure rate.[51,58] A significant degree of disability is common following spinal schistosomiasis and may require prolonged rehabilitation.[61,65] Signs and symptoms can recur in patients who do not receive adequate antiparasitic chemotherapy.[64]

### Conclusion

Correlation of the clinical, epidemiologic, and neuroimaging features together with the demonstration of eggs in the urine or feces and positive serology may be helpful in diagnosing neuroschistosomiasis. Surgical treatment should be considered when the lesion causes a mass effect, the signs and symptoms worsen despite anthelmintic medication, or diagnostic uncertainty exists. Cerebral involvement is associated with a better outcome than disease affecting the spinal cord. Preventive campaigns are urgently needed in areas of endemicity to reduce this disease.

## ◼ Amebiasis

Amebiasis is a widespread parasitic disease caused by the protozoa *Entamoeba histolytica*, *Naegleria fowleri*, *Acanthamoeba* species, and *Balamuthia* species.[70,71] *E. histolytica* is a causative agent of amebic dysentery and invasive extraintestinal amebiasis. CNS infections are rare but have been uniformly fatal.[70,72–75] The various clinicopathologic entities associated with CNS amebiasis include the following: (1) amebic abscess (AMA) due to *E. histolytica*, (2) granulomatous amebic encephalitis (GAE) due to *Acanthamoeba* species and *Balamuthia mandrillaris* (order Leptomyxida), (3) primary amebic meningoencephalitis (PAM) due to *N. fowleri*, and (4) necrotizing hemorrhagic encephalitis due to *Sappinia diploidea*, which is rare.[53,71,76]

### Incidence and Demographics

Amebiasis is a global disease, although most cases are seen in developing countries in the tropics.[72,76] *E. histolytica* is a major human pathogen that is estimated to cause more than 100,000 deaths per year.[77,78] The incidence of amebic brain abscesses due to *Entamoeba* species in patients with confirmed amebic liver abscesses varies from 0.6 to 8.1%.[77,78] More than 200 cases of GAE have been reported worldwide, and approximately 300 cases of PAM.[70,73] CNS amebiasis has been reported to represent 0.27% of all mass lesions of the brain.[74] Both immunocompetent and immunocompromised hosts may be involved.[70,79–82]

### Etiology and Pathogenesis

Usually, humans acquire amebiasis by ingesting cysts of *E. histolytica* in contaminated food, by drinking contaminated water, or by swimming in the infested water of lakes. *E. histolytica* and *B. mandrillaris* reach the brain by hematogenous spread from the colon through the hepatic, pulmonary, or vertebral veins or ascend directly along the nasal mucosa, olfactory nerves, or traumatized skin (mainly in the case of *B. mandrillaris)* to the brain, leading to cerebral vasculitis, hemorrhagic necrosis, meningoencephalitis, or intraparenchymal abscess.[74,80,83,84] Abscesses are usually in the distribution of the middle cerebral artery. The abscess consists of a central area of necrosis that contains amebic trophozoites in the periphery.[73,76]

*Acanthamoeba* infection reaches the CNS via the bloodstream from a site of pulmonary involvement or skin lesions. The brain shows reactive gliosis, acute and chronic inflammation, and areas of necrosis surrounded by trophozoites and cysts.[53,84] Although typical granulomas are not seen, several multinucleated giant cells of the foreign body or Langhans type are found. In PAM, hemorrhagic necrosis is seen involving the inferior frontal lobe along the olfactory nerve.[71]

## Presentation

In cerebral abscess due to *E. histolytica*, most symptoms results from increased intracranial pressure, local mass effect, and meningismus, with fever an uncommon finding. Liver abscesses may be associated with brain abscesses.[85,86] Infections with *Acanthamoeba* are more indolent and often occur in both immunocompetent and immunocompromised hosts, resulting in a subacute granulomatous encephalitis.[70,79,82] The patient often presents with nonspecific symptoms of fever, malaise, and headache. As the disease progresses, seizures, nausea, vomiting, lethargy, and an altered level of consciousness result.[71,83] As is the case with brain abscess, signs and symptoms of a space-occupying lesion develop in patients with large granulomatous lesions.[87] Infections due to *B. mandrillaris* can also cause chronic granulomatous meningoencephalitis, occurring mostly in immuno-

competent individuals and children.[74,81,84] Many patients with GAE present with typical skin lesions, such as a purple nodule.[70,75,80,83] *N. fowleri* can produce a fulminant PAM resembling bacterial meningitis, with death occurring within 72 hours after presentation.[76] Victims tend to be young and healthy, typically with a recent history of swimming in a warm body of water.[71]

## Diagnosis

Diagnosis is made by culture, serology, or immunofluorescence of CSF or brain specimens to demonstrate the trophozoites.[73,75] Recently, the usefulness of molecular analysis and polymerase chain reaction in diagnosing CNS amebiasis has been reported.[86] Skin biopsy and liver abscess with granulomatous infection would aid in the diagnosis.[75,76,86] In cases of GAE, the CSF profile may reveal mildly low to normal glucose concentrations. Pleocytosis with a predominant lymphocytosis and high protein levels are commonly seen.[75] The immune status of the patient should be investigated. Amebic encephalitis involves the cerebral hemispheres, mainly the frontal and parietal lobes and basal ganglia. On MR imaging, T1-weighted imaging demonstrates a centrally hypointense mass with surrounding cerebral edema and heterogeneous or ring enhancement after Gd injection. T2-weighted imaging can show a centrally hyperintense lesion with possible hemorrhage that is surrounded by hyperintense edema.[19,85,88] On diffusion-weighted imaging, a slight area of restricted diffusion and increased signal on the FLAIR sequence may be seen.[75] To establish a definitive diagnosis, stereotactic biopsy is preferred for multiple and small lesions.

## Treatment

In rare cases, excision of the brain lesion may be curative if the infection is localized and the disease has not evolved into diffuse encephalitis.[70] A decompressive frontal lobectomy has been performed with success.[79] CSF diversion is necessary for patients with symptomatic hydrocephalus, although the shunt tubing may become obstructed by inflammatory debris. Except for brain abscess due to *E. histolytica* (metronidazole therapy), treatment of cerebral amebiasis is usually late and nonspecific. After the diagnosis has been confirmed, aggressive treatment with intravenous (and/or intrathecal) amphotericin B, miconazole, rifampin, sulfa drugs, and tetracycline in combination should be started.[89] However, only rare survivors have been reported with *Naegleria* meningoencephalitis.[90] *Acanthamoeba* infection of the CNS has been treated with sulfadiazine and other sulfa drugs with also fatal outcomes.[79] Treatment of CNS *Balamuthia* infection is empiric. There are reports of treatment with flucytosine, pentamidine, fluconazole, sulfadiazine, and a macrolide.[81] Corticosteroids have been used by some investigators to blunt the previously described intense inflammatory reaction.[91] Prophylactic anticonvulsants may be used if appropriate.

## Outcome

Cerebral amebiasis is the second most common cause of death from parasites and accounts for 4.2 to 8.5% of deaths due to amebiasis.[19,72,76] Although brain abscesses due to *E. histolytica* have a relatively good prognosis,[85,86] most cases of PAM and GEA are fatal.[74,82–84] Only rare survivors have been reported, even in previously healthy patients.[79,81] Prevention of amebiasis through improved public health education and adequate management of dysentery is an important goal.

## Conclusion

CNS amebiasis is rare and difficult to diagnose. This infection should be considered in any patient with subacute and/or chronic meningoencephalitis without evidence of bacterial involvement. Except for *E. histolytica*, all other species cause disease that is difficult to treat and commonly fatal. Early aggressive multidrug therapy offers the best chance of survival and the best possible outcome.

## References

1. Del Brutto OH, Rajshekhar V, White AC Jr, et al. Proposed diagnostic criteria for neurocysticercosis. Neurology 2001;57(2):177–183
2. Garcia HH, Del Brutto OH; Cysticercosis Working Group in Peru. Neurocysticercosis: updated concepts about an old disease. Lancet Neurol 2005;4(10):653–661
3. King CH, Fairley J. Cestodes (tapeworms). In: Mandell GL, Bennett JE, Dolin R, eds. Bennett's Principles and Practice of Infectious Diseases. Philadelphia, PA: Elsevier Churchill Livingstone; 2010:3607–3616
4. Hawk MW, Shahlaie K, Kim KD, Theis JH. Neurocysticercosis: a review. Surg Neurol 2005;63(2):123–132, discussion 132
5. White AC Jr. Neurocysticercosis: updates on epidemiology, pathogenesis, diagnosis, and management. Annu Rev Med 2000;51:187–206
6. Diaz Vasquez PP. Parasitoses of the central nervous system: cysticercosis. In: Sindou M, ed. Practical Handbook of Neurosurgery. Vol 1. Vienna, Austria: Springer-Verlag; 2009:483–498
7. Wallin MT, Kurtzke JF. Neurocysticercosis in the United States: review of an important emerging infection. Neurology 2004;63(9):1559–1564
8. García HH, Gonzalez AE, Evans CAW, Gilman RH; Cysticercosis Working Group in Peru. *Taenia solium* cysticercosis. Lancet 2003;362(9383):547–556
9. Psarros TG, Zouros A, Coimbra C. Neurocysticercosis: a neurosurgical perspective. South Med J 2003;96(10):1019–1022
10. Ahmad FU, Sharma BS. Treatment of intramedullary spinal cysticercosis: report of 2 cases and review of literature. Surg Neurol 2007;67(1):74–77, discussion 77
11. Mohanty A, Venkatrama SK, Das S, Das BS, Rao BR, Vasudev MK. Spinal intramedullary cysticercosis. Neurosurgery 1997;40(1):82–87
12. Escobedo F. Neurosurgical aspects of cysticercosis. In: Schmidek HH, Sweet WH, eds. Operative Neurosurgical Techniques. Indications, Methods, and Results. Vol 1. Orlando, FL: Grune & Stratton; 1988:93–102
13. Rajshekhar V, Jeyaseelan L. Seizure outcome in patients with a solitary cerebral cysticercus granuloma. Neurology 2004;62(12):2236–2240
14. Gaskill SJ, Marlin AE. Tuberculosis and fungal and parasitic infections of the central nervous system. In: Leland A, Pollack I, Adelson P, eds. Principles and Practice of Pediatric Neurosurgery. 2nd ed. New York, NY: Thieme; 2008:1182–1195
15. Ramos-Kuri M, Montoya RM, Padilla A, et al. Immunodiagnosis of neurocysticercosis. Disappointing performance of serology (enzyme-linked immunosorbent assay) in an unbiased sample of neurological patients. Arch Neurol 1992;49(6):633–636
16. Wilson M, Bryan RT, Fried JA, et al. Clinical evaluation of the cysticercosis enzyme-linked immunoelectrotransfer blot in patients with neurocysticercosis. J Infect Dis 1991;164(5):1007–1009

17. Prabhakaran V, Rajshekhar V, Murrell KD, Oommen A. *Taenia solium* metacestode glycoproteins as diagnostic antigens for solitary cysticercus granuloma in Indian patients. Trans R Soc Trop Med Hyg 2004;98(8):478–484

18. Sinha S, Sharma BS. Neurocysticercosis: a review of current status and management. J Clin Neurosci 2009;16(7):867–876

19. Hourani RG, Tamraz JC. Imaging of parasitic diseases of the central nervous system. In: Haddad MC, Abd El Baji ME, Tamraz JC, eds. Imaging of Parasitic Diseases. Berlin, Germany: Springer; 2008:7–31

20. Rangel-Castilla L, Serpa JA, Gopinath SP, Graviss EA, Diaz-Marchan P, White AC Jr. Contemporary neurosurgical approaches to neurocysticercosis. Am J Trop Med Hyg 2009;80(3):373–378

21. Cruz M, Cruz I, Horton J. Albendazole versus praziquantel in the treatment of cerebral cysticercosis: clinical evaluation. Trans R Soc Trop Med Hyg 1991;85(2):244–247

22. Del Brutto OH, Sotelo J, Roman GC. Therapy for neurocysticercosis: a reappraisal. Clin Infect Dis 1993;17(4):730–735

23. Del Brutto OH. Prognostic factors for seizure recurrence after withdrawal of antiepileptic drugs in patients with neurocysticercosis. Neurology 1994;44(9):1706–1709

24. Suastegui Roman RA, Soto-Hernandez JL, Sotelo J. Effects of prednisone on ventriculoperitoneal shunt function in hydrocephalus secondary to cysticercosis: a preliminary study. J Neurosurg 1996;84(4):629–633

25. Eckert J, Deplazes P. Biological, epidemiological, and clinical aspects of echinococcosis, a zoonosis of increasing concern. Clin Microbiol Rev 2004; 17(1):107–135

26. Craig P, Budke CM, Schantz PM, et al. Human echinococcosis: a neglected disease? Trop Med Internat Health 2007;35:283–292

27. Dakkak A. Echinococcosis/hydatidosis: a severe threat in Mediterranean countries. Vet Parasitol 2010;174(1-2):2–11

28. da Silva AM. Human echinococcosis: a neglected disease. Gastroenterol Res Pract 2010; 2010:583297

29. Pawlowski Z, Eckert J, Vuitton D, et al. Echinococcosis in humans: clinical aspects, diagnosis and treatment. In: Eckert J, Gemmel MA, Meslin FX, Pawlowski ZS, eds. WHO/OIE Manual on Echinococcosis in Humans and Animals: a Public Health Problem of Global Concern. Paris, France: World Health Organization and World Organization for Animal Health; 2001:20–66

30. Nourbakhsh A, Vannemreddy P, Minagar A, Toledo EG, Palacios E, Nanda A. Hydatid disease of the central nervous system: a review of literature with an emphasis on Latin American countries. Neurol Res 2010;32(3):245–251

31. Altinörs N, Bavbek M, Caner HH, Erdogan B. Central nervous system hydatidosis in Turkey: a cooperative study and literature survey analysis of 458 cases. J Neurosurg 2000;93(1):1–8

32. Pamir MN, Ozduman K, Elmaci I. Spinal hydatid disease. Spinal Cord 2002;40(4):153–160

33. Arana-Iniguez R. Echinococcus. In: Vinken PJ, Bruyn GW, eds. Infections of the Nervous System. Part III. Handbook of Clinical Neurology 1978; 35:175–208

34. Akhaddar A, Gourinda H, el Alami Z, el Madhi T, Miri A. Hydatid cyst of the sacrum. Report of a case. Rev Rhum Engl Ed 1999;66(5):289–291

35. Akhaddar A, Gourinda H, Aghoutane M, El Alami FZ, El Madhi T, Miri A. L'hydatidose vertébrale chez l'enfant. A propos de 4 cas avec revue de la littérature. Rachis (Clichy) 1999;11:215–220

36. Khaldi M, Mohamed S, Kallel J, Khouja N. Brain hydatidosis: report on 117 cases. Childs Nerv Syst 2000;16(10-11):765–769

37. Limaiem F, Bellil S, Bellil K, et al. Primary hydatidosis of the central nervous system: a retrospective study of 39 Tunisian cases. Clin Neurol Neurosurg 2010;112(1):23–28

38. Khazim R, Fares Y, Heras-Palou C, Ruiz Barnes P. Posterior decompression of spinal hydatidosis: long term results: Fundacion Jimenez Diaz, Madrid, Spain. Clin Neurol Neurosurg 2003; 105(3):209–214

39. Braithwaite PA, Lees RF. Vertebral hydatid disease: radiological assessment. Radiology 1981; 140(3):763–766

40. Chakir N, Akhaddar A, El Quessar A, et al. [Primary intradural extramedullary hydatidosis. Case report and review of the literature]. J Neuroradiol 2002;29(3):177–182

41. Ciurea AV, Fountas KN, Coman TC, et al. Long-term surgical outcome in patients with intracranial hydatid cyst. Acta Neurochir (Wien) 2006; 148(4):421–426

42. Abbassioun K, Amirjamshidi A. Diagnosis and management of hydatid cyst of the central nervous system. Part 2. Hydatid cysts of the skull, orbit and spine. Neurosurg Q 2001;11:10–16

43. Lorenzo C, Ferreira HB, Monteiro KM, et al. Comparative analysis of the diagnostic performance of six major *Echinococcus granulosus* antigens assessed in a double-blind, randomized multicenter study. J Clin Microbiol 2005;43(6): 2764–2770

44. Abbassioun K, Amirjamshidi A. Diagnosis and management of hydatid cyst of the central nervous system. Part 1. General considerations and hydatid disease of the brain. Neurosurg Q 2001;11:1–9

45. Abdel Razek AAK, El-Shamam O, Abdel Wahab N. Magnetic resonance appearance of cerebral cystic echinococcosis: World Health Organization (WHO) classification. Acta Radiol 2009;50(5):549–554

46. Izci Y, Tüzün Y, Seçer HI, Gönül E. Cerebral hydatid cysts: technique and pitfalls of surgical management. Neurosurg Focus 2008;24(6):E15

47. Falagas ME, Bliziotis IA. Albendazole for the treatment of human echinococcosis: a review of comparative clinical trials. Am J Med Sci 2007; 334(3):171–179

48. Ross AG, Bartley PB, Sleigh AC, et al. Schistosomiasis. N Engl J Med 2002;346(16):1212–1220

49. Pittella JE. Neuroschistosomiasis. Brain Pathol 1997;7(1):649–662

50. World Health Organization. Prevention and Control of Schistosomiasis and Soil-Transmitted Helminthiasis: Report of a WHO Expert Committee. Geneva, Switzerland: WHO; 2002. Technical Report Series No. 912

51. Shu K, Zhang S, Han L, Lei T. Surgical treatment of cerebellar schistosomiasis. Neurosurgery 2009;64(5):941–943, discussion 943–944

52. Lucas S, Bell J, Chimelli L. Parasitic and fungal infections. In: Love S, Louis DN, Ellison DW, eds. Greenfield's Neuropathology. London, England: Hodder Arnold; 2008:1447–1487

53. Chacko G. Parasitic diseases of the central nervous system. Semin Diagn Pathol 2010;27(3): 167–185

54. Mackenzie IR, Guha A. Manson's schistosomiasis presenting as a brain tumor. Case report. J Neurosurg 1998;89(6):1052–1054

55. Olson S, Rossato R, Guazzo E. Spinal schistosomiasis. J Clin Neurosci 2002;9(3):317–320

56. Kamel MH, Murphy M, Kelleher M, Aquilina K, Lim C, Marks C. Schistosomiasis of the spinal cord presenting as progressive myelopathy. Case report. J Neurosurg Spine 2005;3(1):61–63

57. Lei T, Shu K, Chen X, Li L. Surgical treatment of epilepsy with chronic cerebral granuloma caused by Schistosoma japonicum. Epilepsia 2008;49(1): 73–79

58. Braga MH, de Carvalho GT, Brandão RA, et al. Pseudotumoral form of cerebral Schistosoma mansoni. World Neurosurg 2011;76(1-2):200–207, discussion 84–86

59. Betting LE, Pirani C Jr, de Souza Queiroz L, Damasceno BP, Cendes F. Seizures and cerebral schistosomiasis. Arch Neurol 2005;62(6):1008–1010

60. Junker J, Eckardt L, Husstedt I. Cervical intramedullar schistosomiasis as a rare cause of acute tetraparesis. Clin Neurol Neurosurg 2001;103(1): 39–42

61. Ferrari TC, Moreira PR, Cunha AS. Spinal cord schistosomiasis: a prospective study of 63 cases emphasizing clinical and therapeutic aspects. J Clin Neurosci 2004;11(3):246–253

62. Nobre V, Silva LC, Ribas JG, et al. Schistosomal myeloradiculopathy due to Schistosoma mansoni: report on 23 cases. Mem Inst Oswaldo Cruz 2001;96(Suppl):137–141

63. Ferrari TCA, Moreira PR, Cunha AS. Clinical characterization of neuroschistosomiasis due to Schistosoma mansoni and its treatment. Acta Trop 2008;108(2-3):89–97

64. Ferrari MLA, Coelho PMZ, Antunes CMF, Tavares CAP, da Cunha AS. Efficacy of oxamniquine and praziquantel in the treatment of Schistosoma mansoni infection: a controlled trial. Bull World Health Organ 2003;81(3):190–196

65. Carod-Artal FJ. Neurological complications of Schistosoma infection. Trans R Soc Trop Med Hyg 2008;102(2):107–116

66. Mehta A, Teoh SK, Schaefer PW, Chew FS. Cerebral schistosomiasis. AJR Am J Roentgenol 1997;168(5):1322

67. Preidler KW, Riepl T, Szolar D, Ranner G. Cerebral schistosomiasis: MR and CT appearance. AJNR Am J Neuroradiol 1996;17(8):1598–1600

68. Sanelli PC, Lev MH, Gonzalez RG, Schaefer PW. Unique linear and nodular MR enhancement pattern in schistosomiasis of the central nervous system: report of three patients. AJR Am J Roentgenol 2001;177(6):1471–1474

69. Fowler R, Lee C, Keystone JS. The role of corticosteroids in the treatment of cerebral schistosomiasis caused by Schistosoma mansoni: case report and discussion. Am J Trop Med Hyg 1999;61(1):47–50

70. Deol I, Robledo L, Meza A, Visvesvara GS, Andrews RJ. Encephalitis due to a free-living amoeba (Balamuthia mandrillaris): case report with literature review. Surg Neurol 2000;53(6):611–616

71. Seidel JS. Naegleria, Acanthamoeba, and Balamuthia. In: Feigin R, Cherry JS, Demmler GJ, Kaplan SL, eds. Textbook of Pediatric Infectious Diseases. Vol 2. Philadelphia, PA: Saunders; 2004:2748–2755

72. Marciano-Cabral F, Puffenbarger R, Cabral GA. The increasing importance of Acanthamoeba infections. J Eukaryot Microbiol 2000;47(1):29–36

73. Martinez AJ, Visvesvara GS. Free-living, amphizoic and opportunistic amebas. Brain Pathol 1997;7(1):583–598

74. Galarza M, Cuccia V, Sosa FP, Monges JA. Pediatric granulomatous cerebral amebiasis: a delayed diagnosis. Pediatr Neurol 2002;26(2): 153–156

75. McKellar MS, Mehta LR, Greenlee JE, et al. Fatal granulomatous Acanthamoeba encephalitis mimicking a stroke, diagnosed by correlation of results of sequential magnetic resonance imaging, biopsy, in vitro culture, immunofluorescence analysis, and molecular analysis. J Clin Microbiol 2006;44(11):4265–4269

76. Petri WA Jr, Haque R. Amebiasis. In: Mandell GL, Bennett JE, Dolin R, eds. Bennett's Principles and Practice of Infectious Diseases. Philadelphia, PA: Elsevier Churchill Livingstone; 2010:3411–3427

77. Campbell S. Amebic brain abscess and meningoencephalitis. Semin Neurol 1993;13(2): 153–160

78. Lombardo L, Alonso P, Saenzarroyo L, Brandt H, Humbertomateos J. Cerebral amebiasis-report of 17 cases. J Neurosurg 1964;21:704–709

79. Fung KT, Dhillon AP, McLaughlin JE, et al. Cure of Acanthamoeba cerebral abscess in a liver transplant patient. Liver Transpl 2008;14(3):308–312

80. Schuster FL, Visvesvara GS. Free-living amoebae as opportunistic and non-opportunistic pathogens of humans and animals. Int J Parasitol 2004;34(9):1001–1027

81. Deetz TR, Sawyer MH, Billman G, Schuster FL, Visvesvara GS. Successful treatment of Balamuthia amoebic encephalitis: presentation of 2 cases. Clin Infect Dis 2003;37(10):1304–1312

82. Velho V, Sharma GK, Palande DA. Cerebrospinal acanthamebic granulomas. Case report. J Neurosurg 2003;99(3):572–574

83. White JM, Barker RD, Salisbury JR, et al. Granulomatous amoebic encephalitis. Lancet 2004;364(9429):220

84. Recavarren-Arce S, Velarde C, Gotuzzo E, Cabrera J. Amoeba angeitic lesions of the central nervous system in Balamuthia mandrilaris amoebiasis. Hum Pathol 1999;30(3):269–273

85. De Villiers JP, Durra G. Case report: amoebic abscess of the brain. Clin Radiol 1998;53(4): 307–309

86. Solaymani-Mohammadi S, Lam MM, Zunt JR, Petri WA Jr. *Entamoeba histolytica* encephalitis diagnosed by PCR of cerebrospinal fluid. Trans R Soc Trop Med Hyg 2007;101(3):311–313

87. Akhaddar A, Elouennass M, Baallal H, Boucetta M. Focal intracranial infections due to *Actinomyces* species in immunocompetent patients: diagnostic and therapeutic challenges. World Neurosurg 2010;74(2-3):346–350

88. Singh P, Kochhar R, Vashishta RK, et al. Amebic meningoencephalitis: spectrum of imaging findings. AJNR Am J Neuroradiol 2006;27(6): 1217–1221

89. Gaskill SJ, Marlin AE. Tuberculosis and fungal and parasitic infections of the central nervous system. In: Albright AL, Pollack IF, Adelson PD. Principles and Practice of Pediatric Neurosurgery. 2nd ed. New York, NY: Thieme; 2008:1182–1195

90. Sharma PP, Gupta P, Murali MV, Ramachandran VG. Primary amebic meningoencephalitis caused by *Acanthamoeba*: successfully treated with cotrimoxazole. Indian Pediatr 1993;30(10): 1219–1222

91. Marciano-Cabral F, Cabral G. *Acanthamoeba* spp. as agents of disease in humans. Clin Microbiol Rev 2003;16(2):273–307

# 8

# Bacterial Brain Abscess

Peter D. Kim and Walter A. Hall

Bacterial brain abscess is a life-threatening entity encountered in a wide variety of clinical settings. The condition is often lethal if not treated, but excellent outcomes may be achieved with proper management. With aggressive multimodal treatment, mortality has fallen but remains at about 10%. Diagnosis is at times elusive, and management requires the nuanced use of surgery, antibiotics, and supportive care. Furthermore, numerous complications can occur. In this chapter, the epidemiology, pathophysiology, diagnosis, and management of bacterial brain abscesses are reviewed. Brain abscesses caused by nonbacterial agents are discussed elsewhere in this volume.

## ■ Epidemiology

Brain abscesses are not uncommon and occur in the United States at a rate of approximately 2,500 per year.[1] The prevalence is highest in young men, and increased rates are also observed in young children and neonates; each of these groups exhibits different risk factors and therefore different microbial profiles. Worldwide, the prevalence probably varies significantly as the percentage of populations with immunocompromise, immunization rates, and prevalence of other risk factors vary. As the number of patients with immunocompromise due to human immunodeficiency virus (HIV) and to iatrogenic causes, such as solid-organ transplant

and chemotherapy, increases, reports of bacterial brain abscess secondary to atypical etiologic agents appear to be on the rise.

## ■ Etiologic Agent

The most likely etiologic agent depends on the risk factors of the patient. In neonates, *Proteus* and *Citrobacter* species are the most frequently cultured organisms,[2,3] whereas in older children and adult patients, the most common isolates in reported series are *Streptococcus* species, in particular *Streptococcus milleri*.[4,5] Staphylococcal infections are most common among intravenous drug users as well as after craniotomy and trauma, as a result of inoculation from contaminated skin. *Bacteroides* species (**Fig. 8.1**), which are anaerobic gram-negative bacilli that are part of the normal flora within the digestive system, are also not infrequently isolated.[5]

Aerobic gram-negative bacilli, including *Escherichia coli*, *Haemophilus influenzae*, *Pseudomonas aeruginosa*, and *Klebsiella pneumoniae*, are also isolated from brain abscesses with some frequency—the latter often in association with diabetes mellitus as a risk factor.[6] *Nocardia* species are atypical bacteria that form branching filaments (**Fig. 8.2**) and can cause brain abscess, particularly in immunocompromised patients. *Nocardia* brain abscesses are generally difficult to treat, and mortality rates are higher than

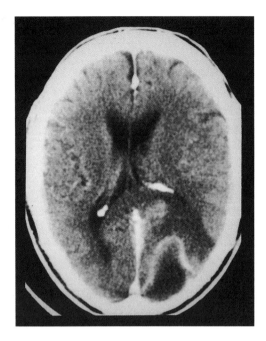

Fig. 8.1 Contrast-enhanced axial computed tomographic scan of the brain shows a left occipital *Bacteroides fragilis* brain abscess that, until the biopsy yielded pus, was thought to represent a brain metastasis in a patient with a long history of smoking.

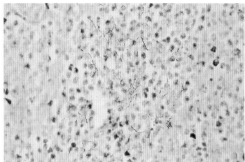

Fig. 8.2 Modified Brown-Brenn stain showing the fine, filamentous bacterium *Nocardia asteroides* in a cardiac transplant recipient with a brain abscess (magnification ×160).

those for other bacterial brain abscesses.[7,8] Spread of *Nocardia* to the brain is most often hematogenous. *Propionibacterium acnes* can cause brain abscess, and as with other cases of *Propionibacterium acnes* CNS involvement, such infections tend to be less severe and may occur in a delayed fashion.[9,10]

A significant percentage of brain abscesses are polymicrobial. Most series also contain a significant number of brain abscesses that are sterile when cultured,[5,6,11,12] which may be due to prior treatment with antibiotics[13] or to issues related to the handling of collected samples.

## ■ Risk Factors

Risk factors for the development of brain abscess may be divided into those resulting from immunologic factors, those due to anatomic issues, and those due to increased exposure to pathogens.

Immunocompromised patients are at a higher risk for brain abscesses. HIV infection is in particular a risk factor for bacterial brain abscess; however, in this population, CNS lymphoma, *Toxoplasma gondii* (**Fig. 8.3**) abscess, and metastatic disease are also relatively common. The evaluation of a ring-enhancing lesion in this population is therefore particularly challenging. Iatrogenic causes of immunocompromise, such as cancer chemotherapy and immunosuppression after solid-organ transplant, are also risk factors for brain abscess development. Transplant patients have an increased risk for developing nocardial brain abscesses,[14–17] which may be part of disseminated infection. Diabetes mellitus and cystic fibrosis result in an increased risk for systemic infections and for brain abscess.

Anatomic risk factors include the presence of cyanotic heart disease and hereditary hemorrhagic telangiectasia (HHT). HHT results in a dramatically increased risk for brain abscess, which is likely the result of paradoxical emboli from pulmonary arteriovenous malformations (**Fig. 8.4**) and most often due to *Streptococcus* species.[18] A higher mortality rate has been reported for brain abscess associated with HHT.[19,20] Cyanotic heart disease is a specific risk factor for pediatric patients.[21,22] Dermoid cysts may contain a sinus tract in communication with the skin that can result in abscess formation, particularly within the cerebellum.[23,24]

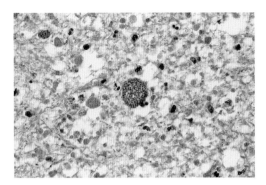

**Fig. 8.3** *Toxoplasma gondii* bradyzoite isolated from a brain abscess in a patient with acquired immunodeficiency syndrome (AIDS) stained with hematoxylin and eosin (magnification ×160).

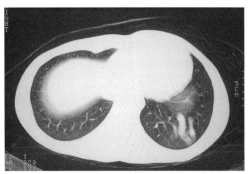

**Fig. 8.4** Contrast-enhanced computed tomographic scan of the chest demonstrating an arteriovenous malformation in the posterior aspect of the left lung in a patient with hereditary hemorrhagic telangiectasia.

Risk factors that derive from increased exposure to pathogens include intravenous drug use, a history of intracranial surgery (including a history of cervical traction or halo pin placement), a history of meningitis, dental surgery, and a history of recurrent sinusitis and otitis media. Otitis media and sinusitis account for the majority of abscesses in several series.[25] Odontogenic abscesses are frequently mentioned in case reports,[26] although the frequency of their true causality is uncertain.

Brain abscess after a neurosurgical procedure is a rare but well-known complication. Two large retrospective studies have been performed and found similar rates of brain abscess after craniotomy that were just under 0.2%.[27,28] Similarly low rates have been described after transnasal endoscopic skull base surgery.[29] Among neurosurgical procedures, the placement of halo pins, such as those used for cervical immobilization, is associated with numerous case reports of brain abscess formation, and the risk may be increased by retightening pins that have become loose after original placement.[30–32]

### ■ Pathophysiology

Brain abscesses may occur anywhere within the brain, although the most frequent sites are the frontal, temporal, and parietal lobes. Their origin is often within the white matter adjacent to the cerebral cortex. Abscesses that result from direct extension of sinus infection are located in the frontal lobe, and the temporal lobe is often the site of abscesses that are the result of mastoiditis (**Fig. 8.5**). Cerebellar abscesses can have an otogenic origin. Abscesses of the brainstem are rare[33] but do occur, and as expected, they carry a poor prognosis.

The stages of brain abscess development, from inoculation of the brain parenchyma to capsule development, have been described.[34] These stages include the early and late cerebritis stages followed by the early and late capsule stages. During the early cerebritis stages, inflammation and edema develop in response to the presence of an infectious inoculum. An area of central necrosis starts to form, with fibroblast deposition of reticulin along the margin during the late cerebritis phase. The formation of a ring-enhancing margin defines the capsule stages (**Fig. 8.6**); it starts as a vascular, gliotic structure (early) and then is sequestered within a completed collagen border (late).

A murine model of staphylococcal brain abscess has suggested that despite the fact that the purulent material is sequestered from the rest of the brain, localized inflammation mediated by tumor necrosis factor-α (TNF-α), interleukin-1b (IL-1b), and macrophage inflammatory protein-2

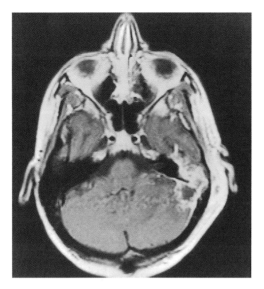

**Fig. 8.5** Axial contrast-enhanced T1-weighted magnetic resonance image of the brain demonstrating *Streptococcus* species mastoiditis with direct extension into the posterior fossa, resulting in a brain abscess in the left cerebellar hemisphere.

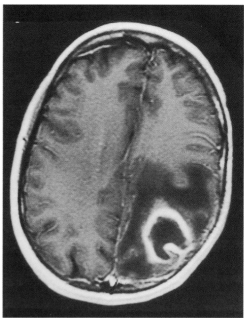

**Fig. 8.6** Contrast-enhanced T1-weighted magnetic resonance image of the brain shows a brain abscess in the late capsular stage with a completed collagen border. The abscess was dental in origin and grew an anaerobic *Streptococcus* species on culture.

(MIP-2) may contribute to damage of the adjacent parenchyma.[35] This inflammation, however, may be necessary for an optimal host response because animals deficient in TNF-α or IL-1 exhibit reduced survival after experimental abscess, the latter of which may be mediated downstream by the chemokines CXCL13 and CCL9.[36] A member of the toll-like receptor family, toll-like receptor-2 (TLR-2), which is expressed on neutrophils and macrophages and recognizes molecular motifs associated with *Staphylococcus* species and other pathogens, appears to be a pathway of inflammatory initiation.[37]

## ■ Diagnosis

The diagnosis of brain abscesses is often delayed because of the nonspecific nature of the presentation. One of the pitfalls in recognition is the incorrect assumption that a patient with a brain abscess will present with signs and symptoms of infection. Because of the immune-privileged nature of the CNS and the size limitations of the intracranial space, brain abscesses most frequently present with signs and symptoms of a mass lesion. As such, headache, nausea, vomiting, lethargy, and focal neurologic deficits may be seen. Fever and meningismus are often absent.[28] Papilledema is occasionally present and adds urgency to the patient assessment. Careful evaluation for the presence of risk factors is crucial in leading to the correct diagnosis. In neonates, signs of abscess may include seizures, enlarging head circumference, decreased feeding, and respiratory difficulties.[2]

Because the presentation is often essentially that of a mass lesion, clues that distinguish the clinical picture from that of a patient presenting with a brain tumor should be sought. A history of intravenous drug use, immunocompromise, or relevant infection is important, and the physical examination then focuses on signs of dental or otologic infection. A history of previous malignancy or tobacco exposure or a strong family history of cancer is similarly more suggestive that a ring-enhancing lesion may be a neoplasm. Finally, the time course is occasionally a clue because intraparenchymal brain abscesses often have a shorter time course than do malignancies.

Laboratory investigations may reveal an elevated white blood cell count and inflammatory markers, in particular C-reactive protein. Serum chemistries should also be obtained to assess for the presence of electrolyte imbalances, and the coagulation profile should be obtained in anticipation of surgical intervention.

Once the diagnosis of brain abscess is suspected, obtaining material for culture is critical in determining appropriate antibiotic therapy. Blood cultures should be obtained in any patient suspected of having a brain abscess, although these are positive in a minority of cases. Lumbar puncture should not be attempted because it carries a risk for neurologic deterioration when performed[12] and is often nondiagnostic. Aspiration of the lesion (as described in the section on treatment) is often necessary to obtain positive cultures (**Fig. 8.7**). Ideally, empiric antibiotic therapy should be delayed until a definitive culture is obtained because sterile cultures may otherwise occur.

## ■ Imaging

Computed tomography (CT) is often the first imaging study obtained and shows evidence of a mass lesion with surrounding cerebral edema. On CT, peripheral rim enhancement is seen on contrast studies with a central area of hypodensity (**Fig. 8.8**). Magnetic resonance (MR) imaging similarly reveals a contrast-enhancing lesion with surrounding edema (see **Fig. 8.6**). Contrast enhancement may be more prominent along the region closer to the ventricle, although this finding is not consistent among patients. The presence of restricted diffusion within the enhancing ring is strongly suggestive of a pyogenic abscess.[38] MR spectroscopy can distinguish abscess from a neoplastic lesion by the presence of increased amino acids and acetate[38]; however, treatment should not be delayed to obtain this test.

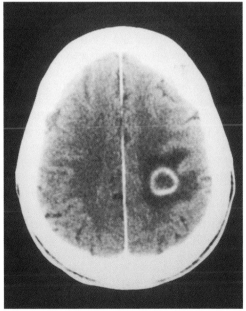

**Fig. 8.8** Axial contrast-enhanced computed tomographic scan of the brain shows a brain abscess with central hypodensity that represents pus and cerebral edema that surrounds a well-established late-stage capsule. The abscess, in a patient who had received a heart transplant, grew *Nocardia asteroides*.

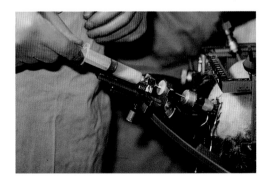

**Fig. 8.7** Intraoperative photograph shows a stereotactic aspiration of a brain abscess. Note the purulent material filling the syringe as a result of gentle aspiration.

## ■ Treatment

Bacterial brain abscesses are treated with antibiotics, which should be started as soon as an adequate specimen is obtained for culture. Prolonged treatment with intravenous antibiotics should be anticipated and arrangements can be made, such as placement of an intravenous catheter for extended use. Empiric antibiotic treatment with broad coverage (e.g., vancomycin, metronidazole, and cefotaxime) is usually started at the time cultures are obtained. The antibiotic regimen is then tailored to the specific pathogen once sensitivities are determined. Anticonvulsant drugs are administered prophylactically to prevent seizures. In most situations, corticosteroids are avoided because of the belief that their presence will diminish the immune response and stabilize the blood–brain barrier, thereby decreasing antibiotic penetration. Corticosteroids can effectively reduce intracerebral swelling secondary to the vasogenic edema associated with brain abscesses (**Fig. 8.9**). Experimental models have differed on whether dexamethasone significantly alters the local immune response to bacterial pathogens.[39,40] Dexamethasone is often administered before it has been determined that the intracranial lesion is an abscess, and occasionally in the presence of a known pyogenic brain abscess to treat life-threatening edema with mass effect and impending herniation.

Medical therapy alone may be contemplated for patients with smaller lesions that are generally less than 2.5 cm in diameter, particularly if the lesion is deep-seated within the brain or if multiple lesions are present. For lesions with a diameter larger than 2.5 cm, surgical treatment is recommended if feasible. The goals of surgery include definitive identification of the causative agent and removal of as much purulent material as possible. Open surgery and stereotactic aspiration have both been advocated. The advantage of open surgery, via craniotomy and corticectomy, is the ability to perform a more extensive removal of infectious material while opening any loculated compartments within

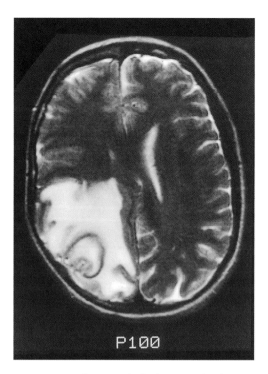

**Fig. 8.9** Significant cerebral edema can develop surrounding a brain abscess, as is apparent on this axial T2-weighted magnetic resonance image of the brain. The ring-shaped area of decreased signal represents the abscess capsule.

the abscess. Stereotactic drainage offers a less invasive surgical approach that is better suited for deep-seated lesions (see **Fig. 8.7**). In cases in which surgery is primarily for diagnostic purposes, stereotactic aspiration may be preferable to craniotomy. Kondziolka et al have described good results with stereotactic drainage, with the failures of this technique occurring in cases that had inadequate antibiotic treatment or insufficient aspiration and in larger abscesses that did not undergo any form of drainage.[41] Open surgery is preferable for lesions located in the cerebellum and for the treatment of recurrent abscesses. Great care must be taken at the time of surgery not to inoculate the ventricular system with infectious material. Unless grossly infected or in the presence of osteomyelitis, the bone flap may be replaced at the time of surgery.

For patients with signs of hydrocephalus or with posterior fossa abscesses exerting mass effect on the fourth ventricle (**Fig. 8.10**), an external ventricular drain should be placed to alleviate or prevent cerebrospinal fluid (CSF) obstruction. The ventriculostomy will be either gradually withdrawn over time and removed or replaced by a shunt at a later time. Permanent shunt hardware is not placed until it has been demonstrated that the CSF is sterile on multiple cultures.

Supportive treatment for the patient includes intubation and mechanical ventilation when necessary and the correction of any electrolyte imbalances when present. Patients often present after an extended period of anorexia, and aggressive fluid resuscitation is necessary to optimize care. Withdrawal from recreational drugs that include alcohol must also be identified and treated appropriately when present because hospitalization may represent an extended absence of such agents. If an infectious source is identified, it must be treated aggressively, as well.

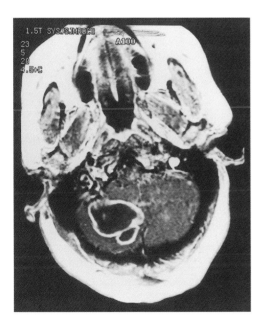

**Fig. 8.10** Axial T1-weighted contrast-enhanced magnetic resonance image of the brain shows a cerebellar brain abscess that caused acute hydrocephalus, requiring emergent placement of an external ventricular drain to relieve cerebrospinal fluid obstruction.

## ■ Complications

### Seizures

Seizures can frequently complicate the treatment of bacterial brain abscess either early or later in the course of the disease. The use of prophylactic antiepileptic drugs is appropriate, although strong evidence for their benefit is lacking and there is no consensus on the duration of treatment. Any patient with an unexplained decline in mental function should receive intensive care unit–based electroencephalographic monitoring for 24 hours once intraventricular rupture and sepsis have been excluded.

### Ventriculitis

Purulent ventriculitis is one of the most feared complications of brain abscess and is the most common cause of death after surgery for brain abscess.[11] Intraventricular extension may occur either spontaneously or as a complication of surgical intervention. Abscess rupture into the ventricle often presents as a sudden deterioration in neurologic function or may be heralded by signs and symptoms of meningismus or sepsis. Once intraventricular rupture does occur, the mortality rate is as high as 80%.[42] Intraventricular purulence should be treated with the placement of an external ventricular drain, the intrathecal administration of antibiotics, and the surgical treatment or re-treatment of the primary abscess if appropriate. With aggressive multimodal treatment, lower mortality rates have been reported for brain abscess.[43]

### Hydrocephalus

Hydrocephalus occurs occasionally as a complication of brain abscesses, in particular in those patients who survive ventricular involvement. Hydrocephalus is also fairly frequently observed in neonates with brain abscesses because many of these occur in conjunction with meningitis. Hydrocephalus in this setting is usually communicating in nature and therefore should be treated with shunt placement as opposed to an endoscopic third ventriculostomy. The shunt is placed after sterile CSF cultures and benign CSF profiles have been demonstrated. Loculi may be present in the ventricles, particularly in survivors of ventriculitis, and in these cases a single ventricular catheter may not be sufficient to treat the resultant hydrocephalus. Endoscopic fenestration may be an option in such complicated cases.

### Recurrent Abscesses

Successful treatment of bacterial brain abscesses requires vigilance for recurrent disease. Abscesses may recur in a delayed fashion after ostensibly successful treatment. For this reason, patients treated for bacterial brain abscess are followed with surveillance MR imaging every 4 to 6 weeks until the lesions have resolved completely. Outpatient follow-up should be for a minimum of 1 year. Predisposing factors that are modifiable must be addressed on a long-term basis.

## ■ Outcome

The survival for brain abscess has improved with the development of more potent antibiotics and a refinement of surgical technique. Mortality in most modern series is approximately 10%. Survivors of neonatal brain abscess often have significant cognitive deficits.[2] This impairment may be due to previous meningitis, postinfectious epilepsy, or both. Adult patients with bacterial brain abscess whose course was complicated by intraventricular rupture are also often severely disabled. In our experience, excellent outcomes in otherwise uncomplicated cases are possible with appropriate treatment.

## ■ Conclusion

Brain abscess is a life-threatening disease entity that is challenging both to diagnose and to treat. A wide array of pathogens may be responsible for the infection, and their successful culture is key to optimizing the medical arm of management. Patients at risk for bacterial brain abscess often present additional challenges by virtue of their medical comorbidities, socioeconomic issues, and neonatal age. Complications such as hydrocephalus, epilepsy, and intraventricular rupture of the abscess can all result in the rapid clinical deterioration of a previously stable patient. Despite these challenges, aggressive, appropriate multispecialty care is often rewarded with an excellent long-term patient outcome.

### References

1. Hall WA, Truwit CL. The surgical management of infections involving the cerebrum. Neurosurgery 2008;62(Suppl 2):519–530, discussion 530–531
2. Renier D, Flandin C, Hirsch E, Hirsch JF. Brain abscesses in neonates. A study of 30 cases. J Neurosurg 1988;69(6):877–882
3. Goodkin HP, Harper MB, Pomeroy SL. Intracerebral abscess in children: historical trends at Children's Hospital Boston. Pediatrics 2004;113(6):1765–1770
4. de Louvois J, Gortavai P, Hurley R. Bacteriology of abscesses of the central nervous system: a multicentre prospective study. BMJ 1977;2(6093):981–984
5. Hakan T, Ceran N, Erdem I, Berkman MZ, Göktaş P. Bacterial brain abscesses: an evaluation of 96 cases. J Infect 2006;52(5):359–366
6. Kao PT, Tseng HK, Liu CP, Su SC, Lee CM. Brain abscess: clinical analysis of 53 cases. J Microbiol Immunol Infect 2003;36(2):129–136
7. Kilincer C, Hamamcioglu MK, Simsek O, et al. Nocardial brain abscess: review of clinical management. J Clin Neurosci 2006;13(4):481–485
8. Sabuncuoğlu H, Cibali Açikgo ZZ, Caydere M, Ustün H, Semih Keskil I. *Nocardia farcinica* brain abscess: a case report and review of the literature. Neurocirugia (Astur) 2004;15(6):600–603
9. Chung S, Kim JS, Seo SW, et al. A case of brain abscess caused by *Propionibacterium acnes* 13 months after neurosurgery and confirmed by 16S rRNA gene sequencing. Korean J Lab Med 2011;31(2):122–126
10. Kranick SM, Vinnard C, Kolson DL. *Propionibacterium acnes* brain abscess appearing 10 years after neurosurgery. Arch Neurol 2009;66(6):793–795
11. Beller AJ, Sahar A, Praiss I. Brain abscess. Review of 89 cases over a period of 30 years. J Neurol Neurosurg Psychiatry 1973;36(5):757–768
12. Nathoo N, Nadvi SS, Narotam PK, van Dellen JR. Brain abscess: management and outcome analysis of a computed tomography era experience with 973 patients. World Neurosurg 2011;75(5-6):716–726, discussion 612–617
13. Mampalam TJ, Rosenblum ML. Trends in the management of bacterial brain abscesses: a re-

view of 102 cases over 17 years. Neurosurgery 1988;23(4):451–458

14. Jimenez-Galanes Marchan S, Meneu Díaz JC, Caso Maestro O, et al. Disseminated nocardiosis: a rare infectious complication following non-heart-beating donor liver transplantation. Transplant Proc 2009;41(6):2495–2497

15. Kalokhe AS, Kraft CS, Lyon GM, Lim P, Wang J. A 35-year-old woman with prior renal transplantation admitted with a temporal brain abscess. Clin Infect Dis 2011;53(8):843–844, 797

16. Moon JH, Cho WS, Kang HS, Kim JE. *Nocardia* brain abscess in a liver transplant recipient. J Korean Neurosurg Soc 2011;50(4):396–398

17. Belhocine W, Purgus R, Almasalma M, et al. *Nocardia carnea* infection in a kidney transplant recipient. Transplant Proc 2010;42(10):4359–4360

18. Sell B, Evans J, Horn D. Brain abscess and hereditary hemorrhagic telangiectasia. South Med J 2008;101(6):618–625

19. Hall WA. Hereditary hemorrhagic telangiectasia (Rendu-Osler-Weber disease) presenting with polymicrobial brain abscess. Case report. J Neurosurg 1994;81(2):294–296

20. Dong SL, Reynolds SF, Steiner IP. Brain abscess in patients with hereditary hemorrhagic telangiectasia: case report and literature review. J Emerg Med 2001;20(3):247–251

21. Goodman ML, Nelson PB. Brain abscess complicating the use of a halo orthosis. Neurosurgery 1987;20(1):27–30

22. Kao KL, Wu KG, Chen CJ, et al. Brain abscesses in children: analysis of 20 cases presenting at a medical center. J Microbiol Immunol Infect 2008; 41(5):403–407

23. Mehnaz A, Syed AU, Saleem AS, Khalid CN. Clinical features and outcome of cerebral abscess in congenital heart disease. J Ayub Med Coll Abbottabad 2006;18(2):21–24

24. Akhaddar A, Jiddane M, Chakir N, El Hassani R, Moustarchid B, Bellakhdar F. Cerebellar abscesses secondary to occipital dermoid cyst with dermal sinus: case report. Surg Neurol 2002; 58(3-4):266–270

25. Roche M, Humphreys H, Smyth E, et al. A twelve-year review of central nervous system bacterial abscesses; presentation and aetiology. Clin Microbiol Infect 2003 Aug;9(8):804–809

26. Karagöz Güzey F, Bas NS, Sencer A, et al. Posterior fossa dermoid cysts causing cerebellar abscesses. Pediatr Neurosurg 2007;43(4):323–326

27. Corson MA, Postlethwaite KP, Seymour RA. Are dental infections a cause of brain abscess? Case report and review of the literature. Oral Dis 2001;7(1):61–65

28. McClelland S III, Hall WA. Postoperative central nervous system infection: incidence and associated factors in 2111 neurosurgical procedures. Clin Infect Dis 2007;45(1):55–59

29. Yang SY. Brain abscess: a review of 400 cases. J Neurosurg 1981;55(5):794–799

30. Kono Y, Prevedello DM, Snyderman CH, et al. One thousand endoscopic skull base surgical procedures demystifying the infection potential: incidence and description of postoperative meningitis and brain abscesses. Infect Control Hosp Epidemiol 2011;32(1):77–83

31. Quiñones-Hinojosa A, Chi JH, Manley GT. Emergent placement of halo orthosis after a traumatic cervical injury leading to a cerebral abscess. J Trauma 2007;62(6):E11–E13

32. Saeed MU, Dacuycuy MA, Kennedy DJ. Halo pin insertion-associated brain abscess: case report and review of literature. Spine 2007;32(8): E271–E274

33. Suzer T, Coskun E, Cirak B, Yagci B, Tahta K. Brain stem abscesses in childhood. Childs Nerv Syst 2005;21(1):27–31

34. Britt RH, Enzmann DR, Placone RC Jr, Obana WG, Yeager AS. Experimental anaerobic brain abscess. Computerized tomographic and neuropathological correlations. J Neurosurg 1984;60(6): 1148–1159

35. Baldwin AC, Kielian T. Persistent immune activation associated with a mouse model of *Staphylococcus aureus*-induced experimental brain abscess. J Neuroimmunol 2004;151(1-2):24–32

36. Kielian T, Bearden ED, Baldwin AC, Esen N. IL-1 and TNF-alpha play a pivotal role in the host immune response in a mouse model of *Staphylococcus aureus*-induced experimental brain abscess. J Neuropathol Exp Neurol 2004;63(4): 381–396

37. Kielian T, Haney A, Mayes PM, Garg S, Esen N. Toll-like receptor 2 modulates the proinflammatory milieu in *Staphylococcus aureus*-induced brain abscess. Infect Immun 2005;73(11):7428–7435

38. Lai PH, Ho JT, Chen WL, et al. Brain abscess and necrotic brain tumor: discrimination with proton MR spectroscopy and diffusion-weighted imaging. AJNR Am J Neuroradiol 2002;23(8): 1369–1377

39. Neuwelt EA, Lawrence MS, Blank NK. Effect of gentamicin and dexamethasone on the natural history of the rat *Escherichia coli* brain abscess model with histopathological correlation. Neurosurgery 1984;15(4):475–483

40. Schroeder KA, McKeever PE, Schaberg DR, Hoff JT. Effect of dexamethasone on experimental brain abscess. J Neurosurg 1987;66(2):264–269

41. Kondziolka D, Duma CM, Lunsford LD. Factors that enhance the likelihood of successful stereotactic treatment of brain abscesses. Acta Neurochir (Wien) 1994;127(1-2):85–90

42. Zeidman SM, Geisler FH, Olivi A. Intraventricular rupture of a purulent brain abscess: case report. Neurosurgery 1995;36(1):189–193, discussion 193

43. Takeshita M, Kawamata T, Izawa M, Hori T. Prodromal signs and clinical factors influencing outcome in patients with intraventricular rupture of purulent brain abscess. Neurosurgery 2001;48(2): 310–316, discussion 316–317

# III

# CNS Locations for Infection

# 9

# Meningeal Infections

## Manika Suryadevara and Joseph B. Domachowske

The clinical presentation of fever, headache, and stiff neck raises the clinical suspicion of meningeal infection in most cases, while biochemical, cellular, and microbiological analysis of the cerebrospinal fluid (CSF) confirms the presence of inflammatory cells and biochemical perturbations and identifies the etiologic agent. Acute bacterial meningitis is a medical emergency, and before the antibiotic era it was almost always a fatal infection. The incidence and demographics of meningeal infections vary by age and geographic location. Many of these differences are the direct result of effective immunization measures for the common causes of bacterial meningitis that have been introduced across the developed world.

demiologic and surveillance studies from the United States, Europe, Brazil, Israel, and Canada show that bacterial meningitis is less common in developed parts of the world but is generally caused by the same groups of microorganisms found in underdeveloped regions.

The development and implementation of vaccines to prevent infections caused by the three most common agents of bacterial meningitis (*Haemophilus influenzae* type B [HIB], *Streptococcus pneumoniae*, and *Neisseria meningitidis*) have had profound effects on the epidemiology of meningitis in children from all regions of the world where these vaccines are routinely available.

## ■ Incidence and Demographics

Bacterial meningitis is a significant global health problem with dramatic differences in infection rates when developed countries are compared with underdeveloped regions of the world. In Senegal, Africa, the average incidence of bacterial meningitis during the 1970s was 50 cases per 100,000 people, with an alarming 1 in 250 children developing meningitis during their first year of life.[1–3] Sub-Saharan Africa is commonly referred to as the meningitis belt because of epidemics of meningococcal meningitis, with incidence rates as high as 100 cases per 100,000 people.[4,5] Epi-

## ■ Etiology and Pathogenesis

Most cases of bacterial meningitis result from hematogenous seeding of the meninges. Direct extension of a bacterial infection from the sinuses, middle ear, or mastoid air cells is another route of spread. Such a source is immediately obvious on neuroimaging. The most common microbiological causes and pathogenesis of bacterial meningitis differ based on the age of the affected patient (**Table 9.1**). Common etiologic agents of bacterial meningitis in the first week of life include *Streptococcus agalactiae* (group B streptococci), *Escherichia coli*, and *Listeria monocytogenes*.[6–10] Late-onset neonatal meningitis occurs after the first

**Table 9.1** Common infecting pathogens and recommended empiric antimicrobial therapy for acute bacterial meningitis by age group

| Age group | Most common pathogens | Recommended empiric antibiotic therapy pending culture result |
|---|---|---|
| Neonates and infants up to 3 mo | Group B streptococci, *Escherichia coli*, *Listeria monocytogenes* | ampicillin[a] + cefotaxime[a] OR ampicillin[a] + gentamicin[a] |
| Older infants, children, and adults younger than 50 years | *Streptococcus pneumoniae*, *Neisseria meningitidis* | vancomycin (60 mg/kg/ d divided every 6 h in children) vancomycin (45 mg/kg/d divided every 8 h in adults) PLUS cefotaxime (300 mg/kg/ d up to 12 g/d divided every 6 h) OR ceftriaxone (100 mg/kg/d up to 4 g/d divided every 12 h) |
| Adults older than 50 years | *S. pneumoniae*, *N. meningitidis*, *L. monocytogenes*, gram-negative bacilli | ampicillin (12 g/d divided every 4 h) + vancomycin + cefotaxime or ceftriaxone as above |

[a] Antibiotic dosing in neonates depends on age and weight. From birth to 7 days, the doses for ampicillin and cefotaxime are the same and are 150 mg/kg per day divided every 8 hours. From days 8 through 28, they are 200 mg/kg per day divided every 6 hours, and after 28 days they are 300 mg/kg per day divided every 6 hours. The gentamicin dose from birth to 7 days is 5 mg/kg per day divided every 12 hours. After 7 days, the dose of gentamicin is 7.5 mg/kg per day divided every 8 hours with therapeutic drug monitoring.

week of life and up to 3 months of age and may be caused by the agents listed above, other enteric gram-negative bacilli, *Pasteurella* after animal exposure,[11] pneumococci, meningococci, and staphylococci.[12]

During late infancy and early childhood, *S. pneumoniae* and *N. meningitidis* account for 80% of cases of bacterial meningitis.[13–16] The remaining 20% are caused by *L. monocytogenes*, *Streptococcus pyogenes* (group A streptococci), *S. agalactiae* (group B streptococci), *H. influenzae* (type B and nontypeable isolates), *E. coli*, and other enteric gram-negative rods (including *Salmonella* species). Bacterial meningitis in adolescents and younger adults is usually caused by either *S. pneumoniae* or *N. meningitidis*[17–19]; however, after the age of 50 years, *L. monocytogenes* becomes more prevalent.[20] In elderly individuals, *S. pneumoniae*, *N. meningitidis*, and *L. monocytogenes* remain the more common microbiological etiologic agents[21]; however, a broad array of other pathogens has been described, depending on the presence of comorbidities, travel, and unusual exposures.[22] Neuroimaging studies of patients with uncomplicated bacterial meningitis will usually demonstrate leptomeningeal enhancement (**Fig. 9.1**) if a contrast image is performed.

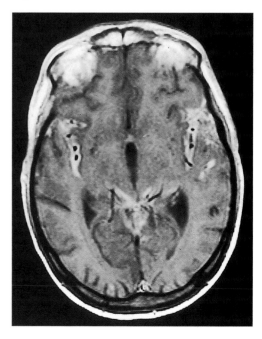

**Fig. 9.1** Diffuse leptomeningeal enhancement seen on a contrast-enhanced magnetic resonance image from a 4-month-old girl with meningococcal meningitis.

## Haemophilus influenzae Type B Meningitis

HIB is a gram-negative organism that invades via the respiratory tract. The primary virulence factor is the polysaccharide capsule, which allows it to evade the host's innate immune defenses. Other encapsulated types of *H. influenzae* (types A, C, D, E, and F) and nontypeable, or unencapsulated, forms of the bacterial species are rare causes of meningitis, usually seen in patients with humoral immune deficiencies. A primary site of infection, such as the lung or middle ear, may precede the bacteremia that is ultimately responsible for hematogenous seeding of the meninges. Once the most common bacterial form of meningitis during childhood, HIB infection is now a rare occurrence in countries where vaccination programs are in place. A diagnosis of HIB meningitis in a vaccinated child merits special attention. Although primary vaccine failure with breakthrough infection can occur, every such child should be evaluated for the possibility of an immunodeficiency condition. Based on the enormous success of HIB vaccination programs in children, HIB meningitis has become a disease found predominately in adults in the United States and Europe.[23–25]

## Pneumococcal Meningitis

*S. pneumoniae* is now the leading cause of bacterial meningitis in the United States and Europe, accounting for more than 60% of all cases.[26] The polysaccharide capsule functions as a primary virulence factor, and more than 90 different capsular serotypes have been described. The serotypes differ in prevalence and their tendency for antibiotic resistance. Some serotypes are more likely to cause invasive disease, including meningitis. Like HIB meningitis, pneumococcal meningitis is usually secondary to hematogenous seeding of the meninges, with a primary focus in the sinopulmonary tract. After introduction of the conjugate vaccine in 2000, U.S. population–based data from the Active Bacterial Core surveillance (ABCs), published by the Centers for Disease Control and Prevention, showed a 59% decline in pneumococcal meningitis in children younger than 2 years of age,[27] and Nationwide Inpatient Sample data showed that the incidence rate fell by 33% in children younger than 5 years of age (from 0.8 to 0.55 cases per 100,000 population).[28]

## Meningococcal Meningitis

*N. meningitidis* is a gram-negative diplococcus. Major virulence factors include the presence of lipopolysaccharide (endotoxin), expression of an immunoglobulin A protease, and the presence of a polysaccharide capsule that allows the organism to evade the host's innate immune response. The 12 serogroups of *N. meningitidis* known to infect humans are characterized by the polysaccharide expressed on the capsule: A, B, C, 29-E, H, I, K, L, W-135, X, Y, and Z. Clinically, the most relevant and most prevalent serogroup types are A, B, C, Y, and W-135. Invasive disease caused by the other types is unusual. Asymptomatic nasopharyngeal carriage of the bacterium is relatively common. In the United States, carrier prevalence in the general population is estimated to be between 5 and 10%. During adolescence, this prevalence can increase to as high as 35%. In situations of close contact, such as military barracks and college dormitories, carriage rates may approach 100%.[29] The balance between carriage and the development of disease is affected by a combination of host and environmental factors, along with the characteristics of the infecting organism.[30,31] Several social factors may also increase risk, such as close contact with an infected person and living or working in crowded conditions. It would appear that changes in behavior are the driving force behind the increased risk for meningococcal carriage in adolescents, particularly with regard to smoking and alcohol consumption.[32,33]

The proportion of cases of meningococcal disease caused by individual serogroups A, B, C, W-135, and Y varies by geographic region. In developed countries, serogroup distribution also differs within regions. In Great Britain, for example, serogroups B and

C account for over 90% of cases, whereas in New Zealand, serogroup B alone causes 87% of all cases. In contrast, meningococcal meningitis diagnosed in the African meningitis belt is usually caused by serogroup A. Attack rates during epidemics in Africa approach 1% of the population.[34–36] In Saudi Arabia, where serogroup W-135 predominates, attack rates have been described at 25 cases per 100,000 population during the Hajj.[37–40] The country of Niger has recently experienced the emergence of serogroup X, where it caused half of 1,139 cases in 2006.[41] In the United States, between 1,200 and 3,500 cases of meningococcal disease occur annually (0.9 to 1.5 cases per 100,000 population). Data for 2006 through 2008 show that serogroups B, Y, and C account for most of the U.S. cases.[42]

## Meningitis Caused by *Streptococcus agalactiae* (Group B Streptococci)

Group B streptococci are gram-positive organisms possessing several virulence factors, including a polysaccharide capsule, several adherence proteins, and cytolytic toxins. The organism remains a common cause of meningitis in newborns, with more than two-thirds of these infections occurring during the first 3 months of life.[43] Several studies have shown that administration of intravenous antibiotics to women in labor who are known to be colonized by group B streptococci is highly effective at reducing subsequent neonatal colonization. A meta-analysis of seven clinical trials demonstrated a 30-fold reduction of neonatal group B streptococcal invasive disease when antibiotics were delivered in this manner.[44] In the United States during the decade of the 1990s, the incidence of neonatal group B streptococcal infection dropped from 1.7 to 0.6 cases per 1,000 live births, likely as a result of the increased use of peripartum antibiotics in women in labor.[45,46] By 2004, rates dropped further, to approximately 0.3 per 1,000 following the implementation of formal obstetric screening guidelines.[47] Meningitis caused by group B streptococci is unusual beyond infancy but has been described.

## Meningitis Caused by *Streptococcus pyogenes* (Group A Streptococci)

*S. pyogenes* accounts for approximately 1% of all cases of bacterial meningitis in children and adults.[48] Primary infection of the middle ear, lung, or sinuses is the rule, with bacteremic spread to the central nervous system (CNS), but cases also occur following recent head injury, after neurosurgical procedures, in the presence of a neurosurgical device, and in patients with CSF leaks.[49,50] Reported mortality rates vary from 4 to 27%, with neurologic sequelae in 28%. Common complications in children include learning difficulties and other cognitive deficits, visual field defects, and hearing loss.[51] The largest published adult series demonstrated a rate of neurologic sequelae (43%) higher than that reported in children.[48]

## Meningitis Caused by *Staphylococcus aureus*

Unlike the community-acquired meningitis caused by *H. influenzae*, pneumococci, meningococci, and group A streptococci, *S. aureus* meningitis is almost always a nosocomial infection, occurring most commonly after a neurosurgical procedure, such as CSF shunt placement.[52,53] In the unusual circumstance of community-acquired *S. aureus* meningitis, the patient should be questioned about possible intravenous drug use and assessed for the presence of an underlying immunodeficiency. In addition, patients with staphylococcal endocarditis frequently develop metastatic infection of the CNS, including brain abscess and meningeal infection.[54,55] The mortality rate for nosocomial *S. aureus* meningitis is approximately 14%.[56] Mortality secondary to community-acquired *S. aureus* meningitis exceeds 50% because of underlying, predisposing diseases.[54]

## Meningitis Caused by *Listeria monocytogenes*

*L. monocytogenes* is a food-borne bacterium responsible for causing meningitis and other serious invasive illness in humans and other animals. *L. monocytogenes* is a gram-positive bacillus with the unusual ability to thrive intracellularly based on a host of characterized virulence factors.[57] *L. monocytogenes* causes approximately 2% of all cases of meningitis in the United States, a proportion that has grown smaller in recent years, likely as a result of a decrease in the contamination of ready-to-eat foods.[58] Infection is often associated with the presence of infectious foci in the brain parenchyma, especially in the brainstem.[59] The organism remains one of the principal causes of bacterial meningitis in neonates.[60–63]

## Meningitis Caused by Enteric Gram-Negative Bacteria

*E. coli*, *Klebsiella* species, *Acinetobacter baumannii*, *Pseudomonas aeruginosa*, and other aerobic gram-negative bacteria have been shown to cause meningitis following head trauma or neurosurgical procedures.[64–67] Meningitis caused by members of this group of organisms tends to occur late after surgery, with a median time until presentation of 12 days. Some infections may be detected more than a month after craniotomy. Community-acquired meningitis caused by aerobic gram-negative rods is unusual in adults but can occur in the context of immune-compromising conditions such as human immunodeficiency virus (HIV) infection. In contrast, enteric gram-negative bacteria as a group are second in frequency to group B streptococci during the neonatal period.[68] Most of these infections are caused by *E. coli*, *Klebsiella* species, and *Citrobacter* species. *Citrobacter koseri* infections are almost universally complicated by the development of parenchymal abscesses. Young infants may also develop meningitis caused by *Pasteurella multocida*, almost always after direct or indirect exposure to cats or dogs in the household.[11] *Salmonella* species have also been shown to cause meningitis. Approximately 15% of pediatric and adult patients who develop bacteremia during gastrointestinal salmonellosis will develop a metastatic infection of the joints, bone, or CNS. CNS seeding may cause meningitis but can also be complicated by subdural empyema and brain abscess.[69,70]

## Lyme Meningitis

Lyme disease is an infection caused by the spirochete *Borrelia burgdorferi*. This infection is transmitted via an infected tick bite in areas of endemicity. The pathogenesis of Lyme meningitis is secondary to spirochetemia during the early disseminated stage of infection.

## Tuberculous Meningitis

Worldwide, tuberculous meningitis remains a serious health threat, particularly in children residing in resource-poor areas of the world. Morbidity among survivors is the rule; death occurs in approximately 60% of patients.[71] The agent of tuberculosis, *Mycobacterium tuberculosis*, is an extremely common cause of pulmonary infection. CNS complications occur following dissemination in the highest-risk groups, including children and patients infected with HIV. Prediction of outcome early in the illness is difficult because the infection runs a protracted course. Clinical indices such as cranial nerve palsy or other focal findings, seizures, and coma at the time of presentation have been assessed as predictors of long-term morbidity. Radiologic findings of hydrocephalus, cerebral infarction, or tuberculomas[65] may offer a more realistic predictive value for long-term sequelae, particularly among children.[72–75]

## ■ Specific Risk Factors for the Development of Bacterial Meningitis

Alcoholism, diabetes mellitus, asplenia, cancer, and other secondary immune compromising conditions all increase the risk for invasive CNS infections, including meningitis. Other risk factors for the development of meningitis can be divided into two broad categories: anatomic and immunologic. Patients who present with recurrent bacterial meningitis need to be evaluated for underlying factors because direct surgical or medical intervention for the underlying cause may be required to prevent further episodes.

## Anatomic Risk Factors

Anatomic abnormalities that predispose patients to bacterial meningitis include neural tube defects, epidermoid cysts, dermoid cysts, dermal sinus tracts, neurenteric cysts, and congenital inner ear malformation, including Mondini defects.[76] Most of these defects become evident during a careful physical examination and/or fairly routine neuroimaging; however, the detection of inner ear malformations requires specialized high-resolution images when suspicion is strong.

### Mondini Dysplasia

The Mondini defect consists of three main features: (1) instead of a cochlea with the normal two and one-half turns, a cochlea with one and one-half turns, comprising a normal basal turn and a cystic apex in place of the distal one and one-half turns;

(2) an enlarged vestibule with normal semicircular canals; and (3) an enlarged vestibular aqueduct containing a dilated endolymphatic sac[77] (**Fig. 9.2**). In most cases, Mondini dysplasia is associated with some degree of hearing impairment and can be associated with CSF otorrhea and meningitis.[78,79] It is thought that a fistula between the CSF spaces and the middle ear predisposes patients to the development of meningitis. The underlying CSF fistula in some patients with Mondini defects can occur in such places as through a deficient oval window or stapes footplate.

### Cochlear Implant

In most cases of meningitis in patients with a cochlear implant, the initial infection is acute otitis media on the side of the implant. Bacteria enter the inner ear through the surgical cochleostomy. Pathways of bacterial access to the CSF from the inner ear include

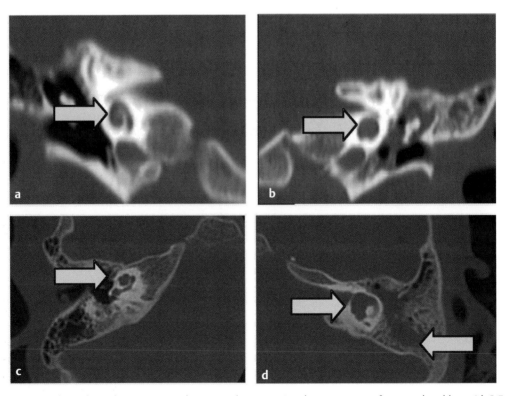

**Fig. 9.2a–d** High-resolution computed tomography comparing the appearance of a normal cochlea, with 2.5 turns (a) and a vestibule (c), with the abnormal findings seen in Mondini dysplasia; (b) shows a dilated cochlea with only 1.5 turns, and (d) shows a dilated vestibule. There is superimposed mastoiditis in this patient, who developed pneumococcal meningitis secondary to the anatomic defect.

entry into the labyrinth, infiltration of the cochlea along the implanted electrode, and/or perivascular pathways into the internal auditory canal to the meninges.[80] In a case-control study performed in children younger than 6 years of age, 26 cases of meningitis were identified among 4,264 patients with cochlear implants.[81] During a 2-year follow-up of the same cohort, an additional 12 episodes of meningitis occurred.[82] This finding represents a more than 30-fold increase in the risk for meningitis compared with the general population. The mortality rate of meningitis in the context of a cochlear implant is approximately 16%. Not surprisingly, *S. pneumoniae* is the most commonly identified etiologic agent of implant-associated bacterial meningitis.

## Immunologic Risk Factors

Primary immune deficiencies, particularly those that impair humoral immunity, and secondary immune deficiencies resulting from alcoholism, HIV infection, diabetes mellitus, asplenia, the use of immunosuppressive medications, and malignancy all increase a patient's risk for developing an invasive systemic infection, including meningitis.[83–85] The most common infecting bacterial pathogen in patients with immunodeficiency is *S. pneumoniae*,[86] but other bacterial, viral, fungal, and even parasitic opportunistic infections must be considered based on the degree of the patient's immunocompromised state. Specifically, HIV-infected individuals have up to a 324-fold higher risk for invasive pneumococcal infection.[87–89] Even following therapy with highly active antiretroviral medications, when HIV replication is controlled, the risk for developing pneumococcal meningitis remains approximately 35-fold higher than that in the general population.[90,91] This increased risk has a profound public health effect in the underdeveloped world, where up to 95% of patients with pneumococcal meningitis are also infected with HIV.[92–95] Opportunistic infections are seen more frequently in those individuals with severe immunodeficiencies, but some immune defects are directly associated with an increased risk for specific offending organisms.

## Hypogammaglobulinemia

Patients with humoral immunodeficiencies are especially prone to develop sinopulmonary infections and meningitis caused by encapsulated bacterial pathogens (pneumococci, meningococci, *H. influenzae*). Although patients with hypogammaglobulinemia have no increased susceptibility to most viral infections, there is one exception. Although immunologically normal individuals develop a self-limited "aseptic meningitis" when enteroviruses infect the CNS, patients with hypogammaglobulinemia can develop chronic meningoencephalitis.[96] Enterovirus-directed therapies are not available, and despite aggressive supportive care, many of these patients lose substantial neurologic function, and some die.

## IRAK-4 and MyD88 Deficiency

Impairments in innate immune responses are also known to increase the risk for developing meningitis. The autosomal recessive interleukin-1 receptor–associated kinase (IRAK)-4 and myeloid differentiation (MyD) factor 88 deficiencies impair toll-like receptor (TLR)–mediated and interleukin-1 receptor–mediated immunity. These defects lead to a predisposition to the development of recurrent life-threatening bacterial diseases, especially during infancy and early childhood. In the single largest clinical report of infections in patients with these deficiencies, approximately half of all invasive bacterial infections were meningitis, although the frequency and types of long-term sequelae were similar to those seen in immunocompetent patients.[97] Infecting agents included *S. pneumoniae*, HIB, *S. aureus*, and group B streptococci.

## Complement Deficiency

Complement deficiencies are rare disorders of immune function afflicting 0.03% of the population. Because complement activation pathways converge at the activation of C3, patients who are deficient in C3 have serious deficiencies in complement-mediated opsonization, phagocyte recruitment, and bacteriolysis. Such patients are prone to invasive infection caused by encapsulated bacteria such as pneumococci, meningococci, and *H. influenzae*. Most infections in patients with C3 deficiency involve the sinopulmonary tract (otitis, sinusitis, and pneumonia), but C3-deficient patients are also predisposed to the development of sepsis and meningitis.[98] An increased incidence of invasive meningococcal disease has been observed in patients with deficiencies or defects in terminal complement components C5–C9 and dysfunctional properdin.[99-101] Any patient who presents with recurrent infections (including meningitis) caused by *Neisseria* species should be evaluated for a terminal complement defect.

## ■ Clinical Presentation

The clinical presentation of acute bacterial meningitis varies by patient age and immune status as well as the etiology of the infection.[102] The classic triad of fever, neck stiffness, and altered mental status is not always present. Only in patients with severe meningeal inflammation (white blood cell [WBC] count ≥ 1,000/mL of CSF) is nuchal rigidity 100% sensitive and specific for the diagnosis of acute meningitis.[103]

Neonatal meningitis is difficult to identify because newborns tend to present with nonspecific symptoms, including temperature instability, respiratory distress, jaundice, poor suck, and lethargy.[102,104,105] Approximately 50 to 88% of neonates present with fever, two-thirds with irritability and/or a bulging fontanelle, one-third with lethargy, and 25 to 40% with seizures before admission.[102,104,105] The presence of a bulging fontanelle is strongly predictive of neonatal meningitis.[106]

Infants beyond the neonatal period and children younger than 5 years of age with meningitis present with fever, irritability, altered mental status, and decreased oral intake.[104,107-109] Seizures occur in 42 to 81% of these children.[104,107] Other symptoms may include neck stiffness, headache, vomiting, lethargy, "staring eyes," and rash.[104,107-109] Children older than 5 years of age are more likely to present with classic meningismus.[104,110]

Other symptoms that are seen include a petechial or purpuric rash, change in muscle tone, vomiting, and decreased oral intake. Of note, a change in a child's state of alertness is one of the most important signs of meningitis, although the finding may be subtle.[102]

A nationwide study in the Netherlands prospectively evaluated 696 episodes of community-acquired bacterial meningitis in adults. They found that the classic triad of fever, neck stiffness, and altered mental status was present in only 44% of the episodes. However, when headache was added to this list, 95% of the patients had at least two of the four symptoms.[19] The classic triad was more likely to be present in pneumococcal meningitis than in meningococcal meningitis.[19,111] Rash was present in 26% of cases and focal neurologic deficit in 33%. Seizures were present in 5% of patients.[19] Neurologic abnormalities seen on presentation in adults with meningitis can include generalized deficits, such as confusion, lethargy, and unresponsiveness, as well as focal neurologic signs, such as cranial nerve palsies, hemiparesis, aphasia, and visual field defects.[17,112]

Elderly patients are another group whose clinical diagnosis can be challenging. Presenting signs and symptoms are quite variable and are often nonspecific.[22] It is important to note that nuchal rigidity can be present for reasons other than meningitis in elderly patients, such as previous cerebrovascular accidents, Parkinson disease, and cervical spondylosis.[113] The elderly are more likely to present with depressed mental status, hemiparesis, and seizures than with headache, nausea, vomiting, and nuchal rigidity.[20,113] Acute complications of pyogenic bacterial meningitis include the development of cerebritis with parenchymal infarcts, subdural empyema, ventriculitis, and hydrocephalus (**Fig. 9.3**). Neuroimaging should not be delayed because emergent surgical intervention may be necessary.

Unlike the other common types of bacterial meningitis, Lyme disease is associated with aseptic meningitis, more closely mimicking mild forms of viral meningitis rather than fulminant, pyogenic bacterial meningitis. One study showed that the

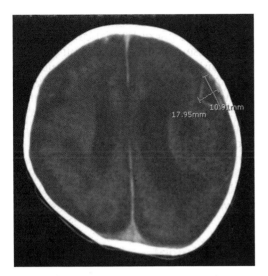

**Fig. 9.3** Contrast-enhanced computed tomographic scan of the brain demonstrating several severe complications of pneumococcal meningitis. The patchy enhancement of the leptomeninges is often seen during bacterial meningitis. The areas of hypodensity, most pronounced in the two frontal and the left parietal lobes, represent diffuse cerebritis with secondary areas of infarction. The pronounced dilatation of the ventricular system is obvious. Finally, an extra-axial ring-enhancing lesion overlying the left cerebral convexity represents a subdural empyema.

duration of headache secondary to Lyme meningitis was three times longer, lasting on average for more than a week.[114] More than half of adults with Lyme meningitis will exhibit symptoms of parenchymal involvement, such as somnolence, memory loss, poor concentration, emotional lability, and behavioral changes. In contrast, a series in children with CNS Lyme infection showed that most young patients have a fairly benign, mild course of aseptic meningitis.[115] Seventh nerve palsy is seen in approximately half of patients with Lyme meningitis but can also be an isolated neurologic finding of *Borrelia* infection.[116] Rare complications and some less common presentations of CNS Lyme infection include other cranial nerve palsies, particularly cranial nerves III and VI, pseudotumor cerebri, chorea, cerebellar ataxia, mononeuritis multiplex, myelitis, and opsoclonus-mycolonus.[117–119]

## Diagnosis

In patients with suspected meningitis, a lumbar puncture is indicated to obtain CSF for biochemical, cellular, and microbiological evaluation. At the time of lumbar puncture, an opening pressure should be obtained, and CSF should be collected and analyzed for cell count and differential, protein and glucose concentrations, Gram stain, and bacterial culture.[120] Additional diagnostic tests may also be considered based on the clinical suspicion for viral, fungal, or parasitic infection. In neonates, CSF glucose concentrations are normally lower than ranges typically observed in older children and adults because of the immaturity of the glucose transport mechanisms and the increased permeability of the blood–brain barrier. In healthy older children and adults, CSF glucose concentrations should remain higher than two-thirds of the serum glucose.[102,121] CNS bacterial infections alter glucose transport across the blood–brain barrier, thereby decreasing CSF concentrations. Effective antimicrobial treatment of the infection results in rapid normalization of the glucose concentration, usually days before the protein concentration normalizes, and the CSF pleocytosis resolves.

Ranges for normal CSF protein concentrations are age-dependent. The normal mean CSF protein concentration is 90 mg/dL in full-term infants and 115 mg/dL in premature infants. Normal CSF protein concentrations decrease to approximately 40 mg/dL by the second month of life.[102,121] Infections of the CNS disrupt the tight junctions between the endothelial cells of the venules, resulting in an increased presence of protein in the CSF.

The presence of leukocytes in the CSF should raise suspicion for meningitis. The WBC count in CSF from healthy neonates is approximately 8/mm$^3$, with upper limits of normal ranging from 22 to 26/mm$^3$.[102,121–123] By 1 month of age, the upper limit of normal decreases to less than 10/ mm$^3$.[102,122] In general, bacterial meningitis results in a substantial CSF pleocytosis (leukocyte count ranging from 100/mm$^3$ to 10,000/mm$^3$), generally higher than leukocyte counts in patients with aseptic meningitis. The leukocyte differential count in cases of bacterial meningitis shows a predominance of neutrophils, whereas aseptic meningitis has a lymphocytic predominance.[124] **Table 9.2** compares the classic CSF findings in bacterial, viral, Lyme disease, and tuberculous meningitis.

CSF Gram stain is positive in 50 to 90% of cases of community-acquired bacterial meningitis. Culture is positive in 70 to 85% of untreated patients with bacterial meningitis, but up to 48 hours may be required for organism identification.[125,126] Some patients who present with meningitis have already received antibiotics (particularly oral antibiotics) before lumbar puncture and CSF analysis. Pretreatment with antibiotics will not normalize CSF perturbations immediately; however, the yield of positive Gram stains decreases by approximately 20%, and CSF cultures may be sterilized. Therefore, patients who have been pretreated with antibiotics and whose clinical picture and CSF analysis are consistent with bacterial meningitis, yet who have negative CSF cultures, should receive a complete course of empiric parenteral antibiotics.[121,125,126]

CSF findings in Lyme meningitis typically include a leukocyte count of 100 to 200/mm³, with a predominance of mononuclear cells (lymphocytes), and a modest elevation in CSF protein. Serologic testing is performed to confirm the diagnosis.[127]

Tuberculous meningitis is confirmed by a positive mycobacterial culture or CSF polymerase chain reaction result in a patient with specific risk factors for tuberculosis. A Mantoux skin test (purified protein derivative [PPD]) should be placed and a chest radiograph obtained. The diagnosis of tuberculous meningitis requires a high index of suspicion and early initiation of empiric therapy because PPD testing is unreliable in this clinical situation, and mycobacterial culture results are often delayed for weeks.[128]

## ■ Treatment

Empiric antibiotic therapy must be initiated promptly even if the lumbar puncture cannot be performed in a timely manner because any delay can be associated with progressive neurologic complications and increased mortality.[125,126,129,130]

Empiric antibiotic choices are determined by the patient's age, immune status, and risk factors and by local antimicrobial resistance rates.[125,126,131] A summary of recommended empiric antibiotic therapy for community-acquired meningitis is included in **Table 9.1**. Previously healthy children and adults should be treated with vancomycin and a third-generation cephalosporin. Neonates, who are at higher risk for infection with *L. monocytogenes* and gram-negative bacilli, should be treated

**Table 9.2** Cerebrospinal fluid findings in bacterial, viral, and tuberculous meningitis

| | Bacterial Meningitis | Viral (Aseptic) Meningitis | Lyme Meningitis | Tuberculous Meningitis |
|---|---|---|---|---|
| Opening pressure | Elevated | Normal to elevated | Normal to elevated | Elevated |
| WBC count (cells/mm³) | ≥ 100–10,000 | 10–300 | 100–200 | 50–500 |
| WBC differential | Predominance of neutrophils | Predominance of lymphocytes | Predominance of lymphocytes | Predominance of lymphocytes |
| Glucose (mg/dL) | Low | Normal | Normal | Low |
| Protein (mg/dL) | Elevated | Normal to high | Mildly elevated | Elevated |

Abbreviation: WBC, white blood cell

with both ampicillin and a third-generation cephalosporin (or gentamicin). Adults past the age of 50 require the combination of ampicillin, vancomycin, and a third-generation cephalosporin.[19,22,102,126,132]

In 1988, studies from the United States showed that children with HIB meningitis who were treated with adjunctive dexamethasone were less likely to develop hearing loss as a complication of meningitis,[133] an observation that was supported in later studies.[134] Adjunctive dexamethasone has also been studied in the context of pneumococcal meningitis. In 1997, a meta-analysis of 10 clinical trials was the first to show borderline benefit in reducing neurologic sequelae, including hearing loss.[134] Subsequently, a multicenter adult trial performed in Europe showed that dexamethasone prevented serious sequelae.[135] Among the most impressive observations was a reduction in mortality from 34 to 14%. In direct contrast, two large clinical trials were performed in patients from Malawi with pneumococcal meningitis. These trials failed to demonstrate any reduction in mortality or neurologic sequelae following pediatric or adult pneumococcal meningitis.[2,136] A Cochrane meta-analysis of trials showing beneficial effects of adjunctive corticosteroids in high-income countries but not in resource-poor countries suggested that differences in baseline characteristics could explain the variable results found in clinical trials done in different regions of the world.[137] Current guidelines from the Infectious Diseases Society of America, the European Federation of Neurological Sciences, and the British Infection Society all recommend adjunctive dexamethasone for patients with suspected or proven pneumococcal meningitis.[138–140] The use of adjunctive dexamethasone has also been studied in the context of meningococcal meningitis. A 2004 meta-analysis showed no decrease in mortality in dexamethasone-treated adult patients.[141] When used, dexamethasone should be administered before or with the first dose of antibiotics at a dose of 0.15 mg/kg intravenously every 6 hours for 4 days.[126,132]

Once a pathogen has been identified as the cause of meningitis, it is important that susceptibility testing be performed before the antimicrobial regimen is de-escalated. Optimizing antibiotic therapy requires an understanding of antibiotic susceptibilities and the ability of the chosen medication to penetrate the blood–brain barrier and achieve a sufficiently high concentration in the CSF. Alternative antimicrobial regimens for antibiotic-resistant bacteria or for patients allergic to penicillins and cephalosporins might include meropenem, trimethoprim-sulfamethoxazole, and other newer classes of drugs. Such cases should be managed with the help of an infectious disease expert.

Seven days of parenteral therapy with penicillin G or ceftriaxone is sufficient for the treatment of meningococcal meningitis. Infections due to a β-lactamase-negative H. influenzae can be treated with ampicillin for 7 days; however, if the organism produces β-lactamase, a third-generation cephalosporin should be used. Uncomplicated meningitis due to S. pneumoniae should be treated for 10 to 14 days. Infections due to group B streptococci, L. monocytogenes, or gram-negative bacilli require longer treatment of at least 14 to 21 days. Ampicillin plus gentamicin is the combination of choice for group B streptococcal meningitis, whereas ampicillin alone is recommended for treatment of listeriosis.[102,125,126,131,132] Lyme meningitis, unlike other manifestations of Lyme disease, requires therapy with 2 weeks of intravenous ceftriaxone.[128]

Tuberculous meningitis requires combination therapy for a year or more. Treatment should begin as soon as the infection is suspected because of high morbidity and mortality rates with untreated infection. It is important to determine antibiotic susceptibility results from infecting isolates because of the increasing prevalence of drug-resistant strains. The recommended first-line antibiotic regimen for M. tuberculosis meningitis includes isoniazid, rifampin, pyrazinamide, and ethambutol or streptomycin. This combination can be altered once the results of antimicrobial susceptibility testing are available. Corticosteroids given as adjunctive therapy for tuberculous meningitis have been shown to decrease neurologic sequelae and improve survival.[120,128,142]

## Complications, Sequelae, and Prognosis

Despite the availability of preventive vaccines and effective antibiotics, bacterial meningitis remains a significant cause of morbidity and mortality in both developed and resource-poor areas of the world. A spectrum of sequelae has been noted in survivors of meningitis, including seizure disorders, focal neurologic deficits, hearing loss, vision loss, and impaired cognitive function.[143] Sequelae vary based on the etiologic agent and age of the infection, but taken together, roughly one in four patients will experience moderate to severe long-term consequences of bacterial meningitis.[144]

### Sequelae of *Haemophilus influenzae* Type B Meningitis

Reported mortality rates for HIB meningitis range from 3 to 42%.[15,145,146] A meta-analysis of studies done in children showed a mortality rate of 4%,[147] while mortality in adults is generally reported to be higher.[54,145,148,149] The most common sequela of HIB meningitis is sensorineural hearing loss, which has been described in up to 16% of children and between 10 and 25% of adults.[54,145]

### Sequelae of Pneumococcal Meningitis

Pneumococcal meningitis has a higher mortality rate than HIB meningitis. In children, mortality is between 8 and 37%, with the highest mortality rates seen in the poorest areas of the world.[15,147,150,151] Adults fare worse, with mortality rates between 20 and 37% in developed countries and as high as 51% in parts of Africa.[3,151–155] Causes of death in patients with pneumococcal meningitis include cardiovascular failure, stroke, status epilepticus, and cerebral edema with herniation. Independent predictors for an unfavorable outcome include a low Glasgow Coma Score on presentation, cranial nerve palsies, a CSF leukocyte count of less than 1,000/mm$^3$, and elevated CSF protein.[21] Neurologic sequelae occur in up to half of all survivors. Permanent consequences include deafness, focal neurologic deficits, seizure disorders, and cognitive impairment.[21,147,156] The loss of cognitive speed appears stable over time; however, early physical impairments generally regress with time.[157]

### Sequelae of Meningococcal Meningitis

The highest number of cases of meningococcal infection occurs in infants, but mortality in this age group is less than 5%. A second peak in the number of cases occurs in adolescents and young adults between 15 and 24 years old, in whom mortality rates are higher than 20%.[158] Case-fatality rates are also higher in patients with serogroup C than in those with serogroup B disease. Mortality is higher among patients with meningococcal septicemia than in those with meningococcal meningitis[159] and is usually the result of endotoxic shock with cardiovascular collapse. As many as 19% of survivors experience serious sequelae, including sensorineural hearing loss, skin and soft tissue necrosis requiring amputation, seizures, ataxia, hemiplegia, and septic or immune complex arthritis.[160–162]

### Sequelae of *Listeria* Meningitis

*Listeria* meningitis is usually a very severe infection in adults. Mean mortality rates are 30% or higher despite early antibiotic treatment.[163,164] The mortality of late-onset neonatal listeriosis is slightly lower (10 to 20%), but survivors of infection may have sequelae such as hydrocephalus and psychomotor retardation.[165]

## Conclusion

Bacterial meningitis remains a major public health problem in both developed and underdeveloped parts of the world. The three most common causes of acute bacterial meningitis, *S. pneumoniae*, *N. meningitidis*, and HIB, are largely vaccine-preventable in areas of the world that are able to implement effective public health programs. The diagnostic approach and treatment regimens are largely straightforward, but challenges emerge when patients have received prior antibiotics or when the infection is caused by unusual or antibiotic-resistant bacteria. Despite the availability of safe and effective antibiotics, and major progress in supportive care for patients with serious CNS infections, the morbidity and mortality associated with meningitis remain substantial. Future efforts at more effective prevention, better access to existing vaccines, and further understanding on how to best avoid long-term complications continue to be explored.

## References

1. Greenwood BM. The epidemiology of acute bacterial meningitis in tropical Africa. In: Williams JD, Burnie J, eds. Bacterial Meningitis. London, England: Academic Press; 1987:93–113

2. Scarborough M, Gordon SB, Whitty CJ, et al. Corticosteroids for bacterial meningitis in adults in sub-Saharan Africa. N Engl J Med 2007;357(24): 2441–2450

3. Scarborough M, Thwaites GE. The diagnosis and management of acute bacterial meningitis in resource-poor settings. Lancet Neurol 2008; 7(7):637–648

4. Campagne G, Schuchat A, Djibo S, Osséini A, Cissé L, Chippaux JP. Epidemiology of bacterial meningitis in Niamey, Niger, 1981-96. Bull World Health Organ 1999;77(6):499–508

5. Decosas J, Koama JB. Chronicle of an outbreak foretold: meningococcal meningitis W135 in Burkina Faso. Lancet Infect Dis 2002;2(12): 763–765

6. Andersen J, Christensen R, Hertel J. Clinical features and epidemiology of septicaemia and meningitis in neonates due to *Streptococcus agalactiae* in Copenhagen County, Denmark: a 10 year survey from 1992 to 2001. Acta Paediatr 2004; 93(10):1334–1339

7. Heath PT, Nik Yusoff NK, Baker CJ. Neonatal meningitis. Arch Dis Child Fetal Neonatal Ed 2003;88(3):F173–F178

8. Hristeva L, Booy R, Bowler I, Wilkinson AR. Prospective surveillance of neonatal meningitis. Arch Dis Child 1993;69(1 Spec No):14–18

9. May M, Daley AJ, Donath S, Isaacs D; Australasian Study Group for Neonatal Infections. Early onset neonatal meningitis in Australia and New Zealand, 1992-2002. Arch Dis Child Fetal Neonatal Ed 2005;90(4):F324–F327

10. Mulder CJ, Zanen HC. *Listeria monocytogenes* neonatal meningitis in The Netherlands. Eur J Pediatr 1986;145(1-2):60–62

11. Kobayaa H, Souki RR, Trust S, Domachowske JB. *Pasteurella multocida* meningitis in newborns after incidental animal exposure. Pediatr Infect Dis J 2009;28(10):928–929

12. Pong A, Bradley JS. Bacterial meningitis and the newborn infant. Infect Dis Clin North Am 1999;13(3):711–733, viii

13. Franco-Paredes C, Lammoglia L, Hernández I, Santos-Preciado JI. Epidemiology and outcomes of bacterial meningitis in Mexican children: 10-year experience (1993-2003). Int J Infect Dis 2008;12(4):380–386

14. Nigrovic LE, Kuppermann N, Malley R; Bacterial Meningitis Study Group of the Pediatric Emergency Medicine Collaborative Research Committee of the American Academy of Pediatrics. Children with bacterial meningitis presenting to the emergency department during the pneumococcal conjugate vaccine era. Acad Emerg Med 2008;15(6):522–528

15. Pelkonen T, Roine I, Monteiro L, et al. Risk factors for death and severe neurological sequelae in childhood bacterial meningitis in sub-Saharan Africa. Clin Infect Dis 2009;48(8):1107–1110

16. Sáez-Llorens X, McCracken GH Jr. Bacterial meningitis in children. Lancet 2003;361(9375): 2139–2148

17. Durand ML, Calderwood SB, Weber DJ, et al. Acute bacterial meningitis in adults. A review of 493 episodes. N Engl J Med 1993;328(1): 21–28

18. Sigurdardóttir B, Björnsson OM, Jónsdóttir KE, Erlendsdóttir H, Gudmundsson S. Acute bacterial meningitis in adults. A 20-year overview. Arch Intern Med 1997;157(4):425–430

19. van de Beek D, de Gans J, Spanjaard L, Weisfelt M, Reitsma JB, Vermeulen M. Clinical features and prognostic factors in adults with bacterial meningitis. N Engl J Med 2004;351(18): 1849–1859

20. Cabellos C, Verdaguer R, Olmo M, et al. Community-acquired bacterial meningitis in elderly patients: experience over 30 years. Medicine (Baltimore) 2009;88(2):115–119

21. Choi C. Bacterial meningitis in aging adults. Clin Infect Dis 2001;33(8):1380–1385

22. Weisfelt M, van de Beek D, Spanjaard L, Reitsma JB, de Gans J. Community-acquired bacterial meningitis in older people. J Am Geriatr Soc 2006;54(10):1500–1507

23. Brouwer MC, van de Beek D, Heckenberg SG, Spanjaard L, de Gans J. Community-acquired *Haemophilus influenzae* meningitis in adults. Clin Microbiol Infect 2007;13(4):439–442

24. Dworkin MS, Park L, Borchardt SM. The changing epidemiology of invasive *Haemophilus influenzae* disease, especially in persons > or = 65 years old. Clin Infect Dis 2007;44(6):810–816

25. Farhoudi D, Löfdahl M, Giesecke J. Invasive *Haemophilus influenzae* type b disease in Sweden 1997-2003: epidemiological trends and pat-

terns in the post-vaccine era. Scand J Infect Dis 2005;37(10):717–722

26. Arda B, Sipahi OR, Atalay S, Ulusoy S. Pooled analysis of 2,408 cases of acute adult purulent meningitis from Turkey. Med Princ Pract 2008;17(1): 76–79

27. Whitney CG, Farley MM, Hadler J, et al; Active Bacterial Core Surveillance of the Emerging Infections Program Network. Decline in invasive pneumococcal disease after the introduction of protein-polysaccharide conjugate vaccine. N Engl J Med 2003;348(18):1737–1746

28. Tsai CJ, Griffin MR, Nuorti JP, Grijalva CG. Changing epidemiology of pneumococcal meningitis after the introduction of pneumococcal conjugate vaccine in the United States. Clin Infect Dis 2008;46(11):1664–1672

29. van Deuren M, Brandtzaeg P, van der Meer JW. Update on meningococcal disease with emphasis on pathogenesis and clinical management. Clin Microbiol Rev 2000;13(1):144–166

30. Caugant DA, Tzanakaki G, Kriz P. Lessons from meningococcal carriage studies. FEMS Microbiol Rev 2007;31(1):52–63

31. Dull PM, Abdelwahab J, Sacchi CT, et al. *Neisseria meningitidis* serogroup W-135 carriage among US travelers to the 2001 Hajj. J Infect Dis 2005;191(1):33–39

32. MacLennan J, Kafatos G, Neal K, et al; United Kingdom Meningococcal Carriage Group. Social behavior and meningococcal carriage in British teenagers. Emerg Infect Dis 2006;12(6): 950–957

33. Imrey PB, Jackson LA, Ludwinski PH, et al. Meningococcal carriage, alcohol consumption, and campus bar patronage in a serogroup C meningococcal disease outbreak. J Clin Microbiol 1995;33(12):3133–3137

34. Pinner RW, Gellin BG, Bibb WF, et al; Meningococcal Disease Study Group. Meningococcal disease in the United States—1986. J Infect Dis 1991;164(2):368–374

35. Moore PS. Meningococcal meningitis in sub-Saharan Africa: a model for the epidemic process. Clin Infect Dis 1992;14(2):515–525

36. Moore PS, Reeves MW, Schwartz B, Gellin BG, Broome CV. Intercontinental spread of an epidemic group A *Neisseria meningitidis* strain. Lancet 1989;2(8657):260–263

37. Rosenstein NE, Perkins BA, Stephens DS, Popovic T, Hughes JM. Meningococcal disease. N Engl J Med 2001;344(18):1378–1388

38. Pollard AJ. Global epidemiology of meningococcal disease and vaccine efficacy. Pediatr Infect Dis J 2004;23(12, Suppl):S274–S279

39. Wilder-Smith A, Barkham TMS, Ravindran S, Earnest A, Paton NI. Persistence of W135 *Neisseria meningitidis* carriage in returning Hajj pilgrims: risk for early and late transmission to household contacts. Emerg Infect Dis 2003;9(1): 123–126

40. Wilder-Smith A, Goh KT, Barkham T, Paton NI. Hajj-associated outbreak strain of *Neisseria meningitidis* serogroup W135: estimates of the attack rate in a defined population and the risk of invasive disease developing in carriers. Clin Infect Dis 2003;36(6):679–683

41. Boisier P, Nicolas P, Djibo S, et al. Meningococcal meningitis: unprecedented incidence of serogroup X-related cases in 2006 in Niger. Clin Infect Dis 2007;44(5):657–663

42. Centers for Disease Control and Prevention. Active Bacterial Core surveillance (ABCs) Report: *Neisseria meningitidis*, 2009. http://www.cdc.gov/abcs/reports-findings/survreports/mening09.html. Accessed December 17, 2012

43. Phares CR, Lynfield R, Farley MM, et al; Active Bacterial Core surveillance/Emerging Infections Program Network. Epidemiology of invasive group B streptococcal disease in the United States, 1999-2005. JAMA 2008;299(17):2056–2065

44. Allen UD, Navas L, King SM. Effectiveness of intrapartum penicillin prophylaxis in preventing early-onset group B streptococcal infection: results of a meta-analysis. CMAJ 1993;149(11): 1659–1665

45. Schrag S, Gorwitz R, Fultz-Butts K, Schuchat A. Prevention of perinatal group B streptococcal disease. Revised guidelines from CDC. MMWR Recomm Rep 2002;51(RR-11):1–22

46. Schrag SJ, Zywicki S, Farley MM, et al. Group B streptococcal disease in the era of intrapartum antibiotic prophylaxis. N Engl J Med 2000; 342(1):15–20

47. Johri AK, Paoletti LC, Glaser P, et al. Group B *Streptococcus*: global incidence and vaccine development. Nat Rev Microbiol 2006;4(12): 932–942

48. van de Beek D, de Gans J, Spanjaard L, Sela S, Vermeulen M, Dankert J. Group A streptococcal meningitis in adults: report of 41 cases and a review of the literature. Clin Infect Dis 2002;34(9): e32–e36

49. Perera N, Abulhoul L, Green MR, Swann RA. Group A streptococcal meningitis: case report and review of the literature. J Infect 2005;51(2): E1–E4

50. Baraldés MA, Domingo P, Mauri A, et al. Group A streptococcal meningitis in the antibiotic era. Eur J Clin Microbiol Infect Dis 1999;18(8): 572–578

51. Arnoni MV, Berezin EN, Sáfadi MA, Almeida FJ, Lopes CR. *Streptococcus pyogenes* meningitis in children: report of two cases and literature review. Braz J Infect Dis 2007;11(3):375–377

52. Federico G, Tumbarello M, Spanu T, et al. Risk factors and prognostic indicators of bacterial meningitis in a cohort of 3580 postneurosurgical patients. Scand J Infect Dis 2001;33(7): 533–537

53. Jensen AG, Espersen F, Skinhøj P, Rosdahl VT, Frimodt-Møller N. *Staphylococcus aureus* meningitis. A review of 104 nationwide, consecutive cases. Arch Intern Med 1993;153(16): 1902–1908

54. Brouwer MC, Keizerweerd GD, De Gans J, Spanjaard L, Van De Beek D. Community acquired *Staphylococcus aureus* meningitis in adults. Scand J Infect Dis 2009;41(5):375–377

55. Pintado V, Meseguer MA, Fortún J, et al. Clinical study of 44 cases of *Staphylococcus aureus* meningitis. Eur J Clin Microbiol Infect Dis 2002; 21(12):864–868

56. Korinek AM, Golmard JL, Elcheick A, et al. Risk factors for neurosurgical site infections after craniotomy: a critical reappraisal of antibiotic prophylaxis on 4,578 patients. Br J Neurosurg 2005;19(2):155–162

57. Vázquez-Boland JA, Kuhn M, Berche P, et al. *Listeria* pathogenesis and molecular virulence determinants. Clin Microbiol Rev 2001;14(3): 584–640

58. Voetsch AC, Angulo FJ, Jones TF, et al; Centers for Disease Control and Prevention Emerging Infections Program Foodborne Diseases Active Surveillance Network Working Group. Reduction in the incidence of invasive listeriosis in foodborne diseases active surveillance network sites, 1996-2003. Clin Infect Dis 2007;44(4):513–520

59. Nieman RE, Lorber B. Listeriosis in adults: a changing pattern. Report of eight cases and review of the literature, 1968-1978. Rev Infect Dis 1980;2(2):207–227

60. Lorber B. Listeriosis. Clin Infect Dis 1997;24(1): 1–9, quiz 10–11

61. Rocourt J, Brosch R. Human listeriosis 1990. Document WHO/ HPP/FOS/92.4. Geneva, Switzerland: World Health Organization; 1992

62. Schuchat A, Swaminathan B, Broome CV. Epidemiology of human listeriosis. Clin Microbiol Rev 1991;4(2):169–183

63. Synnott MB, Morse DL, Hall SM. Neonatal meningitis in England and Wales: a review of routine national data. Arch Dis Child 1994;71(2): F75–F80

64. Kim BN, Peleg AY, Lodise TP, et al. Management of meningitis due to antibiotic-resistant *Acinetobacter* species. Lancet Infect Dis 2009;9(4): 245–255

65. Reichert MC, Medeiros EA, Ferraz FA. Hospital-acquired meningitis in patients undergoing craniotomy: incidence, evolution, and risk factors. Am J Infect Control 2002;30(3):158–164

66. Tang LM, Chen ST. Klebsiella ozaenae meningitis: report of two cases and review of the literature. Infection 1994;22(1):58–61

67. Tang LM, Chen ST. *Klebsiella oxytoca* meningitis: frequent association with neurosurgical procedures. Infection 1995;23(3):163–167

68. Unhanand M, Mustafa MM, McCracken GH Jr, Nelson JD. Gram-negative enteric bacillary meningitis: a twenty-one-year experience. J Pediatr 1993;122(1):15–21

69. Tabarani CM, Bennett NJ, Kiska DL, Riddell SW, Botash AS, Domachowske JB. Empyema of pre-existing subdural hemorrhage caused by a rare *Salmonella* species after exposure to bearded dragons in a foster home. J Pediatr 2010;156(2): 322–323

70. Mahapatra AK, Pawar SJ, Sharma RR. Intracranial *Salmonella* infections: meningitis, subdural collections and brain abscess. A series of six surgically managed cases with follow-up results. Pediatr Neurosurg 2002;36(1):8–13

71. Kent SJ, Crowe SM, Yung A, Lucas CR, Mijch AM. Tuberculous meningitis: a 30-year review. Clin Infect Dis 1993;17(6):987–994

72. Hosoglu S, Geyik MF, Balik I, et al. Predictors of outcome in patients with tuberculous meningitis. Int J Tuberc Lung Dis 2002;6(1):64–70

73. Uysal G, Köse G, Güven A, Diren B. Magnetic resonance imaging in diagnosis of childhood central nervous system tuberculosis. Infection 2001;29(3):148–153

74. Yasar KK, Pehlivanoglu F, Sengoz G. Predictors of mortality in tuberculous meningitis: a multivariate analysis of 160 cases. Int J Tuberc Lung Dis 2010;14(10):1330–1335

75. Springer P, Swanevelder S, van Toorn R, van Rensburg AJ, Schoeman J. Cerebral infarction and neurodevelopmental outcome in childhood tuberculous meningitis. Eur J Paediatr Neurol 2009;13(4):343–349

76. Tebruegge M, Curtis N. Epidemiology, etiology, pathogenesis, and diagnosis of recurrent bacterial meningitis. Clin Microbiol Rev 2008;21(3):519–537

77. Mondini C. Minor works of Carlo Mondini: the anatomical section of a boy born deaf. Am J Otol 1997;18(3):288–293

78. Lo WW. What is a 'Mondini' and what difference does a name make? AJNR Am J Neuroradiol 1999;20(8):1442–1444

79. Ohlms LA, Edwards MS, Mason EO, Igarashi M, Alford BR, Smith RJ. Recurrent meningitis and Mondini dysplasia. Arch Otolaryngol Head Neck Surg 1990;116(5):608–612

80. Arnold W, Bredberg G, Gstöttner W, et al. Meningitis following cochlear implantation: pathomechanisms, clinical symptoms, conservative and surgical treatments. ORL J Otorhinolaryngol Relat Spec 2002;64(6):382–389

81. Reefhuis J, Honein MA, Whitney CG, et al. Risk of bacterial meningitis in children with cochlear implants. N Engl J Med 2003;349(5): 435–445

82. Biernath KR, Reefhuis J, Whitney CG, et al. Bacterial meningitis among children with cochlear implants beyond 24 months after implantation. Pediatrics 2006;117(2):284–289

83. Mourtzoukou EG, Pappas G, Peppas G, Falagas ME. Vaccination of asplenic or hyposplenic adults. Br J Surg 2008;95(3):273–280

84. Muller LM, Gorter KJ, Hak E, et al. Increased risk of common infections in patients with type 1 and type 2 diabetes mellitus. Clin Infect Dis 2005;41(3):281–288

85. Nelson S, Kolls JK. Alcohol, host defence and society. Nat Rev Immunol 2002;2(3):205–209

86. Brouwer MC, van de Beek D, Heckenberg SG, Spanjaard L, de Gans J. Community-acquired *Listeria monocytogenes* meningitis in adults. Clin Infect Dis 2006;43(10):1233–1238

87. Bliss SJ, O'Brien KL, Janoff EN, et al. The evidence for using conjugate vaccines to protect HIV-infected children against pneumococcal disease. Lancet Infect Dis 2008;8(1):67–80

88. Frankel RE, Virata M, Hardalo C, Altice FL, Friedland G. Invasive pneumococcal disease: clinical features, serotypes, and antimicrobial resistance patterns in cases involving patients with and without human immunodeficiency virus infection. Clin Infect Dis 1996;23(3):577–584

89. Janoff EN, Breiman RF, Daley CL, Hopewell PC. Pneumococcal disease during HIV infection. Epidemiologic, clinical, and immunologic perspectives. Ann Intern Med 1992;117(4):314–324

90. Grau I, Pallares R, Tubau F, et al; Spanish Pneumococcal Infection Study Network (G03/103). Epidemiologic changes in bacteremic pneumococcal disease in patients with human immunodeficiency virus in the era of highly active antiretroviral therapy. Arch Intern Med 2005;165(13):1533–1540

91. Heffernan RT, Barrett NL, Gallagher KM, et al. Declining incidence of invasive *Streptococcus pneumoniae* infections among persons with AIDS in an era of highly active antiretroviral therapy, 1995-2000. J Infect Dis 2005;191(12):2038–2045

92. Gordon SB, Chaponda M, Walsh AL, et al. Pneumococcal disease in HIV-infected Malawian adults: acute mortality and long-term survival. AIDS 2002;16(10):1409–1417

93. Gordon SB, Walsh AL, Chaponda M, et al. Bacterial meningitis in Malawian adults: pneumococcal disease is common, severe, and seasonal. Clin Infect Dis 2000;31(1):53–57

94. Klugman KP, Madhi SA, Feldman C. HIV and pneumococcal disease. Curr Opin Infect Dis 2007;20(1):11–15

95. Molyneux EM, Tembo M, Kayira K, et al. The effect of HIV infection on paediatric bacterial meningitis in Blantyre, Malawi. Arch Dis Child 2003;88(12):1112–1118

96. Cunningham CK, Bonville CA, Ochs HD, et al. Enteroviral meningoencephalitis as a complication of X-linked hyper IgM syndrome. J Pediatr 1999;134(5):584–588

97. Picard C, von Bernuth H, Ghandil P, et al. Clinical features and outcome of patients with IRAK-4 and MyD88 deficiency. Medicine (Baltimore) 2010;89(6):403–425

98. Figueroa JE, Densen P. Infectious diseases associated with complement deficiencies. Clin Microbiol Rev 1991;4(3):359–395

99. Fijen CA, Kuijper EJ, Tjia HG, Daha MR, Dankert J. Complement deficiency predisposes for meningitis due to nongroupable meningococci and *Neisseria*-related bacteria. Clin Infect Dis 1994;18(5):780–784

100. Ross SC, Densen P. Complement deficiency states and infection: epidemiology, pathogenesis and consequences of neisserial and other infections in an immune deficiency. Medicine (Baltimore) 1984;63(5):243–273

101. Sjöholm AG, Kuijper EJ, Tijssen CC, et al. Dysfunctional properdin in a Dutch family with meningococcal disease. N Engl J Med 1988;319(1):33–37

102. Klein JO, Feigin RD, McCracken GH Jr. Report of the task force on diagnosis and management of meningitis. Pediatrics 1986;78(5 Pt 2):959–982

103. Thomas KE, Hasbun R, Jekel J, Quagliarello VJ. The diagnostic accuracy of Kernig's sign, Brudzinski's sign, and nuchal rigidity in adults with suspected meningitis. Clin Infect Dis 2002;35(1):46–52

104. Molyneux E, Walsh A, Phiri A, Molyneux M. Acute bacterial meningitis in children admitted to the Queen Elizabeth Central Hospital, Blantyre, Malawi in 1996-97. Trop Med Int Health 1998;3(8):610–618

105. Chang CJ, Chang WN, Huang LT, et al. Neonatal bacterial meningitis in southern Taiwan. Pediatr Neurol 2003;29(4):288–294

106. Berkley JA, Versteeg AC, Mwangi I, Lowe BS, Newton CR. Indicators of acute bacterial meningitis in children at a rural Kenyan district hospital. Pediatrics 2004;114(6):e713–e719

107. Chinchankar N, Mane M, Bhave S, et al. Diagnosis and outcome of acute bacterial meningitis in early childhood. Indian Pediatr 2002;39(10):914–921

108. Weber MW, Herman J, Jaffar S, et al. Clinical predictors of bacterial meningitis in infants and young children in The Gambia. Trop Med Int Health 2002;7(9):722–731

109. Lehmann D, Yeka W, Rongap T, et al. Aetiology and clinical signs of bacterial meningitis in children admitted to Goroka Base Hospital, Papua New Guinea, 1989-1992. Ann Trop Paediatr 1999;19(1):21–32

110. Curtis S, Stobart K, Vandermeer B, Simel DL, Klassen T. Clinical features suggestive of meningitis in children: a systematic review of prospective data. Pediatrics 2010;126(5):952–960

111. Wiberg K, Birnbaum A, Gradon J. Causes and presentation of meningitis in a Baltimore community hospital 1997-2006. South Med J 2008;101(10):1012–1016

112. Weisfelt M, van de Beek D, Spanjaard L, Reitsma JB, de Gans J. Clinical features, complications, and outcome in adults with pneumococcal meningitis: a prospective case series. Lancet Neurol 2006;5(2):123–129

113. Miller LG, Choi C. Meningitis in older patients: how to diagnose and treat a deadly infection. Geriatrics 1997;52(8):43–44, 47–50, 55

114. Avery RA, Frank G, Glutting JJ, Eppes SC. Prediction of Lyme meningitis in children from a Lyme disease-endemic region: a logistic-regression model using history, physical, and laboratory findings. Pediatrics 2006;117(1):e1–e7

115. Belman AL, Iyer M, Coyle PK, Dattwyler R. Neurologic manifestations in children with North

American Lyme disease. Neurology 1993; 43(12):2609–2614

116. Clark JR, Carlson RD, Sasaki CT, Pachner AR, Steere AC. Facial paralysis in Lyme disease. Laryngoscope 1985;95(11):1341–1345

117. Peter L, Jung J, Tilikete C, Ryvlin P, Mauguiere F. Opsoclonus-myoclonus as a manifestation of Lyme disease. J Neurol Neurosurg Psychiatry 2006; 77(9):1090–1091

118. Sarff LD, Platt LH, McCracken GH Jr. Cerebrospinal fluid evaluation in neonates: comparison of high-risk infants with and without meningitis. J Pediatr 1976;88(3):473–477

119. Raucher HS, Kaufman DM, Goldfarb J, Jacobson RI, Roseman B, Wolff RR. Pseudotumor cerebri and Lyme disease: a new association. J Pediatr 1985;107(6):931–933

120. Bamberger DM. Diagnosis, initial management, and prevention of meningitis. Am Fam Physician 2010;82(12):1491–1498

121. Bonadio WA. The cerebrospinal fluid: physiologic aspects and alterations associated with bacterial meningitis. Pediatr Infect Dis J 1992;11(6): 423–431

122. Chadwick SL, Wilson JW, Levin JE, Martin JM. Cerebrospinal fluid characteristics of infants who present to the emergency department with fever: establishing normal values by week of age. Pediatr Infect Dis J 2011;30(4):e63–e67

123. Darras BT, Annunziato D, Leggiadro RJ. Lyme disease with neurologic abnormalities. Pediatr Infect Dis 1983;2(1):47–49

124. Lee BE, Chawla R, Langley JM, et al. Paediatric Investigators Collaborative Network on Infections in Canada (PICNIC) study of aseptic meningitis. BMC Infect Dis 2006;6:68

125. Lin AL, Safdieh JE. The evaluation and management of bacterial meningitis: current practice and emerging developments. Neurologist 2010;16(3):143–151

126. Tunkel AR, Hartman BJ, Kaplan SL, et al. Practice guidelines for the management of bacterial meningitis. Clin Infect Dis 2004;39(9): 1267–1284

127. Eppes SC, Nelson DK, Lewis LL, Klein JD. Characterization of Lyme meningitis and comparison with viral meningitis in children. Pediatrics 1999;103(5 Pt 1):957–960

128. Ginsberg L, Kidd D. Chronic and recurrent meningitis. Pract Neurol 2008;8(6):348–361

129. Proulx N, Fréchette D, Toye B, Chan J, Kravcik S. Delays in the administration of antibiotics are associated with mortality from adult acute bacterial meningitis. QJM 2005;98(4):291–298

130. Namani S, Koci R, Dedushi K. The outcome of bacterial meningitis in children is related to the initial antimicrobial therapy. Turk J Pediatr 2010;52(4):354–359

131. DE Gaudio M, Chiappini E, Galli L, DE Martino M. Therapeutic management of bacterial meningitis in children: a systematic review and comparison of published guidelines from a European perspective. J Chemother 2010;22(4):226–237

132. Hoffman O, Weber RJ. Pathophysiology and treatment of bacterial meningitis. Ther Adv Neurol Disord 2009;2(6):1–7

133. Lebel MH, Freij BJ, Syrogiannopoulos GA, et al. Dexamethasone therapy for bacterial meningitis. Results of two double-blind, placebo-controlled trials. N Engl J Med 1988;319(15): 964–971

134. McIntyre PB, Berkey CS, King SM, et al. Dexamethasone as adjunctive therapy in bacterial meningitis. A meta-analysis of randomized clinical trials since 1988. JAMA 1997;278(11): 925–931

135. de Gans J, van de Beek D; European Dexamethasone in Adulthood Bacterial Meningitis Study Investigators. Dexamethasone in adults with bacterial meningitis. N Engl J Med 2002; 347(20):1549–1556

136. Molyneux EM, Walsh AL, Forsyth H, et al. Dexamethasone treatment in childhood bacterial meningitis in Malawi: a randomised controlled trial. Lancet 2002;360(9328):211–218

137. van de Beek D, de Gans J, McIntyre P, Prasad K. Corticosteroids for acute bacterial meningitis. Cochrane Database Syst Rev 2007;(1):CD004405

138. Chaudhuri A, Martinez-Martin P, Kennedy PG, et al; EFNS Task Force. EFNS guideline on the management of community-acquired bacterial meningitis: report of an EFNS Task Force on acute bacterial meningitis in older children and adults. Eur J Neurol 2008;15(7):649–659

139. Heyderman RS, Lambert HP, O'Sullivan I, Stuart JM, Taylor BL, Wall RA. Early management of suspected bacterial meningitis and meningococcal septicaemia in adults. J Infect 2003;46(2): 75–77

140. Tunkel AR, Hartman BJ, Kaplan SL, et al. Practice guidelines for the management of bacterial meningitis. Clin Infect Dis 2004;39(9): 1267–1284

141. van de Beek D, de Gans J, McIntyre P, Prasad K. Steroids in adults with acute bacterial meningitis: a systematic review. Lancet Infect Dis 2004;4(3):139–143

142. Sinner SW. Approach to the diagnosis and management of tuberculous meningitis. Curr Infect Dis Rep 2010;12(4):291–298

143. Mace SE. Acute bacterial meningitis. Emerg Med Clin North Am 2008;26(2):281–317, viii

144. Chandran A, Herbert H, Misurski D, Santosham M. Long-term sequelae of childhood bacterial meningitis: an underappreciated problem. Pediatr Infect Dis J 2011;30(1):3–6

145. Pedersen TI, Howitz M, Ostergaard C. Clinical characteristics of *Haemophilus influenzae* meningitis in Denmark in the post-vaccination era. Clin Microbiol Infect 2010;16(5):439–446

146. Anh DD, Kilgore PE, Kennedy WA, et al. *Haemophilus influenzae* type B meningitis among children in Hanoi, Vietnam: epidemiologic patterns and estimates of *H. Influenzae* type B disease burden. Am J Trop Med Hyg 2006;74(3): 509–515

147. Baraff LJ, Lee SI, Schriger DL. Outcomes of bacterial meningitis in children: a meta-analysis. Pediatr Infect Dis J 1993;12(5):389–394

148. Domingo P, Pericas R, Mirelis B, Nolla J, Prats G. *Haemophilus influenzae* meningitis in adults: analysis of 12 cases [in Spanish]. Med Clin (Barc) 1998;111(8):294–297

149. Schuchat A, Robinson K, Wenger JD, et al; Active Surveillance Team. Bacterial meningitis in the United States in 1995. N Engl J Med 1997;337(14):970–976

150. Arditi M, Mason EO Jr, Bradley JS, et al. Three-year multicenter surveillance of pneumococcal meningitis in children: clinical characteristics, and outcome related to penicillin susceptibility and dexamethasone use. Pediatrics 1998;102(5):1087–1097

151. Casado-Flores J, Aristegui J, de Liria CR, Martinón JM, Fernández C; Spanish Pneumococcal Meningitis Study Group. Clinical data and factors associated with poor outcome in pneumococcal meningitis. Eur J Pediatr 2006;165(5):285–289

152. Kornelisse RF, Westerbeek CM, Spoor AB, et al. Pneumococcal meningitis in children: prognostic indicators and outcome. Clin Infect Dis 1995;21(6):1390–1397

153. Stanek RJ, Mufson MA. A 20-year epidemiological study of pneumococcal meningitis. Clin Infect Dis 1999;28(6):1265–1272

154. Weightman NC, Sajith J. Incidence and outcome of pneumococcal meningitis in northern England. Eur J Clin Microbiol Infect Dis 2005;24(8):542–544

155. Weisfelt M, van de Beek D, Spanjaard L, Reitsma JB, de Gans J. Clinical features, complications, and outcome in adults with pneumococcal meningitis: a prospective case series. Lancet Neurol 2006;5(2):123–129

156. Østergaard C, Konradsen HB, Samuelsson S. Clinical presentation and prognostic factors of *Streptococcus pneumoniae* meningitis according to the focus of infection. BMC Infect Dis 2005;5:93

157. Hoogman M, van de Beek D, Weisfelt M, de Gans J, Schmand B. Cognitive outcome in adults after bacterial meningitis. J Neurol Neurosurg Psychiatry 2007;78(10):1092–1096

158. Sharip A, Sorvillo F, Redelings MD, Mascola L, Wise M, Nguyen DM. Population-based analysis of meningococcal disease mortality in the United States: 1990-2002. Pediatr Infect Dis J 2006;25(3):191–194

159. Kaplan SL, Schutze GE, Leake JAD, et al. Multicenter surveillance of invasive meningococcal infections in children. Pediatrics 2006;118(4):e979–e984

160. Weisfelt M, van de Beek D, Spanjaard L, de Gans J. Arthritis in adults with community-acquired bacterial meningitis: a prospective cohort study. BMC Infect Dis 2006;6:64

161. Erickson L, De Wals P. Complications and sequelae of meningococcal disease in Quebec, Canada, 1990-1994. Clin Infect Dis 1998;26(5):1159–1164

162. Harrison LH, Pass MA, Mendelsohn AB, et al. Invasive meningococcal disease in adolescents and young adults. JAMA 2001;286(6):694–699

163. McLauchlin J. Human listeriosis in Britain, 1967-85, a summary of 722 cases. 1. Listeriosis during pregnancy and in the newborn. Epidemiol Infect 1990;104(2):181–189

164. McLauchlin J. Human listeriosis in Britain, 1967-85, a summary of 722 cases. 2. Listeriosis in non-pregnant individuals, a changing pattern of infection and seasonal incidence. Epidemiol Infect 1990;104(2):191–201

165. Evans JR, Allen AC, Bortolussi R, Issekutz TB, Stinson DA. Follow-up study of survivors of fetal and early onset neonatal listeriosis. Clin Invest Med 1984;7(4):329–334

# 10

# Epidural and Subdural Infections

Sandi Lam and Peter C. Warnke

Subdural empyema is a focal purulent infection between the dura mater and arachnoid mater. More than 95% of cases of subdural empyema occur in the intracranial space rather than the spinal neuraxis.[1] Subdural empyemas make up 15 to 22% of focal intracranial infections. The historically high mortality rate of more than 80% before the widespread availability of antibiotics was reduced to 15.6 to 41% after the advent of antimicrobial therapy.[1] Once an empyema is established within the subdural space, there are few anatomic barriers to the spread of infection. From 70 to 80% of these cases occur over the cerebral convexities, although they can also have a parafalcine, tentorial, or infratentorial location. Concomitant intracerebral abscess is present in up to 6 to 22% of cases, whereas epidural abscess is found in 9 to 17% of cases.[2–4]

Epidural abscess develops between the skull and the dura mater. The adherence of the dura mater to the calvaria can limit the expansion of an intracranial epidural abscess. Autopsy studies reveal evidence of the spread of epidural infection into the subdural space in 80% of cases.[5]

## ■ Epidemiology and Pathophysiology

A majority of cases of subdural empyema develop by the direct local extension of infection rather than by hematogenous spread. In infants, most cases of subdural empyema re-

sult from the infection of subdural effusions associated with meningitis.[4] Local spread of infection most commonly occurs from frontal, ethmoid, or sphenoid sinusitis; osteomyelitis; and retrograde thrombophlebitis of the valveless diploic veins.

Rarely do mastoid infections lead to epidural abscess or subdural empyema. The vascularity of the diploic system is at its most prominent in men in their second and third decades of life. The frontal sinus also continues to develop during this period. Most cases of complicated sinusitis occur in otherwise healthy men in this age group. There is a predisposition for subdural empyema to develop in males, with a male-to-female ratio of 3:1.[2,4,6–8]

Direct extension of infection into the subdural space occurs in chronic otitis media and rarely as a consequence of mastoiditis. Infection can be introduced after the application of cranial pins and traction devices, neurosurgical or otolaryngologic procedures, and penetrating head trauma. Infection can also occur as a complication of preexisting subdural collections and with rare pulmonary and hematogenous diseases. Tuberculous subdural empyema has been reported.[1,4,5,8–11]

Like subdural empyema, epidural abscesses occur most frequently in males during the second and third decades of life, corresponding to the population with the highest likelihood of developing complicated sinusitis. Intracranial epidural abscesses arise from direct extension in association with sinusitis, osteomyelitis, cranial pin and traction device placement, penetrating head trauma, or postoperative infection.[4,5,8,10]

The focus of this chapter is limited to intracranial epidural abscess and subdural empyema. However, it is important to note that the spine, in contrast to the intracranial compartment, provides a relatively large space that can allow significant extension of a spinal epidural abscess. The spread can be hematogenous by direct extension of a contiguous local infection, and the pathophysiology of spinal epidural abscess is different from that of intracranial epidural abscess. Epidural abscess is estimated to occur nine times more frequently in the spine than intracranially.[5]

# Clinical Features

In cases of subdural empyema, the most common presenting features are fever and headache. Clinical symptoms of sinusitis or a history of sinusitis may or may not be present. Altered mental status is frequent. Other presenting features of subdural empyema include meningismus, hemiparesis, nausea, vomiting, sinus tenderness, local swelling/inflammation, speech difficulty, homonymous hemianopsia, decreased visual acuity, photophobia, cranial nerve palsies, and papilledema. Seizures occur in 8 to 20%. Neurologic symptoms are typically due to inflammation of the cerebrum and meninges, mass effect, and thrombophlebitis of the cerebral venous drainage. Focal deficits and seizures develop as disease progression increases the mass effect or causes cerebritis.[1,12]

Patients with intracranial epidural abscess generally present with signs and symptoms of infection and an expanding extra-axial intracranial mass. These may include fever, headache, altered mental status, malaise, nausea, vomiting, focal neurologic deficits, seizures, sinus tenderness, or local inflammation. In cases of postoperative infection after craniotomy, over 90% of patients with epidural abscess have evidence of a wound infection.[5,12] Compared with that of subdural empyema, the clinical presentation of intracranial epidural abscess is generally described as more indolent, although cases may vary.[12]

# Work-Up and Diagnosis

## Laboratory Studies

Laboratory studies apply to both subdural empyema and epidural abscess. They include complete blood counts, which reveal a leukocytosis with a predominance of polymorphonuclear neutrophils. Abnormalities of the erythrocyte sedimentation rate and C-reactive protein level are nonspecific findings, with an ESR that is elevated but generally less than 100 mm/h.[4,12–14] Blood, urine, and sputum should be cultured to identify potential organisms and sources of infection. A metabolic panel should be obtained to allow correction of any electrolyte abnormalities, such as hyponatremia, and to screen for underlying metabolic dysfunction in light of medical and antibiotic treatment.[1,14,15] Lumbar puncture is typically not recommended for subdural empyema or intracranial epidural abscess because of the risk for brain herniation due to increased intracranial pressure. Cerebrospinal fluid (CSF) studies are often nonspecific and show a moderate pleocytosis with predominantly polymorphonuclear neutrophils, moderately elevated protein, and normal to low glucose levels. Gram stain and CSF studies are negative in over 75% cases of both epidural abscess and subdural empyema. Normal or sterile CSF samples do not exclude the diagnosis of intracranial epidural abscess or subdural empyema.[4,12] Causative organisms vary with the etiology of the primary infection (**Tables 10.1** and **10.2**). Sterile intraoperative cultures are reported in up to 50% of cases of epidural abscess and subdural empyema, presumably as a result of the preoperative administration of antibiotics. For this reason, empiric administration of antibiotics before the collection of a specimen for culture should be avoided.[4,12–14]

## Imaging

Although magnetic resonance (MR) imaging is recognized to be more sensitive for showing morphological detail, detecting intraparenchymal abnormalities, and delineating the extent of infection, computed tomography (CT) is still the imag-

**Table 10.1** Common causative organisms: subdural empyema

| Associated Source | Organisms |
| --- | --- |
| Paranasal sinusitis (frontal, ethmoid, sphenoid) | α-Hemolytic streptococci |
| | Staphylococci |
| | Anaerobic/microaerophilic streptococci |
| | Aerobic gram-negative bacilli |
| | *Bacteroides* species |
| Otitis media/mastoiditis | Aerobic and anaerobic streptococci |
| | *Pseudomonas aeruginosa* |
| | *Bacteroides* species |
| | *Enterobacter* species |
| | Staphylococci |
| Postoperative infection | Staphylococci |
| | *Enterobacter* species |
| | *P. aeruginosa* |
| | *Propionibacterium* species |
| Penetrating head trauma | Staphylococci |
| | Aerobic gram-negative bacilli |
| | *Clostridium* species |
| Meningitis (neonate) | Group B streptococci |
| | *Enterobacter* species |
| | *Listeria monocytogenes* |
| Meningitis (child) | *Streptococcus pneumoniae* |
| | *Haemophilus influenzae* |
| | *Neisseria meningitidis* |
| | *Escherichia coli* |

ing modality most widely available and accessible in a timely manner. CT is most helpful when obtained with and without intravenous contrast, allowing differentiation between chronic subdural or epidural hematoma, postoperative changes, and infectious processes. CT findings for subdural empyema typically demonstrate a hypodense subdural lesion with enhance-ment, particularly along the medial border of the lesion at the pial surface, inward displacement of the gray–white junction, and effacement of the ventricles, cortical sulci, and basal cisterns (**Fig. 10.1**). Mass effect is often caused more by edema than by the empyema collection itself. Vasogenic edema is prominent in cases of subdural empyema that are complicated by cerebritis,

**Table 10.2** Common causative organisms: epidural abscess

| Associated Source | Organisms |
| --- | --- |
| Paranasal sinusitis (frontal, ethmoid, sphenoid) | α-Hemolytic streptococci |
| | Staphylococci |
| | Anaerobic/microaerophilic streptococci |
| | Aerobic gram-negative bacilli |
| | *Bacteroides* species |
| Otitis media/mastoiditis | Aerobic and anaerobic streptococci |
| | *Pseudomonas aeruginosa* |
| | *Bacteroides* species |
| | *Enterobacter* species |
| | Staphylococci |
| Postoperative infection | Staphylococci |
| | *Enterobacter* species |
| | *P. aeruginosa* |
| | *Propionibacterium* species |
| Penetrating head trauma | Staphylococci |
| | Aerobic gram-negative bacilli |
| | *Clostridium* species |

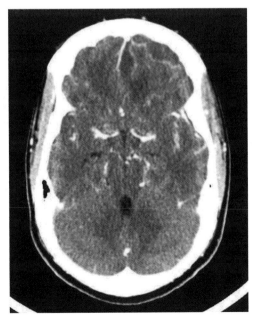

**Fig. 10.1** Computed tomographic scan with contrast of left frontal and interhemispheric subdural empyema in a 15-year-old boy with frontal and ethmoid sinusitis. Note the hypodense subdural collection with enhancement along the pial surface, underlying effacement of the cortical sulci, and mass effect from the purulent lesion and from cerebral edema.

sinusitis, skull osteomyelitis, compound skull fracture, or craniotomy defect.[6,8,13,16] On MR imaging, subdural empyemas generally appear hypointense or variable on T1-weighted images and hyperintense on T2-weighted images; they have high signal on diffusion-weighted images, indicating restricted diffusion. Rim enhancement is seen following gadolinium administration. Intracranial epidural abscesses exhibit hyperintensity on T2-weighted images, variable intensity on T1-weighted images, and restricted diffusion, and they most often demonstrate contrast enhancement at the periphery[1,4,13,17] (**Fig. 10.2**).

## Treatment and Management

For both subdural empyema and epidural abscess, broad-spectrum antibiotics should be administered as soon as possible with coverage for aerobic and anaerobic organ-isms after a specimen is obtained. These should subsequently be tailored according to culture and sensitivity results. Initial empiric antimicrobial therapy should provide coverage for gram-positive cocci, gram-negative bacilli, and anaerobes. The standard recommended empiric antibiotic regimen includes vancomycin, metronidazole, and a third-generation cephalosporin. The duration of antibiotic therapy is typically recommended to be 4 to 6 weeks and is extended to 6 to 8 weeks or longer in the presence of osteomyelitis. For neonates and children, empiric antibiotic choices may vary according to local rates of microbial resistance; particularly in cases of subdural empyema, they may mirror the antibiotic regimens that are used for meningitis treatment.[4,10,14,15,18] Prophylaxis for seizures is recommended, and anticonvulsants are mandatory if seizure activity is observed.[4,12,18]

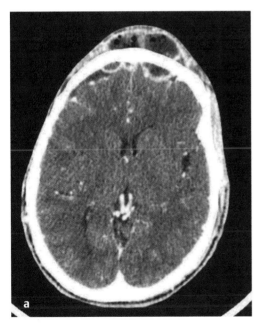
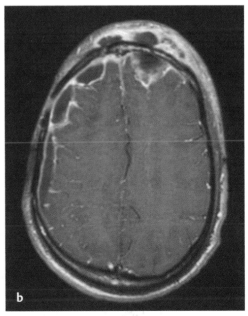

**Fig. 10.2a,b** Computed tomographic (CT) scan with contrast and magnetic resonance (MR) image (T1-weighted image with contrast, T2-weighted image, and diffusion-weighted image sequence) of right frontal epidural abscess and of left frontal and parietal subdural empyema in a 19-year-old man with associated frontal sinusitis and subgaleal abscess. This patient had a history of surgical cosmetic craniofacial reconstruction for congenital craniofacial abnormalities. **(a)** CT scan with contrast shows an enhancing lenticular extra-axial mass representing the left frontal epidural abscess. The right frontal area harbors multiple subdural hypodense collections with enhancement, particularly along the pial surfaces, representing the subdural empyemas. Note also the subgaleal collection of pus. **(b)** MR T1-weighted image with contrast shows the enhancing lesions and delineates the anatomy and extent of disease involvement with more detail than the CT scan. *(Continued on page 130)*

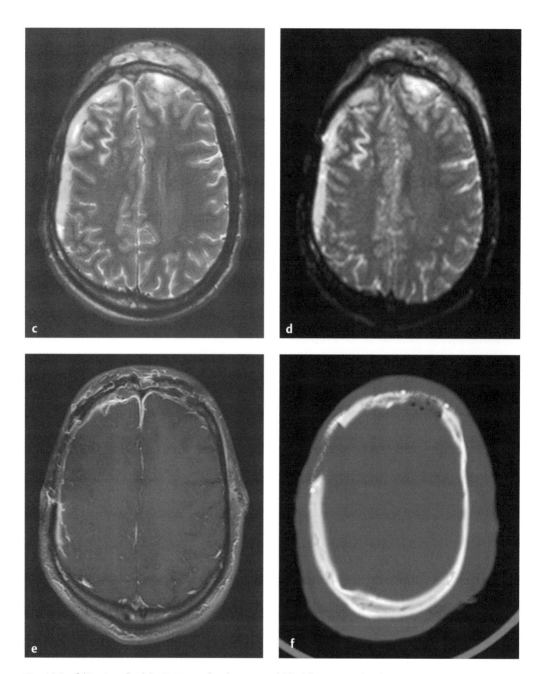

**Fig. 10.2c–f** *(Continued)* **(c)** MR T2-weighted image and **(d)** diffusion-weighted image sequence shows hyperintense signal within the purulent areas. **(e)** Postoperative MR T1-weighted image with contrast and **(f)** CT scan of the head with bone windows. **(f)** After surgical drainage of the right frontal epidural abscess and left frontoparietal subdural empyema as well as right frontal sinus exenteration, image shows evacuation of the purulent material and the craniotomy sites repaired with titanium mesh.

Surgical management is indicated in almost all cases of subdural empyema for cerebral decompression, drainage of purulent material, and identification of the causative organism(s). There is no consensus regarding the optimal surgical approach. Interventions include burr hole drainage, stereotactic drainage for deep-seated parafalcine or tentorial empyemas, and craniotomy for irrigation, débridement, and drainage. Purulent material tends to be in a fluid state early in the disease process and may produce loculate as time passes. Repeat surgical procedures may be required. Burr holes or craniotomy for decompression with irrigation, débridement, and drainage is warranted in a majority of cases of epidural abscess. A delay in surgical intervention has been associated with higher morbidity and mortality rates. Repeat surgical procedures may be necessary in cases of persistent or recurrent suppurative infection.[2,12,15,18–21] For both subdural empyema and epidural abscess, definitive surgical management of complicated sinusitis should also be undertaken in conjunction with the otolaryngology service.[4]

Surgery per se is not curative, but it is an essential component of treatment in the vast majority of cases to create those pharmacokinetic conditions (reduced diffusion distance, sink effect, and improved perfusion) that will allow antibiotics to penetrate the infected areas, helping to provide curative therapy.[14,15,19] In a limited number of scenarios, subdural empyema and epidural abscess can be managed nonoperatively. This treatment strategy is usually not considered except for patients with very limited disease extension, no mass effect, no neurologic symptoms or deficits, and an early favorable response to antibiotics.[2–4,12]

### Prognosis

Neurologic status at the time of presentation is a predictor of neurologic outcome. Delays in diagnosis or treatment are associated with increased morbidity and mortality. Mortality is estimated to be 10% in patients with treated intracranial epidural abscess.[4,5] Unfavorable prognostic indicators include age older than 60 years, poor neurologic status at the time of presentation, rapid disease progression, delay in initiating antibiotics, and subdural empyema resulting from trauma or surgery. Mortality in treated cases of subdural empyema reaches 5 to 20%. Up to half of patients have neurologic deficits at the time of discharge from the hospital, with 15 to 35% having hemiparesis and up to 30% having persistent seizures.[1,4,12,13]

## ■ Conclusion

Intracranial epidural abscess and subdural empyema are surgical emergencies that carry significant morbidity, even in the context of prompt appropriate treatment. Recognition of risk factors and a strong degree of suspicion aid in the diagnosis. In both of these entities, treatment with broad-spectrum antibiotics should be started as soon as a sample for culture is obtained. Surgery is performed in most cases with the goal of treating mass effect and reducing the size of purulent collections to optimize antibiotic penetration.

### References

1. Lam S, Nguyen T. Subdural empyema. In: Lisak R, Truong D, Carroll W, Bhidayasiri R, eds. International Neurology: a Clinical Approach. Oxford, England: Blackwell Publishing; 2009:245–247
2. Bok AP, Peter JC. Subdural empyema: burr holes or craniotomy? A retrospective computerized tomography-era analysis of treatment in 90 cases. J Neurosurg 1993;78(4):574–578
3. Dill SR, Cobbs CG, McDonald CK. Subdural empyema: analysis of 32 cases and review. Clin Infect Dis 1995;20(2):372–386
4. Osborn MK, Steinberg JP. Subdural empyema and other suppurative complications of paranasal sinusitis. Lancet Infect Dis 2007;7(1):62–67
5. Lam S, Nguyen T. Epidural abscess. In: Lisak R, Truong D, Carroll W, Bhidayasiri R, eds. International Neurology: a Clinical Approach. Oxford, England: Blackwell Publishing; 2009:248–249
6. Kombogiorgas D, Seth R, Athwal R, Modha J, Singh J. Suppurative intracranial complications of sinusitis in adolescence. Single institute experience and review of literature. Br J Neurosurg 2007; 21(6):603–609
7. Nathoo N, Nadvi SS, van Dellen JR, Gouws E. Intracranial subdural empyemas in the era of

computed tomography: a review of 699 cases. Neurosurgery 1999;44(3):529–535, discussion 535–536

8. Pradilla G, Ardila GP, Hsu W, Rigamonti D. Epidural abscesses of the CNS. Lancet Neurol 2009; 8(3):292–300

9. Hlavin ML, Kaminski HJ, Fenstermaker RA, White RJ. Intracranial suppuration: a modern decade of postoperative subdural empyema and epidural abscess. Neurosurgery 1994;34(6):974–980, discussion 980–981

10. Krauss WE, McCormick PC. Infections of the dural spaces. Neurosurg Clin N Am 1992;3(2): 421–433

11. van Dellen A, Nadvi SS, Nathoo N, Ramdial PK. Intracranial tuberculous subdural empyema: case report. Neurosurgery 1998;43(2):370–373

12. Tunkell A. Subdural empyema, epidural abscess, and suppurative intracranial thrombophlebitis. In: Mandell GL, Bennett JE, Dolin R, eds. Mandell, Douglas, and Bennett's Principles and Practices of Infectious Diseases. Philadelphia, PA: Elsevier Churchill Livingstone; 2005:1165–1168

13. Anslow P. Cranial bacterial infection. Eur Radiol 2004;14(Suppl 3):E145–E154

14. Bernardini GL. Diagnosis and management of brain abscess and subdural empyema. Curr Neurol Neurosci Rep 2004;4(6):448–456

15. Amar AP, Ghosh S, Apuzzo ML. Treatment of central nervous system infections: a neurosurgical perspective. Neuroimaging Clin N Am 2000; 10(2):445–459

16. Foerster BR, Thurnher MM, Malani PN, Petrou M, Carets-Zumelzu F, Sundgren PC. Intracranial infections: clinical and imaging characteristics. Acta Radiol 2007;48(8):875–893

17. Baum PA, Dillon WP. Utility of magnetic resonance imaging in the detection of subdural empyema. Ann Otol Rhinol Laryngol 1992;101(10): 876–878

18. Hall WA, Truwit CL. The surgical management of infections involving the cerebrum. Neurosurgery 2008;62(Suppl 2):519–530, discussion 530–531

19. Feuerman T, Wackym PA, Gade GF, Dubrow T. Craniotomy improves outcome in subdural empyema. Surg Neurol 1989;32(2):105–110

20. Ziai WC, Lewin JJ III. Advances in the management of central nervous system infections in the ICU. Crit Care Clin 2006;22(4):661–694, abstract viii–ix

21. Ziai WC, Lewin JJ III. Update in the diagnosis and management of central nervous system infections. Neurol Clin 2008;26(2):427–468, viii

# 11

# Infectious Intracranial Aneurysms

Hoon Choi, Walter A. Hall, and Eric M. Deshaies

The earliest published case of an infectious aneurysm dates back to 1869, when Church described a 13-year-old boy with left hemiparesis who was found to have a ruptured right middle cerebral artery aneurysm and mitral valve endocarditis.[1] The term *mycotic aneurysm* was introduced by Sir William Osler in 1885 to describe an aortic aneurysm in the setting of bacterial endocarditis.[2] This term was subsequently used to describe all intra- and extracranial aneurysms of an infectious etiology. Because of the inaccuracy of this term in describing a condition most commonly due to bacterial involvement, several alternative terms have been suggested, such as *infected, infectious, infective, inflammatory, septic, bacterial,* and *microbial*. More recently, the term *infectious intracranial aneurysm* (IIA) has gained popularity. For this chapter, we reviewed the literature and found a total of 303 patients with 390 aneurysms from 1966 to 2008 that were associated with infection[3-34] (**Table 11.1**). These cases will help to illustrate the pathogenesis, presentation, microbiology, aneurysmal characteristics, natural history, and treatment strategies for IIA.

## ■ Epidemiology

The autopsy review of Fearnsides in 1916 estimated that 30% of all intracranial aneurysms were infectious in origin.[35] More recent reviews have put the estimate at 2 to 6%.[36-38] This decrease in the incidence is likely due to the introduction of antibiotic therapy. The difficulty in estimating the true incidence of IIA stems from the somewhat protean natural history of the disease. Bacterial IIAs have been observed to form and regress spontaneously with antibiotic therapy, whereas IIAs associated with fungal and tuberculous infections have been observed to be more persistent than bacterial infections.[20,35,39-42] The increasing number of patients immunocompromised as a consequence of acquired immunodeficiency syndrome (AIDS), steroid therapy, chemotherapeutic regimens, or organ transplant presents a potential source for an increase in the number of IIAs in susceptible populations.

Although intracranial aneurysms are less common in children than in adults, those diagnosed in children are more likely to be infectious. Approximately 10% of an-

**Table 11.1** List of case reviews and reports included in the analysis

| Case Series or Report | Year | No. of Patients | No. of Aneurysms | Mean Age | Medical Therapy | Surgical Therapy | Endovascular Therapy | NR | Mortality |
|---|---|---|---|---|---|---|---|---|---|
| Ojemann et al[24] | 1966 | 1 | 4 | 46 | 1 | | | | |
| Suwanwela[32] | 1972 | 6 | 12 | 13 | 5 | 1 | | | 1 |
| Bingham[6] | 1977 | 2 | 5 | 19.5 | 2 | | | | |
| Bohmfalk et al[7] | 1978 | 4 | 6 | 32.8 | 3 | 1 | | | 2 |
| Frazee et al[14] | 1980 | 13 | 19 | 40 | 8 | 5 | | | 6 |
| Day[12] | 1981 | 2 | 2 | 44 | | 2 | | | |
| Mielke et al[22] | 1981 | 1 | 1 | 58 | 1 | | | | 1 |
| Pootrakul and Carter[27] | 1982 | 1 | 1 | 40 | | 1 | | | |
| Rout et al[29] | 1984 | 6 | 6 | 20.5 | 4 | 2 | | | |
| Kikuchi et al[18] | 1985 | 1 | 4 | 61 | | 1 | | | 1 |
| Hart et al[16] | 1987 | 2 | 2 | 25.5 | 1 | 1 | | | 1 |
| Salgado et al[30] | 1987 | 68 | 68 | 31.4 | 66 | 2 | | | NR |
| Hadley et al[15] | 1988 | 1 | 1 | 28 | | 1 | | | |
| Monsuez et al[23] | 1989 | 12 | 12 | 30.7 | 7 | 5 | | | 3 |
| Barrow and Prats[4] | 1990 | 12 | 15 | 26.5 | 6 | 6 | | | 4 |
| Brust et al[8] | 1990 | 17 | 29 | 35 | 5 | 12 | | | 4 |

| Study | | | | | | | | |
|---|---|---|---|---|---|---|---|---|
| Lee et al[20] | 1990 | 1 | 2 | 7 mo | | 1 | | | 1 |
| Aspoas and de Villiers[3] | 1993 | 25 | 33 | 23 | 3 | 21 | | 1 | 1 |
| Kurino et al[19] | 1994 | 1 | 1 | 63 | ` | 1 | | | 1 |
| Corr et al[11] | 1995 | 14 | 18 | 27.3 | 6 | 8 | | | 1 |
| Lin and Vieco[21] | 1995 | 1 | 1 | 35 | | 1 | | | |
| Scotti et al[31] | 1996 | 3 | 4 | 40 | | | 3 | | 1 |
| Powell and Rijhsinghani[28] | 1997 | 1 | Multiple | 38 | 1 | | | | |
| Piastra et al[26] | 2000 | 1 | 1 | 2 mo | | 1 | | | 1 |
| Venkatesh et al[34] | 2000 | 17 | 22 | 29.7 | 12 | 5 | | | 2 |
| Chun et al[10] | 2001 | 20 | 27 | 33.5 | 5 | 10 | 5 | | 2 |
| Bartakke et al[5] | 2002 | 1 | 1 | 5 | 1 | | | | |
| Chapot et al[9] | 2002 | 14 | 18 | 43.6 | | | 14 | | |
| Phuong et al[25] | 2002 | 16 | 29 | 48.9 | 4 | 10 | | 2[a] | 3 |
| Kannoth et al[17] | 2007 | 25 | 29 | 24.8 | 10 | 11 | | 4 | 8 |
| Dhomne et al[13] | 2008 | 13 | 14 | 33.8 | | | 13 | | 2 |
| Trivedi et al[33] | 2008 | 1 | 1 | 35 | 1 | 1 | | | 1 |
| Total | | 303 | 390+ | 34.3 | 151 | 110 | 35 | 7 | 45 |

*Abbreviations:* NR, not reported

[a]One patient died before receiving any treatment.

eurysms in children are estimated to be infectious in origin.[43–47] Endocarditis, especially left-sided valve disease, is frequently associated with IIA. In the present analysis, 76% of patients with IIA had a diagnosis of infective endocarditis (**Table 11.2**). Extravascular infections, such as meningitis, orbital cellulitis, and postcraniotomy infections, have been reported to lead to IIA.

## ■ Pathogenesis

The pathogenesis of IIA can be conceptualized into three different processes: intravascular, extravascular, and cryptogenic. The intravascular mechanism is the most common, involves septic emboli, and is commonly secondary to bacterial endocarditis. IIAs due to septic emboli are often located at vessel branch points in the distal vasculature. Showers of septic emboli can lead to the formation of multiple IIAs, seen in 17% of the reviewed cases (**Table 11.3**). This result was consistent with the previously reported rate of 20%.[48]

### Intravascular

In 1887, Eppinger[49] described the infectious and inflammatory processes leading to weakening of the arterial wall and subsequent aneurysm formation. He observed that the inflammation involved the adventitia initially and then spread inward to the internal elastic membrane. This notion was confirmed in a mongrel dog model involving silicone rubber emboli.[50,51] Although vasa vasorum play a role in aortic aneurysm formation after infection in a dog model,[52] vasa vasorum are rarely present in intracranial vessels.[53] Molinari and col-

**Table 11.2** Associated infections

| Associated Infection | Number | Percentage |
|---|---|---|
| IE | 231 | 76 |
| Mitral IE | 84 | 28 |
| Aortic IE | 23 | 8 |
| Septal defect | 4 | 1 |
| Tricuspid IE | 2 | 0.7 |
| Meningitis | 31 | 10 |
| CST | 19 | 6 |
| Dental infection | 12 | 4 |
| Orbital cellulitis | 11 | 3.6 |
| Abscess | 5 | 1.7 |
| UTI | 3 | 1 |
| Vasculitis | 2 | 0.7 |
| Post-craniotomy | 2 | 0.7 |
| Cellulitis | 1 | 0.3 |
| DVT phlebitis | 1 | 0.3 |

*Abbreviations*: CST, cavernous sinus thrombosis; DVT, deep vein thrombosis; IE, infective endocarditis; UTI, urinary tract infection

**Table 11.3** Aneurysm location

| Aneurysm Location | Number | Percentage |
|---|---|---|
| MCA | 167 | 43 |
| PCA | 37 | 9 |
| ACA | 30 | 8 |
| ICA | 23 | 6 |
| BA | 8 | 2 |
| PICA | 8 | 2 |
| SCA | 6 | 1.5 |
| VA | 4 | 1 |
| AICA | 1 | 0.3 |
| Other | 10 | 2.5 |
| NR | 96 | 25 |
| Total aneurysms | 390 | 100 |
| No. of patients with multiple aneurysms | 52 | 17 |

*Abbreviations*: ACA, anterior cerebral artery; AICA, anterior inferior cerebellar artery; BA, basilar artery; ICA, internal cerebral artery; MCA, middle cerebral artery; NR, not reported; PCA, posterior cerebral artery; PICA, posterior inferior cerebellar artery; SCA, superior cerebellar artery; VA, vertebral artery

leagues have suggested that in the absence of vasa vasorum, bacteria can escape from the lumen of the vessel through the occluded origins of the thin-walled penetrating vessels into the Virchow-Robin space and from there to the adventitia of the occluded vessel.

In the experimental model by Molinari et al,[51] aneurysm formation occurred at the proximal end of the occluded segment, overlapping the embolus and the adjacent segment with a patent lumen, indicating the importance of arterial pulse pressure in the dilation of the diseased, weakened arterial wall. Chronic aneurysms were also induced by subtherapeutic doses of antibiotics. These aneurysms were found to be firmly adherent to both the leptomeninges and pachymeninges and had intact, indurated, fibrotic walls. Inadequate antibiotic treatment permitted microorganisms to disseminate through penetrating vessels into the infarcted intraparenchymal area, causing brain abscess.

### Extravascular

IIAs can also form as a result of primary extravascular infections, such as meningitis, postcraniotomy infections, orbital cellulitis, skull osteomyelitis, sinusitis, tonsillitis, and pharyngitis (see **Table 11.2**). Orbital cellulitis, sinusitis (**Fig. 11.1**), and skull base infections often lead to cavernous sinus thrombosis, which in turn can lead to the formation of cavernous internal carotid artery aneurysms. The histologic changes that develop are similar to the changes seen after septic embolic occlusion. There is a progressive infiltration of the adventitia and media by polymorphonuclear leukocytes, followed by prominent intimal inflammation (**Fig. 11.2**). There is often thrombosis of the involved arteries and venous structures. The infective arteritis results in a weakened vessel wall, leading to aneurysm formation and rupture. Upon macroscopic examination, the aneurysm wall is very friable and often adherent to the adjacent brain parenchyma.

### Cryptogenic

The third type of IIA is described as cryptogenic or primary IIA. This category represents a presumptive diagnosis based on the clinical situation and angiographic appearance of the abnormality.[54] These aneurysms occur in the absence of an obvious inflammatory process in the rest of the body, and blood cultures are frequently negative.

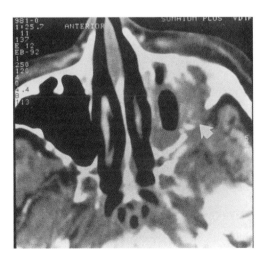

**Fig. 11.1** Axial computed tomographic scan with contrast shows maxillary sinusitis (*arrow*) due to *Aspergillus fumigatus* in a patient with diabetes mellitus.

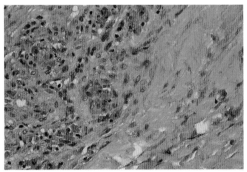

**Fig. 11.2** Photomicrograph showing inflammatory cells infiltrating the wall of an infectious intracranial aneurysm (magnification unknown).

## ■ Microbiology

In the present analysis of 303 patients with IIAs spanning more than 42 years, the most common causative organisms were *Streptococcus* species, present in 102 patients (**Table 11.4**). Of these patients, 40 were found to have *Streptococcus viridans* (*S. sanguinis, S. mutans,* and *S. mitis*). The second most common causative organisms were *Staphylococcus* species, found in 48 patients (16%). Of the 48 patients, 41 were found to be infected with *S. aureus. Enterococcus* species were seen in 10 patients. Gram-negative bacteria were rare, isolated in only four cases, three of which were *Pseudomonas aeruginosa. Mycobacterium* species were isolated in four patients. Other bacteria isolated in patients with IIA have included *Staphylococcus epidermidis, Streptococcus pneumoniae, Streptococcus bovis, Streptococcus pyogenes,* α- and γ-hemolytic streptococci, *Peptostreptococcus, Klebsiella* species, *Escherichia coli, Diphtheria* species, and *Serratia marcescens.*

A true mycotic (fungal) etiology was verified in 13 of 303 patients with IIA (4%). At least seven of these patients were immunocompromised. Fungal IIA tended to involve more proximal segments of the arterial vasculature, and an associated thrombosis of the neighboring arteries could be seen in some cases of fungal IIA. These patients were often afebrile at presentation and had a more indolent clinical course. A combination of difficulty in making a diagnosis, poor response to antimicrobial treatment, proximal location of fungal IIA, adjacent thrombosis, immunosuppression, medical comorbidities, and often a friable arterial wall led to a poor outcome compared with patients who had bacterial IIA. The mortality rate for fungal IIA was 92%. *Aspergillus fumigatus, Candida albicans,* and *Mucor* species are the three most common IIA-causing fungi (**Fig. 11.3**). Other reported fungi include *Petriellidium boydii, Pseudallescheria boydii,* and organisms causing chromoblastomycosis.[4,22,54,55]

Blood cultures were positive in only 55% of the reviewed cases (**Table 11.5**). Ojemann's review found negative blood cultures in 12.5%, which was comparable with the 10% in the review of Bohmfalk et al.[7,37] The high rate of negative blood cultures in the present review may be due to the lack of information on the absence of growth from blood cultures. In two cases in which the cerebrospinal fluid culture was positive for *Staphylococcus* species in the presence of negative blood cultures, the result was likely due to early antibiotic treatment.[29,32] In one case, the only positive culture result was from a sputum sample, which grew *Klebsiella pneumoniae* and *E. coli.*[29]

**Table 11.4**  Causative microorganisms

| Microorganism | Number | Percentage |
|---|---|---|
| *Streptococcus* | 102 | 34 |
| Viridans group | 40 | 13 |
| *Enterococcus* | 10 | 3 |
| *Staphylococcus* | 48 | 16 |
| *S. aureus* | 41 | 14 |
| Fungi | 13 | 4 |
| *Candida* | 4 | 1 |
| Gram-negative rods | 4 | 1 |
| *Pseudomonas* | 3 | 1 |
| *Mycobacterium* | 4 | 1 |

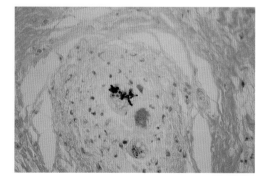

**Fig. 11.3**  Gomori methenamine silver stain showing the fungal hyphae of *Aspergillus fumigatus* within the wall of a mycotic aneurysm (magnification unknown).

**Table 11.5** Presentation

| Presentation | Number | Percentage |
|---|---|---|
| Positive blood culture | 168 | 55 |
| Fever | 156 | 51 |
| Headache | 99 | 33 |
| Malaise | 84 | 28 |
| Motor deficit | 83 | 27 |
| LOC/MS change | 46 | 15 |
| Seizure | 39 | 13 |
| Nausea, vomiting | 35 | 12 |
| Cranial nerve palsy | 34 | 11 |
| Meningitis | 31 | 10 |
| Behavioral change | 25 | 8 |
| Petechiae | 12 | 4 |
| Speech deficit | 9 | 3 |

*Abbreviations*: LOC, loss of consciousness; MS, mental status

**Table 11.6** Predisposing factors

| Predisposing Factor | Number | Percentage |
|---|---|---|
| Valvular disease | 83 | 27 |
| Rheumatic heart disease | 46 | 15 |
| Congenital heart disease | 16 | 5 |
| Intravenous drug use | 20 | 7 |
| Immunocompromise | 9 | 3 |

## ■ Presentation

Of 303 patients with IIA found in the literature review, 146 (48%) were female, and the average age was 34.5 years (see **Table 11.1**). The most common clinical finding was fever, which was present in 156 patients (51%). Blood cultures were positive in 168 patients (55%) (see **Table 11.5**). A total of 231 (76%) patients had a concurrent diagnosis of infective endocarditis (see **Table 11.2**). The mitral valve was the most commonly involved site, with evidence of documented vegetations in 84 patients, followed by the aortic valve in 23 patients. Evidence of preexisting valvular disease was present in 83 patients (27%) (**Table 11.6**). The most common cause of an underlying valvular abnormality was rheumatic heart disease, which was reported in 46 cases. Congenital heart disease was documented in 16 patients and was found to be an important factor in the pediatric

cases of IIA. Conditions found to be associated with fungal IIA included intravenous drug use (20 cases) and immunosuppression (9 cases).

Headache was part of the initial presentation in 99 patients (33%) (see **Table 11.5**). Loss of consciousness or altered mental status was present in 46 cases (15%). Thirty-nine patients (13%) presented with seizures. Motor deficit was present in 83 cases (27%), followed by cranial nerve palsy in 34 (11%) and speech deficit in 9 (3%).

Of 303 patients in the present analysis, 208 (69%) experienced aneurysmal rupture (**Table 11.7**). Thirty-one percent of these

**Table 11.7** Aneurysmal rupture and intracranial hemorrhage on presentation

| Presentation | Number | Percentage |
|---|---|---|
| Ruptured aneurysm | 208 | 69 |
| SAH | 64 | 21 |
| IPH | 78 | 26 |
| IVH | 15 | 5 |
| EDH | 1 | 0.3 |
| Unruptured | 84 | 28 |
| NR | 11 | 3 |

*Abbreviations*: EDH, epidural hemorrhage; IPH, intraparenchymal hemorrhage; IVH, intraventricular hemorrhage; NR, not reported; SAH, subarachnoid hemorrhage patients had subarachnoid hemorrhage (**Fig. 11.4**). Seventy-eight patients experienced intraparenchymal hemorrhage (**Fig. 11.5**); a majority of these cases were the result of aneurysmal rupture, but a small number were the result of hemorrhagic transformation after an ischemic stroke due to septic emboli. Intraventricular hemorrhage was seen in 15 patients. The presence of infarction was not consistently documented throughout the 303 reviewed cases. In Ojemann's review of 81 patients from 1959 and 1980, the clinical presentation was hemorrhage in 52%, infarction in 20%, infarction followed by hemorrhage in 6%, and headache in 2%.[37]

There were 45 deaths, all but three of which occurred in the patients with ruptured aneurysm (see **Table 11.1**). Of 303 IIA cases, 84 (28%) had no aneurysmal rupture (see **Table 11.7**). Generally, these patients had better outcomes than the patients with ruptured IIA.

Patients with IIA arising from an extravascular source had a different clinical presentation than those with an intravascular etiology. Articles by Rout et al and by Suwanwela et al describe IIA associated with cavernous sinus thrombosis resulting from local infection, such as orbital cellulitis.[29,32] These patients presented predominantly with ocular pain, ophthalmoplegia, proptosis, fever, and meningismus and tended to have unruptured cavernous internal carotid artery aneurysms.

## ■ Location

A total of 390 IIAs were found in 303 patients in the current review (see **Table 11.3**). Of these IIAs, 167 were located on the middle cerebral artery (43%). Of the reviewed IIAs, 9.5% were located on the posterior cerebral artery, followed closely by 8% on the anterior cerebral artery and 6% on the internal carotid artery. Most of these aneurysms were located distally, consistent with their pathogenesis, in which septic emboli

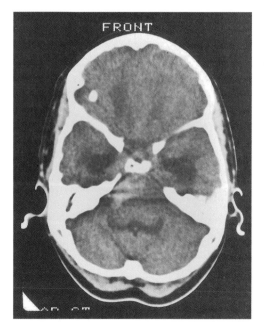

**Fig. 11.4** Axial computed tomographic scan showing a subarachnoid hemorrhage to the right of the brainstem that was due to the rupture of a basilar trunk mycotic aneurysm caused by *Aspergillus* species.

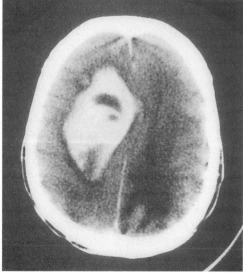

**Fig. 11.5** Axial computed tomographic scan showing an intracerebral hemorrhage presumed to be due to a mycotic aneurysm in a patient with systemic aspergillosis.

lodge within the blood vessel. Proximally located aneurysms were seen in cavernous sinus thrombosis, tuberculous meningitis (**Fig. 11.6**), and locally angioinvasive fungal infections. Posterior circulation aneurysms that involved the vertebrobasilar artery and posterior and anterior inferior cerebellar arteries occurred in 7%. Fox reported on 175 bacterial aneurysms in 140 patients and found that 64% of these were located on the middle cerebral artery, 11% on the anterior cerebral artery, 11% on the internal carotid artery, 8% on the posterior cerebral artery, and 6% on the vertebrobasilar arteries.[50] Multiple aneurysms were seen in 52 of 303 patients (17%) in the present analysis, consistent with Fox's finding of 18%. Information on the morphology of the aneurysms was not readily available, but when it was described, the numbers of fusiform and saccular aneurysms appeared to be similar.

## ■ Natural History

Autopsy reports and clinical series have varying incidence rates of IIA because of the presence of clinically dormant and un-

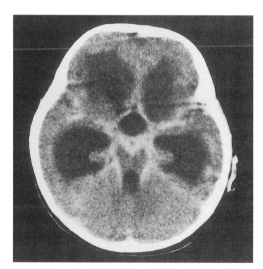

**Fig. 11.6** Contrast-enhanced axial computed tomographic scan in a child with tuberculous meningitis. Notice the presence of severe hydrocephalus.

diagnosed aneurysms.[56] Depending on the degree of inflammation, virulence of the causative organism, and whether there has been antibiotic treatment, the natural history of IIA can be variable. Antibiotic administration interferes with the efforts to determine the incidence rates accurately and limits clinical projections. In Ojemann's retrospective review of 27 patients with IIA who were subjected to serial angiography with concurrent antibiotic treatment, 30% of the aneurysms resolved, 19% diminished in size, 15% did not change in size, and 22% enlarged; new aneurysms developed in 15%.[57] Other series have noted similar general outcome patterns with variations that would be expected given the differences in patient populations and specific treatment algorithms.

The overall mortality rate in the present review was 15% (45 of 303 patients) (see **Table 11.1**). Of 208 patients with ruptured IIA, 42 (20%) died, which was an underestimate because of the lack of data on mortality in 68 patients from the review by Salgado et al.[30] With this study eliminated, the mortality rate in patients with ruptured IIA increased to 27%. This rate is in contrast to the rate in patients with unruptured IIA, in whom the mortality rate was 3.6%. Bohmfalk et al noted that 42% of patients presenting to the hospital with evidence of subarachnoid hemorrhage due to an intracranial bacterial aneurysm died.[7] Patients with fungal IIA had the worst outcome, with 12 of 13 cases progressing to death.[4,10,17–19,22,26] These results are consistent with the reported fungal mortality rate of greater than 90% despite medical or surgical treatment.[36] This mortality rate is likely influenced by the immunocompromised status of these patients.

## ■ Treatment

In patients with IIA, it is imperative to start appropriate antibiotic therapy as early as possible. The animal experiments by Molinari et al revealed that within 24 hours after the administration of septic emboli, intense inflammation and disruption of the adventitia and muscularis occurred.[51,52] Of 303 patients, 151 (50%) in this analysis received only medical treatment (**Table 11.8**), whereas 110 patients (36%) received medical treatment and underwent surgical intervention. Endovascular techniques, which became available for patients who were treated in the later years covered by our review, were performed in conjunction with antibiotic therapy in 35 patients (12%). Of the 45 deaths in the current analysis, 29 occurred in the patients who received medical treatment (19%), 5 in patients who received surgical treatment (4.5%), 4 in patients who had endovascular treatment (11%), 6 in patients with unknown treatment, and 1 in a patient who was untreated. These numbers are likely influenced by the fact that the medically unstable patients were deemed unsuitable for surgical intervention or died before surgical intervention could be performed.

Medical treatment can result in complete resolution of aneurysms in approximately 30% of cases.[7,11,37,58] Broad-spectrum antibiotic treatment, covering *Streptococcus* species and *Staphylococcus* species, should be started as early as possible. Patients should be receive at least 6 weeks of therapy, although there is no prospective randomized clinical trial to determine the optimal duration of treatment. The antibiotic of choice should be governed by its ability to cross the blood–brain barrier and the sensitivity results of the causative organism. Unruptured aneurysms should be initially treated conservatively with antibiotic therapy unless the aneurysms fail to resolve or enlarge after at least 6 weeks of treatment.[4,39,57,58] Conservative medical treatment may be the only safe option if the patient is medically unstable for surgery or the location and morphology of the IIA do not permit safe surgery. Serial angiography is important in monitoring the progression of the aneurysm (**Fig. 11.7**). The presence of fungal IIA is a relative indication for conservative, nonsurgical management.[58]

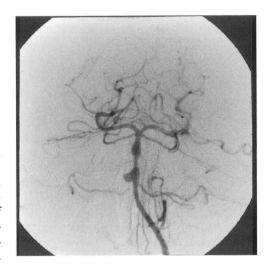

**Fig. 11.7** Cerebral angiogram illustrating an aneurysm of the basilar artery in a patient with *Aspergillus fumigatus* pneumonia.

**Table 11.8** Management

| Management | Number | Percentage | Mortality, No. | Mortality, % |
|---|---|---|---|---|
| Medical | 151 | 50 | 29 | 19 |
| Surgical | 110 | 36 | 5 | 4.5 |
| Endovascular | 35 | 12 | 4 | 11 |
| NR | 6 | 2 | 6 | 100 |
| No treatment | 1 | 0.3 | 1 | 100 |

*Abbreviations*: NR, died before treatment

Surgical intervention may initially be indicated in patients with ruptured IIA for the treatment of intracranial hypertension and herniation syndromes. Surgery for the purpose of definitively treating aneurysms was performed in 36% of patients in the current analysis (see **Table 11.8**). Surgery was more likely to be performed if there was an enlargement or persistence of the IIA despite appropriate antibiotic therapy, aneurysms were located distally, or neurologic decline was noted. Antibiotic therapy can help reduce the risk for surgical complications because antimicrobials can lead to reparative fibrosis in aneurysm walls, making them less likely to rupture.[4,40] Because of the friable nature of the IIA, clip ligation may not always be possible. In this case, wrapping the aneurysm dome is a surgical treatment option, as is trapping the parent artery. Another therapeutic alternative is surgical excision of the aneurysm and a segment of the parent vessel, which has the advantage of removing the intracranial nidus of infection.[12] This procedure can be combined with a primary vascular anastomosis, such as an extracranial–intracranial bypass.[15] For proximal lesions, such as intracavernous internal carotid artery aneurysms, carotid ligation with distal revascularization is an option.[29] Multiple aneurysms should be closely monitored with serial angiography, then managed in the same manner as solitary aneurysms. Consideration should be given to the treatment of the aneurysm that has most likely bled and any other easily accessible adjacent lesions.

The sophistication and efficacy of endovascular options for aneurysm treatment have increased over the last two decades. Chapot et al treated all 18 IIAs in 14 patients with endovascular methods.[9] Distal or fusiform aneurysms were treated with parent vessel occlusion in which cyanoacrylate, autologous clot, polyvinyl alcohol microparticles, or a combination of a straight coil and cyanoacrylate was used; proximal saccular aneurysms were selec-

tively treated by means of latex balloons and coils. Follow-up angiography showed stable occlusion of 16 aneurysms and refilling of 2, which were subsequently successfully treated. Chun et al demonstrated a multimodality approach to IIA treatment, with 5 of 27 aneurysms treated by endovascular means.[10] In the 4 surviving patients, follow-up angiography showed no aneurysmal recurrence.

## ■ Conclusion

IIAs are a relatively rare entity. They are most commonly due to septic emboli, often in association with infective endocarditis, that lodge in the distal vasculature, where they cause inflammation and disruption of the arterial wall from the adventitia inward. A majority of patients with IIA present with signs of infection and aneurysmal rupture, although the clinical presentation may vary for those with an extravascular source of infection. The most common causative microorganisms are *Streptococcus* species, followed by *Staphylococcus* species. Patients with immunosuppression are at risk for fungal IIA and have a mortality rate of over 90%. Multiple aneurysms may be present, but this has not been proven to be a negative prognostic indicator. The middle cerebral artery is by far the most frequently affected intracranial blood vessel. Management strategy should begin with the early institution of antibiotic therapy (**Fig. 11.8**). Serial angiography should be performed to monitor the progression of the aneurysms closely. When unruptured aneurysms do not respond to conservative therapy, or when the patient displays signs of intracranial hypertension, surgery should be considered. Ruptured IIAs should be treated with appropriate antibiotics and either surgical or endovascular intervention to prevent rebleeding. Endovascular options should be explored when open surgical treatment is being considered.

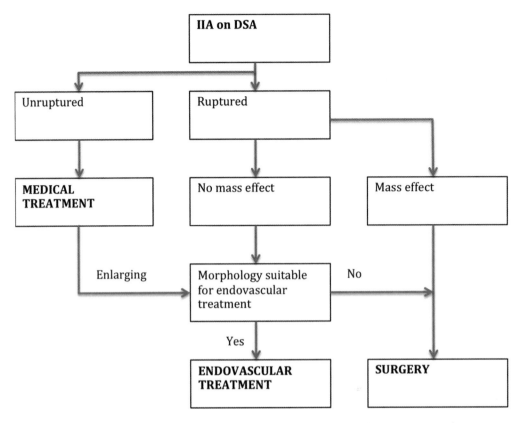

**Fig. 11.8** Management algorithm for infectious intracranial aneurysms. IIA, infectious intracranial aneurysm

### References

1. Church WS. Aneurysm of the right cerebral artery in a boy of thirteen. Trans Pathol Soc London 1869;20:109–110
2. Osler W. Gulstonian lecture on malignant endocarditis. BMJ 1885;1(1264):577–579
3. Aspoas AR, de Villiers JC. Bacterial intracranial aneurysms. Br J Neurosurg 1993;7(4):367–376
4. Barrow DL, Prats AR. Infectious intracranial aneurysms: comparison of groups with and without endocarditis. Neurosurgery 1990;27(4):562–572, discussion 572–573
5. Bartakke S, Kabde U, Muranjan MN, Bavdekar SB. Mycotic aneurysm: an uncommon cause for intracranial hemorrhage. Indian J Pediatr 2002;69(10):905–907
6. Bingham WF. Treatment of mycotic intracranial aneurysms. J Neurosurg 1977;46(4):428–437
7. Bohmfalk GL, Story JL, Wissinger JP, Brown WE Jr. Bacterial intracranial aneurysm. J Neurosurg 1978;48(3):369–382
8. Brust JC, Dickinson PC, Hughes JE, Holtzman RN. The diagnosis and treatment of cerebral mycotic aneurysms. Ann Neurol 1990;27(3):238–246
9. Chapot R, Houdart E, Saint-Maurice JP, et al. Endovascular treatment of cerebral mycotic aneurysms. Radiology 2002;222(2):389–396
10. Chun JY, Smith W, Halbach VV, Higashida RT, Wilson CB, Lawton MT. Current multimodality management of infectious intracranial aneurysms. Neurosurgery 2001;48(6):1203–1213, discussion 1213–1214
11. Corr P, Wright M, Handler LC. Endocarditis-related cerebral aneurysms: radiologic changes with treatment. AJNR Am J Neuroradiol 1995; 16(4):745–748
12. Day AL. Extracranial-intracranial bypass grafting in the surgical treatment of bacterial aneurysms: report of two cases. Neurosurgery 1981; 9(5):583–588
13. Dhomne S, Rao C, Shrivastava M, Sidhartha W, Limaye U. Endovascular management of ruptured cerebral mycotic aneurysms. Br J Neurosurg 2008; 22(1):46–52

14. Frazee JG, Cahan LD, Winter J. Bacterial intracranial aneurysms. J Neurosurg 1980;53(5): 633–641
15. Hadley MN, Spetzler RF, Martin NA, Johnson PC. Middle cerebral artery aneurysm due to *Nocardia asteroides*: case report of aneurysm excision and extracranial-intracranial bypass. Neurosurgery 1988;22(5):923–928
16. Hart RG, Kagan-Hallet K, Joerns SE. Mechanisms of intracranial hemorrhage in infective endocarditis. Stroke 1987;18(6):1048–1056
17. Kannoth S, Iyer R, Thomas SV, et al. Intracranial infectious aneurysm: presentation, management and outcome. J Neurol Sci 2007;256(1-2):3–9
18. Kikuchi K, Watanabe K, Sugawara A, Kowada M. Multiple fungal aneurysms: report of a rare case implicating steroid as predisposing factor. Surg Neurol 1985;24(3):253–259
19. Kurino M, Kuratsu J, Yamaguchi T, Ushio Y. Mycotic aneurysm accompanied by aspergillotic granuloma: a case report. Surg Neurol 1994; 42(2):160–164
20. Lee KS, Liu SS, Spetzler RF, Rekate HL. Intracranial mycotic aneurysm in an infant: report of a case. Neurosurgery 1990;26(1):129–133
21. Lin BH, Vieco PT. Intracranial mycotic aneurysm in a patient with endocarditis caused by *Cardiobacterium hominis*. Can Assoc Radiol J 1995;46(1):40–42
22. Mielke B, Weir B, Oldring D, von Westarp C. Fungal aneurysm: case report and review of the literature. Neurosurgery 1981;9(5):578–582
23. Monsuez JJ, Vittecoq D, Rosenbaum A, et al. Prognosis of ruptured intracranial mycotic aneurysms: a review of 12 cases. Eur Heart J 1989; 10(9):821–825
24. Ojemann RG, New PF, Fleming TC. Intracranial aneurysms associated with bacterial meningitis. Neurology 1966;16(12):1222–1226
25. Phuong LK, Link M, Wijdicks E. Management of intracranial infectious aneurysms: a series of 16 cases. Neurosurgery 2002;51(5):1145–1151, discussion 1151–1152
26. Piastra M, Chiaretti A, Tortorolo L. Ruptured intracranial mycotic aneurysm presenting as cerebral haemorrhage in an infant: case report and review of the literature. Childs Nerv Syst 2000;16(3): 190–193
27. Pootrakul A, Carter LP. Bacterial intracranial aneurysm: importance of sequential angiography. Surg Neurol 1982;17(6):429–431
28. Powell S, Rijhsinghani A. Ruptured bacterial intracranial aneurysm in pregnancy. A case report. J Reprod Med 1997;42(7):455–458
29. Rout D, Sharma A, Mohan PK, Rao VR. Bacterial aneurysms of the intracavernous carotid artery. J Neurosurg 1984;60(6):1236–1242
30. Salgado AV, Furlan AJ, Keys TF. Mycotic aneurysm, subarachnoid hemorrhage, and indications for cerebral angiography in infective endocarditis. Stroke 1987;18(6):1057–1060
31. Scotti G, Li MH, Righi C, Simionato F, Rocca A. Endovascular treatment of bacterial intracranial aneurysms. Neuroradiology 1996;38(2): 186–189
32. Suwanwela C, Suwanwela N, Charuchinda S, Hongsaprabhas C. Intracranial mycotic aneurysms of extravascular origin. J Neurosurg 1972;36(5): 552–559
33. Trivedi MP, Carroll C, Rutherford S. Infective endocarditis complicated by rupture of intracranial mycotic aneurysm during pregnancy. Int J Obstet Anesth 2008;17(2):182–187
34. Venkatesh SK, Phadke RV, Kalode RR, Kumar S, Jain VK. Intracranial infective aneurysms presenting with haemorrhage: an analysis of angiographic findings, management and outcome. Clin Radiol 2000;55(12):946–953
35. Fearnsides EG. Intracranial aneurysms. Brain 1916;39:224
36. Kojima Y, Saito A, Kim I. The role of serial angiography in the management of bacterial and fungal intracranial aneurysms—report of two cases and review of the literature. Neurol Med Chir (Tokyo) 1989;29(3):202–216
37. Ojemann RG. Infectious intracranial aneurysms. In: Ojemann RG, Ogilvy CS, Crowell RM, Heros RC, eds. Surgical Management of Cerebrovascular Disease. 3rd ed. Baltimore, MD: Williams & Wilkins; 1995:369–375
38. Stengel A, Wolforth CC. Mycotic (bacterial) aneurysms of intravascular origin. Arch Intern Med 1923;31:527–554
39. Baldwin HZ, Zabramski JM, Spetzler RF. Infectious intracranial aneurysms. In: Carter LP, Spetzler RF, Hamilton MG, eds. Neurovascular Surgery. New York, NY: McGraw-Hill; 1998:777–778
40. Cantu RC, LeMay M, Wilkinson HA. The importance of repeated angiography in the treatment of mycotic-embolic intracranial aneurysms. J Neurosurg 1966;25(2):189–193
41. McDonald CA, Jorb M. Intracranial aneurysms. Arch Neurol Psychiatry 1939;42:298–328
42. Roach MR, Drake CG. Ruptured cerebral aneuryms caused by micro-organisms. N Engl J Med 1965;273:240–244
43. Daltroff G, Lamit J, Bichet J, Chague D, Jacquet G, Portha C. Intracranial septic aneurysm in an infant. Apropos of a case and review of the literature [in French]. Pediatrie 1984;39(2):125–132
44. Hacker RJ. Intracranial aneurysms of childhood: a statistical analysis of 500 cases from the world literature. Neurosurgery 1982;10:775
45. Humphreys RP. Aneurysms and arteriovenous malformations of the brain. In: Hoffman HJ, Epstein F, eds. Disorders of the Developing Nervous System. Boston, MA: Blackwell Scientific; 1986:
46. Mazza C, Pasqualin A, Da Pian R, Pezzotta S. Intracranial aneurysms and subarachnoid hemorrhage in children and adolescents [in Italian]. Minerva Med 1986;77(25):1145–1151
47. Pasqualin A, Mazza C, Cavazzani P, Scienza R, Da-Pian R. Intracranial aneurysms and subarachnoid hemorrhage in children and adolescents. Childs Nerv Syst 1986;2(4):185–190
48. Shibuya S, Igarashi S, Amo T, Sato H, Fukumitsu T. Mycotic aneurysms of the internal carotid artery. Case report. J Neurosurg 1976;44(1): 105–108
49. Eppinger. Arch f Klin Chir, Berlin, Bd. xxxv. 5.156

50. Molinari GF, Smith L, Goldstein MN, Satran R. Brain abscess from septic cerebral embolism: an experimental model. Neurology 1973;23(11): 1205–1210

51. Molinari GF, Smith L, Goldstein MN, Satran R. Pathogenesis of cerebral mycotic aneurysms. Neurology 1973;23(4):325–332

52. Nakata Y, Shionoya S, Kamiya K. Pathogenesis of mycotic aneurysm. Angiology 1968;19(10): 593–601

53. Clare CE, Barrow DL. Infectious intracranial aneurysms. Neurosurg Clin N Am 1992;3(3):551–566

54. Barker WF. Mycotic aneurysms. Ann Surg 1954;139(1):84–89

55. Weir B. Aneurysms Affecting the Nervous System. Baltimore, MD: Williams & Wilkins; 1987

56. Yao KC, Bederson JB. Infectious intracranial aneurysms. In: Winn HR, ed. Youman's Neurological Surgery. 5th ed. Philadelphia, PA: Saunders; 2003:2101–2106

57. Ojemann RG. Surgical management of bacterial intracranial aneurysms. In: Schmidek HH, Sweet WH, eds. Operative Neurosurgical Techniques. New York, NY: Grune & Stratton; 1988:997–1001

# 12

# Vertebral Column Infections

## Kyle I. Swanson and Daniel K. Resnick

Vertebral column infections involve bone (osteomyelitis), intervertebral disk(s) (diskitis), or a combination of both (spondylodiskitis). Spontaneous infection results from the spread of organisms from other parts of the body to the vertebral column. Infections resulting in instability or neurologic deficit are treated with a combination of antibiotics and surgery, whereas vertebral column infections without instability or deficit are frequently treated with antibiotics alone. When infections are identified early and treated appropriately, the prognosis is generally favorable. The relatively nonspecific signs and symptoms of vertebral column infections are frequently missed, however, resulting in considerable delay in diagnosis. Untreated infection can result in chronic pain, spinal deformity, neurologic deficits, and death.

## ■ Incidence and Demographics

Spontaneous diskitis has an incidence of 0.2 to 2.4 per 100,000, with a bimodal distribution that peaks in early childhood and again at around 60 to 70 years of age.[1,2] The overall incidence of spontaneous vertebral osteomyelitis is approximately 2.4 per 100,000, with an incidence that increases with age. The incidence is 0.3 per 100,000 in those younger than 20 years of age and 6.5 per 100,000 in those older than 70 years of age.[3] Vertebral column infection has a male predominance.[3–5] Patient risk factors for spontaneous diskitis include intravenous drug use, alcoholism, diabetes mellitus, malignancy, immunosuppression, human immunodeficiency virus (HIV) infection, endocarditis, renal failure, and cirrhosis.[1,2,6] Similar risk factors are associated with spontaneous vertebral osteomyelitis.[5,7,8]

Some fungal and atypical bacterial infections are endemic in certain areas. Blastomycosis is more common around the Great Lakes and Ohio and Mississippi River basins. Coccidioidomycosis is localized to the southwestern United States and Central America.[9] In countries around the Mediterranean Sea, brucellosis comprises a sizable portion of vertebral column infections. Spinal tuberculosis, also known as Pott disease, is more common in Southeast Asia and Africa (**Fig. 12.1**).[10]

The overall rate of infection after spine surgery is 2.1% (range, 0.5 to 12%), with the procedure type a main determinant of the postoperative infection rate.[11–20] In general, longer procedures and operations with instrumentation have higher rates of infection. The incidence of infection after procedures involving intervertebral disks is relatively low, at 0.5 to 1%.[21,22] Simple laminectomy without bony fusion has an infection rate of approximately 1.5 to 2%.[22,23] With the addition of instrumentation and grafting, the rate of infection increases significantly to 2.8 to 6%.[22–25] The infection rate is increased still further if the surgery is done in the setting of spine trauma, with a reported risk of 10%.[26]

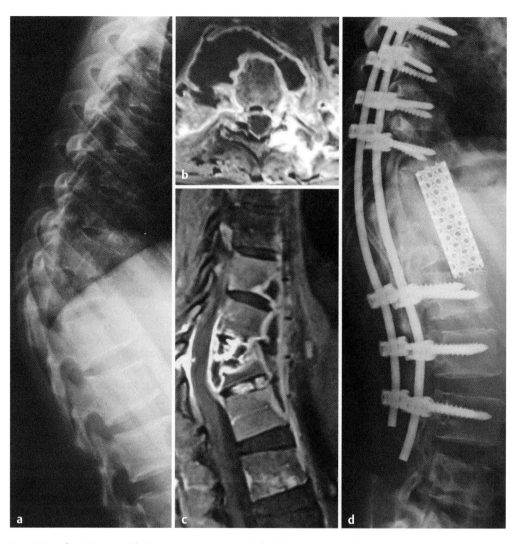

**Fig. 12.1a–d** A 24-year-old Vietnamese man presented with long-standing thoracic back pain and worsening kyphotic deformity. Lateral radiograph **(a)** revealed a gibbous deformity centered on T11. Contrasted T1-weighted magnetic resonance images revealed enhancement consistent with osteomyelitis involving predominantly T10–T12, with an associated large paravertebral abscess and a small epidural abscess **(b,c)**. The patient underwent T10–T12 corpectomies and drainage of the paravertebral abscess via a thoracolumbar approach, with use of a titanium cage and autograft, and a T6–L3 posterior instrumented fusion **(d)**. Intraoperative cultures confirmed the diagnosis of tuberculosis.

A large number of patient characteristics have been associated with an increased risk for spine surgical site infections: obesity, malnutrition, increased age, steroid use, tobacco abuse, alcoholism, diabetes mellitus, malignancy, concomitant urinary tract infection, prior surgery, prior infection, prior radiation therapy, prolonged preoperative hospitalization, trauma, and complete neurologic deficit before surgery.[20,23,24,26–35] The presence of three or more comorbidities further increases the risk for postoperative infection.[20]

## ■ Etiology and Pathogenesis

Infections of vertebral column are most often the result of direct implantation during invasive procedures and surgery. A much less common source of direct implantation is penetrating trauma.[36,37] Spontaneous infections are usually caused by hematogenous spread from a remote infection, such as endocarditis, dental abscess, skin infection, or urinary tract infection. This hematogenous spread can be either arterial or venous. The paravertebral venous plexus (Batson plexus) is a valveless venous system that connects the internal vertebral plexus to the deep pelvic and thoracic veins, thus allowing a conduit for the distant spread of infection to the vertebral column.[38] Finally, infection may spread to the vertebral column from contiguous infected structures, such as overlying infected skin and decubitus ulcers, as well as deep infections, such as pyelonephritis, mediastinitis, and pharyngeal abscesses.

The bimodal distribution of ages seen in patients with spontaneous diskitis is likely due to the differences in vascular anatomy between children and adults. During childhood, end-arteries penetrate the nucleus pulposus of the intervertebral disk, providing a direct channel through which bacteria can enter the disk. Also, the vertebral end plates have more arterial anastomoses in children, allowing better bacterial clearance. By adulthood, the arterial supply reaches only the annulus fibrosus, decreasing the likelihood of direct bacterial embolization into the disk, whereas involvement of the vertebral end plates increases. The rate of diskitis increases again in late adulthood because of the increase of comorbidities with age.[1,39]

*Staphylococcus aureus* is the most common organism to cause diskitis, followed by gram-negative rods, *Streptococcus* species, and *Enterococcus* species.[2,4] The likelihood of gram-negative rod diskitis increases in patients with gastrointestinal or genitourinary infection, diabetes mellitus, intravenous drug use, or a suppressed immune system.[6] Fungal diskitis is uncommon but is more likely in patient populations that are immunocompromised, neutropenic, critically ill, on multiple antibiotics, or that have indwelling central venous catheters.[40] Atypical bacteria, such as those causing tuberculosis or brucellosis, can involve the disk space but are much more likely to involve the vertebrae. Patients with sickle cell disease have an increased risk for infection with *Salmonella* species and *Haemophilus influenzae*.[6]

Spontaneous vertebral osteomyelitis generally begins at the vascular vertebral body end plates; therefore, the vertebral body is almost always involved, whereas the posterior elements are only rarely involved (3 to 12%).[41] The most common source for spontaneous vertebral osteomyelitis is urinary tract infection, followed by skin infection.[5]

As with diskitis, the most frequent organism causing vertebral osteomyelitis is *S. aureus*, followed by gram-negative rod species, especially *Escherichia coli*.[5] *Pseudomonas aeruginosa* is relatively more common in intravenous drug users, but even in this patient population *S. aureus* is the most frequent causative organism.[7] Tuberculosis remains an important cause of osteomyelitis in many developing regions of the world and in certain at-risk populations, such as patients with HIV infection. Brucellosis is another atypical bacterial cause of osteomyelitis that is found in the Mediterranean region and is associated with animal contact or the ingestion of unpasteurized milk.[42] Other causes of spontaneous vertebral osteomyelitis include various fungal infections, such as candidiasis, aspergillosis, coccidioidomycosis, histoplasmosis, and blastomycosis, and rarely parasitic infections such as echinococcosis.[9,40,43]

The distribution of the involved spinal segments is similar for both diskitis and osteomyelitis, with the lumbar spine most frequently involved (60%), followed by the thoracic spine (30%) and the cervical spine (10%).[1,4,5] Usually, one spinal level is involved, but multilevel involvement is seen in 5 to 18% of pyogenic cases and 20% of tuberculosis cases.[1] Vertebral osteomyelitis is frequently associated with adjacent paravertebral abscesses (26%) and epidural abscesses (17%).[8]

Postoperative vertebral column infections are caused by the direct spread of bacteria into the surgical wound from surgical instruments, the surgeon's hands, or airborne transmission. For early-onset infections, the most common organism is *S. aureus*, which accounts for 50 to 75% of cases, followed by *Staphylococcus epidermidis*, gram-negative rod species, and polymicrobial infections.[22,23] *S. epidermidis*, *Propionibacterium acnes*, and *Corynebacterium* species are often the cause of late-onset infections associated with instrumentation.[44]

Decreasing exposure of the surgical wound to bacterial contamination aids in preventing postoperative infection. Adequate cleansing of the skin before the start of surgery is vitally important. Randomized controlled trials have demonstrated that chlorhexidine-alcohol is superior to povidone-iodine for preoperative skin cleansing.[45] Likewise, chlorhexidine-based scrubs and alcohol rubs are superior to povidone-iodine–based scrubs for decolonizing hands before surgery.[46] The practice of double gloving reduces the incidence of glove perforations that can result in cross-contamination.[47] Vertical laminar airflow decreases the exposure of surgical wounds to airborne contamination and decreases the rate of infection in posterior spine fusions.[48] Frequent irrigation decreases the bacterial burden in direct contact with the wound.

During any surgery there will be some bacterial contamination because perfect sterility is not possible. Any factor that prolongs surgery will theoretically increase exposure to contamination and increase the risk for infection. Operative times longer than 3 hours increase postoperative infection rates.[49] Multilevel surgical fusions also increase the risk for infection, in part because of the prolonged operative time, although the addition of a foreign body likely also plays a role.[50]

The ability of the body to defend itself against infection also plays an important role in determining whether a postoperative infection will develop. This is governed in large part by underlying patient conditions, as described previously. Surgical factors that influence the immune response are also critical. A large volume of blood loss that is greater than 1 L or requires blood transfusion has been associated with increased rates of infection.[24,32] Prolonged retraction can devitalize tissue and provide

an environment conducive for bacterial growth. This may explain in part why posterior spinal surgeries, which require the extensive use of retractors, have a significantly higher rate of infection than anterior spinal surgeries.[26,51] Retraction should be periodically relaxed during prolonged surgery. The gentle handling of tissues and meticulous reapproximation of skin edges will also aid in healing.

Finally, perioperative intravenous prophylactic antibiotics can decrease bacterial viability and prevent postoperative infections.[52,53] The appropriate use of prophylactic antibiotics decreases the rate of postoperative spine infections from 5.9 to 2.2%.[54] Prophylactic antibiotics should be given just before incision, should be dosed again during long procedures, and should be continued for no more than 24 hours. Topical prophylactic antibiotics applied to the wound bed may also help prevent postoperative infections. Gentamicin-soaked collagen sponges placed in the disk space may decrease the rate of postoperative diskitis, and vancomycin powder applied to the surgical wound before closure has been shown to decrease infections in instrumented spine fusions; however, irrigation with antibiotic-containing saline has not been proven to have additional benefit over irrigation with normal saline alone.[52,55–58]

## ■ Clinical Presentation

The major presenting symptom of both spontaneous diskitis and osteomyelitis is localized pain, with approximately 90% of patients reporting back or neck pain, depending on the region involved.[1,8] The pain caused by a vertebral column infection is less likely to decrease with rest or recumbency than back or neck pain caused by degenerative conditions and is often more resistant to analgesic medications. Radicular pain related to irritation or compression of adjacent nerve roots can occasionally occur. Patients with lumbar involvement may have pain elicited with a straight leg raise test. The pain associated with diskitis in children can present as a refusal to walk or bear weight.[39] Osteomyelitis may also present with a sudden, severe worsening of pain associated with vertebral body fracture. Localized tenderness to percussion or palpation occurs in approximately one-fifth of patients with osteomyelitis.[59]

Another common symptom of spontaneous vertebral column infection is fever. The association of back or neck pain with fever should always raise the possibility of spine infection; however, fever is not universally present. Only 60 to 70% of patients with diskitis and 35 to 60% of those with osteomyelitis report fever.[2,8,59] Other, less frequent systemic findings include chills, night sweats, general malaise, and anorexia.[59]

Neurologic deficits, including weakness, difficulty walking, sensory abnormality, urinary incontinence or retention, fecal incontinence, and reflex abnormality, can all occur and are reported in approximately one-third of osteomyelitis cases.[59] Neurologic deficits are less likely in diskitis. Paralysis or rapidly progressing deficits are concerning for concurrent spinal epidural abscess. Chronic osteomyelitis may present as a worsening kyphosis, most pronounced in the sharply angled gibbous deformity, which can also cause spinal cord compression and neurologic deficits.[8] Chronic vertebral osteomyelitis may present with a draining sinus tract.[10]

Vertebral column infections are often initially misdiagnosed because the most common presenting symptom, pain, is nonspecific. The mean time to diagnosis for vertebral osteomyelitis is 1.8 months. In one series, the diagnosis of vertebral osteomyelitis was considered in only a quarter of patients at initial evaluation.[8] The differential diagnosis of vertebral column infection includes infections of the spinal canal, vertebral column fracture, degenerative disk disease or herniated disk, metastatic or primary malignancy, inflammatory spondyloarthopathies, neuropathic arthropathy, sarcoidosis, psoas abscess, pancreatitis, and pyelonephritis.[60]

Worsening pain is also a frequent symptom in postoperative vertebral column infections. Differentiation between the expected pain of surgery and the pain caused by infection can be difficult. Pain that returns after initial postoperative relief of preoperative symptoms and worsening localized pain remote from the time of surgery are concerning for infection. Diskitis can present as just worsening pain, more than a month after diskectomy, in a patient with a well-healed incision and no fevers. Recurrent disk herniation is sometimes mistakenly diagnosed, or the patient may be wrongly accused of malingering. An evaluation for infection should be considered in patients with recent spine surgery and worsening pain.

Fever is frequently, but not always, present in postoperative vertebral column infections. Moreover, several other common causes for fever postoperatively must be considered, including atelectasis, pneumonia, urinary tract infection, drug reaction, and deep vein thrombosis.

Wound drainage is the most common sign of postoperative spine infections and can be the only sign or symptom in some patients. Approximately 93% of patients with postoperative spine infection have drainage. Other external signs of infection include erythema, swelling, tenderness, and wound dehiscence. The time from surgery to initial presentation of a postoperative spine infection is around 2 weeks. Infection with aggressive organisms like *Clostridium perfringens,* however, can present in days, and infection with indolent organisms like *P. acnes* can present years after surgery.[22]

The development of new neurologic deficits not initially present postoperatively should warrant urgent evaluation to rule out abscess causing spinal cord or nerve root compression. Treatment of an abscess causing spinal cord compression is a neurosurgical emergency because delay in treatment may dramatically increase morbidity or mortality.[61]

## ■ Diagnosis

### Laboratory

Laboratory markers of inflammation play an important role in the diagnosis of vertebral column infections, especially when the clinical signs and symptoms are not specific. An elevated white blood cell count with neutrophilia is frequently present in spontaneous diskitis and vertebral osteomyelitis, as well as in postoperative infections, but a significant number of cases will have no leukocytosis and a normal white blood cell differential. Approximately two-thirds of patients with vertebral osteomyelitis will have an elevated white blood cell count, and about a third will have neutrophilia.[62] In some series, fewer than half of patients with diskitis have a leukocytosis.[63] The absence of leukocytosis does not rule out the possibility of infection.

An elevated C-reactive protein (CRP) level and erythrocyte sedimentation rate (ESR) are much more sensitive markers for infection than the white blood cell count but are nonspecific, and these parameters can be elevated in the setting of many different types of inflammation. The CRP level and ESR will be elevated in most cases of vertebral column infection.[62–64] The likelihood of infection in a patient with a normal white blood cell count, CRP level, and ESR is quite low, although not impossible. Because the CRP level and ESR are normally elevated after surgery, caution must be exercised when they are used to diagnose infections postoperatively. After surgery, the ESR will be maximal around postoperative day 5 and will often remain elevated for weeks. The CRP level has a much earlier peak, at around 2 days, and will usually normalize within 5 to 14 days after surgery.[64,65] The CRP level can be especially useful in diagnosing late postoperative infections that present with nonspecific symptoms, such as pain. The quicker response time of the CRP level also makes it a more accurate gauge of treatment success or failure than the ESR.[64]

The proper diagnosis and treatment of vertebral column infections depends on identifying the causative organism. Cultures should be obtained before antibiotics are started to maximize yield. All patients with suspected infection should have blood cultures collected because blood culture is a minimally invasive procedure that frequently identifies the causative organism. Ideally, three blood cultures obtained at different locations and times should be collected. Collecting the sample while the patient is febrile increases the yield. Approximately half of all patients with diskitis or osteomyelitis will have positive blood cultures that can be used to guide treatment.[4,5] Echocardiography is usually warranted in patients with bacteremia, especially *S. aureus* bacteremia, as endocarditis is present in a significant number of patients with spontaneous diskitis and vertebral osteomyelitis. Similarly, patients with the new onset of back pain in the setting of known endocarditis should be evaluated for vertebral column infection.[66]

If blood cultures demonstrate no growth after 2 days, a computed tomography (CT)–guided percutaneous biopsy is warranted as the next step in the evaluation of spontaneous vertebral column infections. The diagnostic yield for CT-guided biopsy is between 60 and 70%, and a repeat percutaneous biopsy can increase the yield further if the initial biopsy is negative.[4,63] Biopsy specimens should be routinely sent for aerobic and anaerobic bacterial cultures and fungal culture. Sensitivities should be performed on any identified organism. Histopathology samples should be evaluated with Gram stain and fungal stains. In patients with risk factors associated with tuberculosis or brucellosis, appropriate cultures should be obtained, and histopathology should be evaluated for granulomas and acid-fast bacilli.[60] Blood cultures should also be repeated a few hours after percutaneous biopsy.[1] Open biopsy is warranted if both blood cultures and percutaneous biopsy fail to yield a diagnosis and infection is still suspected. The yield of open biopsy is 77% (range, 47 to 100%).[5]

Serologic testing for specific fungal, parasitic, or atypical bacterial causes of vertebral column infections, such as brucellosis and cat-scratch fever (*Bartonella henselae*), may be warranted in patients who are from regions where these diseases are endemic or who have environmental exposures.[39,67] Antigen testing is another adjunct for the diagnosis of vertebral column infections caused by certain fungi, such as candidiasis, aspergillosis, and cryptococcosis. A tuberculin skin test should be performed in patients suspected of having tuberculous spondylitis.[10]

Blood cultures should also be obtained from patients with suspected postoperative vertebral column infections. A majority of patients with surgical site infections will need surgical débridement, so cultures are best obtained at the time of surgery. Occasionally, percutaneous needle aspiration is used in postoperative infections to drain an abscess or to obtain a diagnosis in situations for which surgery is not indicated, such as isolated diskitis. Cultures from late-onset infections in the setting of instrumentation should be allowed to incubate for a prolonged period of time, up to 7 to 15 days, to increase the likelihood of identifying slow-growing organisms like *P. acnes*.[44] Cultures taken from the incision site or from external drainage are often misleading because they will grow skin flora that may not be related to the underlying infection.

## Imaging

Plain radiographs are not particularly sensitive or specific for the diagnosis of vertebral column infections, and findings may be normal for weeks after the onset of infection. Paravertebral soft tissue swelling, which is more noticeable in the cervical region, can sometimes be the first radiographic sign of vertebral column infection. Disk space narrowing generally takes between 7 and 10 days to develop but is common in degenerative spine disease as well. Vertebral end plate erosion and vertebral body rarefaction take weeks to develop. Vertebral fracture or collapse can develop late and is sometimes confused with osteoporotic fracture. In patients with kyphotic deformity in the setting of vertebral osteomyelitis, the comparison of recumbent and standing radiographs can aid in the determination of overt instability. In general, plain radiographs may be useful as an initial screening study and can also be used as a follow-up study to monitor for new or worsening kyphotic deformity (**Fig. 12.2e,f**).

CT information is similar to that of plain radiographs but is more sensitive to early changes and has markedly increased anatomic detail. CT is the best study for evaluating the features of bony involvement and is vital for preoperative planning in vertebral column infections requiring surgical fixation (**Fig. 12.2a**). Some soft tissue details are also discernible on CT, such as the presence of paravertebral fluid collections. The administration of intravenous iodinated contrast will usually result in the enhancement of infected disk and bone as well as rim enhancement of associated abscesses. Contrasted CT is particularly useful for the imaging guidance of percutaneous biopsies or abscess drainage. Although contrasted CT is not as sensitive or specific for vertebral column infections as contrasted magnetic resonance (MR) imaging, it can often provide adequate diagnostic images in patients who are unable to undergo MR imaging because of implanted devices or morbid obesity.[68]

Myelography is generally avoided because of the availability of adequate noninvasive techniques and the risk for seeding the cerebrospinal fluid by performing a lumbar puncture in the setting of infection.

MR imaging combined with gadolinium contrast administration is the most reliable imaging modality for diagnosing spontaneous vertebral column infections. On noncontrasted T1-weighted images, diskitis and osteomyelitis will demonstrate hypointensity of the disk and vertebral bodies, as opposed to normal hyperintensity in the vertebral bone marrow due to the presence of fat (**Fig. 12.2b**). Intravenous gadolinium will enhance regions of inflammation, especially the vertebral end plates and associated abscesses (**Fig. 12.2c**).[68] The involved bone and disk will usually be hyperintense on T2-weighted images because of increased edema (**Fig. 12.2d**). With diskitis, there is usually a loss of the intranuclear cleft and decreased disk space height.[69] End plate destruction, frank vertebral collapse, and kyphotic deformities are late findings of vertebral column infections. With isolated diskitis, MR imaging has a sensitivity and specificity of over 90%, and with vertebral osteomyelitis, the sensitivity is 96% and the specificity is 93%.[68,70] Imaging the

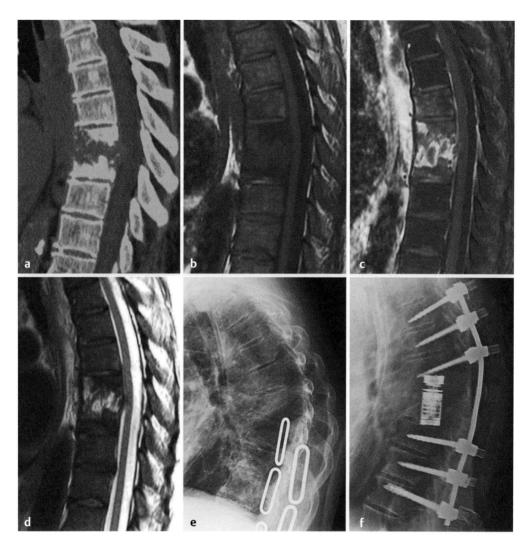

**Fig. 12.2a–f** A 63-year-old woman on dialysis with diabetes mellitus, end-stage renal disease, and obesity presented with 2 months of right upper quadrant pain. She was found to have methicillin-sensitive *Staphylococcus aureus* mitral valve endocarditis and bacteremia. Three days later, she developed thoracic back pain. Thoracic computed tomography **(a)** revealed diskitis and osteomyelitis at T7 and T8. Thoracic magnetic resonance imaging confirmed the diagnosis, with the involved area demonstrating hypointensity on T1-weighted images **(b)**, enhancement on T1-weighted images with contrast **(c)**, and focal hyperintensity on T2-weighted images **(d)**. The patient developed progressive kyphosis on follow-up radiographs **(e)** despite appropriate antibiotics and bracing. She underwent corpectomies of T7 and T8 via a costotransversectomy approach, with use of a titanium expandable cage and autograft, and a T4–T11 posterior instrumented fusion **(f)**. The patient recovered well from the surgery but died 2 months later from complications of endocarditis.

entire spine is recommended by some authors because of the possibility of concomitant distant vertebral column infection.[71]

Radionuclide studies are sometimes useful when MR imaging is either not possible or nondiagnostic, such as in the setting of hardware-induced artifact.[68] They rely on increased uptake of various radioactive tracers in metabolically active regions, such as infection, but will also label inflammation in general. They are less sensitive than MR imaging but more sensitive than contrasted CT. Gallium-67 single-photon emission computed tomography

(SPECT) and combined gallium-67/technetium-99 (bone) SPECT have the highest reported sensitivity (91%) and specificity (92%). SPECT scans are more accurate than scintigraphy.[54] Labeled leukocyte imaging, although useful in the diagnosis of osteomyelitis elsewhere in the body, has been found to be less effective for the diagnosis of vertebral osteomyelitis. [[18]F]Fluorodeoxyglucose positron emission tomography (FDG-PET) is another modality that has, in preliminary studies, identified vertebral osteomyelitis with good accuracy.[72]

Postoperative vertebral column infections have many of the same radiologic characteristics mentioned above, but the interpretation of imaging is often made more difficult because surgery itself causes inflammatory changes that can mimic infection.[73] Contrasted CT and MR imaging can both identify enhancing fluid collections concerning for abscess, although care must be taken not to confuse abscesses with other postoperative fluid collections, such as hematomas and seromas. A plain radiograph can be useful for ruling out retained foreign body. Both radiographs and CT scans can demonstrate the loosening of implants, which can be associated with late-onset infections.[74]

# ■ Treatment

The goal of the treatment of vertebral column infections is to eliminate infection permanently while maintaining spinal stability and neurologic function. In spontaneous infections, the mainstay of treatment is tailored antibiotics, with surgical intervention reserved for selected indications, such as instability or neurologic compression. In isolated diskitis, more than three-quarters of patients can be treated nonoperatively with appropriate antibiotics.[1] Although disease is usually more extensive in vertebral osteomyelitis, the majority of cases can still be successfully treated without surgery. A systematic review found that only 42% of patients with pyogenic osteomyelitis required surgery in addition to antibiotics.[5] Furthermore, medical treatment

alone is successful in a majority of patients with tuberculous vertebral osteomyelitis.[75] Postoperative vertebral column infections, on the other hand, are treated in most cases with a combination of targeted antibiotics and surgical débridement.

## Surgical Treatment

Surgical treatment is indicated for the following reasons: failure to obtain diagnostic cultures via less invasive means, débridement of infected tissue and drainage of associated abscesses in the setting of persistent or recurrent infection despite adequate antimicrobial treatment or in the setting of overt sepsis, intractable pain, decompression of the spinal cord or spinal nerve roots in the setting of severe or worsening neurologic deficits, and stabilization of the spine or correction of significant deformity.[76]

Early treatment of kyphosis caused by tuberculous vertebral osteomyelitis should be considered in patients with risk factors for progression of deformity: kyphotic angle of more than 30 degrees, loss of more than 1.5 times the vertebral body height, involvement of greater than three vertebral bodies, overt radiographic instability, involvement of both anterior and posterior elements, and onset of disease during spinal immaturity.[77]

## Approaches

Surgery for isolated diskitis is rarely required and is most frequently used for identification of the causative organism. In the lumbar spine, the standard posterior microdiskectomy approaches may be utilized. In the cervical spine, anterior cervical diskectomy approaches are preferred. For isolated diskitis in the thoracic spine, a posterolateral approach, such as the transpedicular approach or the transfacet pedicle-sparing approach, can be used. A lateral approach, such as the lateral extracavitary approach or costotransversectomy, is also an option. Associated paravertebral abscesses can be drained percutaneously.

The surgical treatment of vertebral osteomyelitis, when necessary, requires more extensive débridement and usually concurrent stabilization. With adequate surgical débridement and antibiotics, there does not seem to be an increased risk for recurrence of infection when autograft, allograft, or instrumentation is used in the setting of acute infection, even in an immunocompromised patient population.[72,78–81] Anterior surgical approaches are often preferred because vertebral osteomyelitis most often involves the vertebral bodies, with only rare involvement of the posterior elements. Approaching anteriorly allows a more complete débridement of infected tissue and direct reconstruction of the compromised portion of the vertebral column.

Vertebral osteomyelitis involving the upper cervical spine at C1 and C2 is quite rare and may require transoral resection and supplemental posterior instrumented fusion (**Fig. 12.3**). Subaxial cervical vertebral column infections are treated via anterior cervical diskectomy or corpectomy with the use of an autologous graft or cage, with or without ventral plating. Complications associated with plating in this setting have been reported.[71]

The thoracic spine presents a particular challenge for the surgical treatment of vertebral osteomyelitis because of the difficulty of anterior approaches. The cervicothoracic junction can be approached ventrally via cervical exposure, partial sternotomy, or manubrial resection.[82] Posterolateral approaches have also been used to access this region and include the transpedicular, lateral extracavitary, and parascapular extrapleural approaches.[83–85] Posterior instrumented fusion is often used in conjunction with the anterior surgery to prevent cervicothoracic instability.[80,86] The midthoracic spine can be approached anteriorly via a thoracotomy, or it can be accessed posterolaterally by either a costotransversectomy or a lateral extracavitary approach (**Fig. 12.2**).[83,84,87] The lower thoracic spine and thoracolumbar junction can be reached ventrally via a thoracoabdominal approach (**Fig. 12.1**).[88]

The lumbar spine is approached anteriorly by either a retroperitoneal or transperitoneal approach. The retroperitoneal approach also allows drainage of any associated psoas abscess.[10] The upper sacral spine can be accessed ventrally via similar routes.

The correction of severe, fixed kyphotic deformity often requires complex posterior surgical techniques utilizing wedge osteotomies and posterior instrumented fixation. These deformity correction surgeries can have a relatively high level of associated operative morbidity.[75]

The treatment of postoperative vertebral column infections involves exploration of the wound with meticulous débridement of all necrotic and infected material. Sutures from the prior surgery should be removed. In early-onset postoperative infections, intact spinal instrumentation and viable bone graft should be left in situ to increase the chance of fusion.[12–14,22,25,50,51,74,89–91] The wound should be copiously irrigated with liters of normal saline or antibiotic-containing saline.[22,74] Pulse-lavage irrigation may enhance débridement.

The wound can be closed primarily with a drain in place. Alternatively, the wound can initially be left open to heal by secondary intention, or it can be closed in a delayed fashion. Vacuum-assisted closure (VAC) dressings can decrease nursing requirements and may help the healing process, although the benefit of VAC dressings over traditional gauze packing has yet to be definitively demonstrated.[92–94] An irrigation-suction system for continuous irrigation has been reported for the postoperative treatment of infected spine instrumentation.[51] In patients with severe infections, sepsis, extensive associated necrosis, or polymicrobial infections, repeat débridement 2 to 3 days after the initial operation may provide additional benefit.[22,25,74] Nonabsorbable monofilament suture is recommended for skin closure.

When patients with instrumented spine fusions present with late-onset postoperative infection, they should be treated with removal of hardware, in addition to the usual débridement and irrigation.[91,95,96] These late postoperative infections are often caused by organisms capable of creating a glycocalyx covering on instrumentation that increases resistance to antibiotic therapy.[96] Leaving the hardware

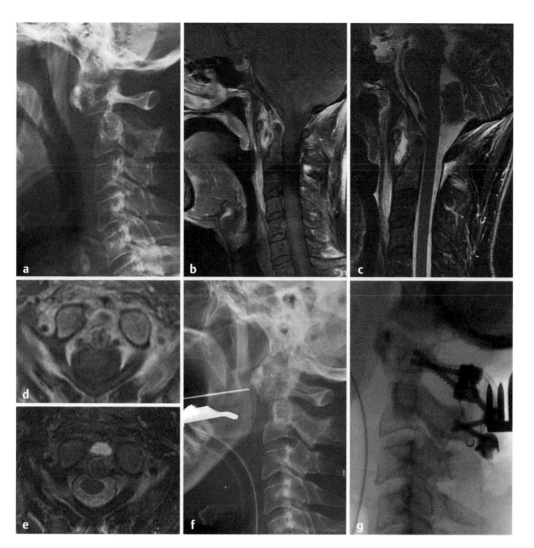

**Fig. 12.3a–g** A 44-year-old man with a history of tobacco abuse presented with 2 months of neck stiffness. The patient described an episode of violent choking, caused by a fish bone, a few weeks before the onset of neck symptoms. His erythrocyte sedimentation rate and C-reactive protein level were elevated, but he was afebrile without leukocytosis. Radiographs revealed erosion of the odontoid process of C2 and 10 mm of anterior displacement of C1 relative to the body of C2 **(a)**. The patient was placed in a halo brace for initial stabilization. Contrasted T1-weighted magnetic resonance images revealed enhancement consistent with osteomyelitis involving the odontoid process and the anterior arch of C1, and a paravertebral abscess **(b,d)**. The paravertebral abscess demonstrated marked T2-weighted hyperintensity **(c,e)**. The patient underwent a transoral resection **(f)**, followed by a posterior fusion involving C1 lateral mass screws and C2 translaminar screws, with wire fixation of an iliac crest autograft between C1 and C2 **(g)**. The infection was polymicrobial, consistent with contamination from a penetrating foreign body.

in place significantly increases the risk for infection relapse.[91] These patients should be monitored closely for worsening deformity that might indicate a need for repeat instrumented fusion, although they often have already achieved stable fusion.

## Medical Treatment

The cornerstone of medical management for vertebral column infections is antibiotic therapy tailored to the causative organism and drug sensitivities. Empiric antibiotics should be withheld if possible until adequate cultures have been obtained. Consultation with infectious disease specialists is advised to help guide antibiotic selection and duration. Spinal immobilization via orthosis or short-term bed rest can aid in pain control. Physical rehabilitation may also be beneficial. Proper nutrition is vital to the successful treatment of vertebral column infections.[27,74] Medical comorbidities, such as diabetes mellitus and HIV infection, should be adequately treated. Steroids are not used in the treatment of vertebral column infections.

### Antimicrobial Therapies

For pyogenic diskitis, intravenous antibiotics are usually continued for 4 to 6 weeks, although some recent reports suggest that a 12-week course of antibiotics, with a switch to oral antibiotics after 6 weeks, may decrease the risk for recurrence.[1,6] A 6-week course of antibiotics is usually recommended for the treatment of pyogenic vertebral osteomyelitis, although reported courses range from 4 weeks to 3 months.[97] In patients with vertebral osteomyelitis, there is an increased risk for relapse with regimens that are less than 4 weeks.[98] Successful treatment of vertebral osteomyelitis with a completely oral regimen (fluoroquinolones and rifampin) has been reported.[99]

For patients with postoperative vertebral column infections who do not have implanted hardware, intravenous antibiotics are continued for 4 to 6 weeks. Postoperative infections involving instrumented fusions are treated with at least 6 weeks of antibiotics. For patients who have implanted hardware, the addition of oral antibiotic suppression therapy, started after the initial intravenous antibiotic course and continued for a minimum of 6 months and occasionally indefinitely, has been found to decrease the risk for late recurrence.[91]

Empiric antibiotics can be started in seriously ill patients after adequate cultures have been obtained. Any empiric regimen should have good gram-positive cocci coverage, especially against *S. aureus*, as well as gram-negative rod coverage. Given the increasing resistance of *S. aureus*

to β-lactam antibiotics, empiric coverage should generally also have activity against methicillin-resistant *S. aureus* (MRSA). One viable combination is vancomycin and ceftriaxone. In patients at high risk for *P. aeruginosa* infections, such as intravenous drug users, ceftriaxone can be switched for a cephalosporin with antipseudomonal coverage, such as cefepime or ceftazidime.

High-dose nafcillin or oxacillin is the preferred treatment for methicillin-sensitive *S. aureus* (MSSA). Vancomycin is used for MRSA and coagulase-negative *Staphylococcus* species. *P. aeruginosa* is usually treated with ceftazidime or cefepime, and in seriously ill patients it is combined initially with either an aminoglycoside or ciprofloxacin. Nonpseudomonal gram-negative rod bacteria, such as *E. coli,* are usually treated with either ceftriaxone or ciprofloxacin. Penicillin G is the first-line treatment for *Streptoccocus* species. Anaerobic infections can be covered by either clindamycin or metronidazole.[100]

The first-line regimen for the treatment of tuberculosis is a combination of isoniazid, rifampicin, ethambutol, and pyrazinamide for 2 months. This is subsequently pared down to just isoniazid and rifampicin to complete a 6- to 9-month total course of treatment.[101] Susceptibility testing is important given the rise of multidrug-resistant tuberculosis. Brucellosis is often treated with a combination of doxycycline and rifampicin for 6 months, although streptomycin or gentamicin may be added for the first 2 to 3 weeks.[10] Amphotercin B is the first-line treatment of many serious fungal infections, including candidiasis and blastomycosis, although voriconazole is now preferred for the treatment of invasive aspergillosis.[10,100]

Patients should be monitored closely for evidence of therapy failure. A lack of symptomatic improvement, continued fevers, or persistent elevation of the CRP level after 4 weeks are all suggestive of treatment failure.[64] Regular laboratory testing is usually indicated to monitor for antimicrobial toxicity. Repeat MR imaging is a poor predictor of outcome after treatment has started and may initially appear worse than pretreatment imaging. New MR imaging may be indicated in the setting of neurologic decline to rule out new or worsening abscess.[60,102] Serial radiographs can be used to monitor for progressive kyphosis.

## Outcome

The reported recurrence rate after an initial course of antibiotics for pyogenic spondylodiskitis is 8% (range, 1 to 22%).[1,63] Recurrence is usually within 6 months, but infection can return years later. Vertebral osteomyelitis relapse is more likely in the setting of an associated paravertebral abscess, a chronically draining sinus tract, or recurrent bacteremia. With adequate treatment, pyogenic vertebral column infections will generally progress to fusion across the involved disk spaces over the course of 6 to 24 months, although pseudarthrosis can develop.[1] In patients with tuberculosis, 65 to 79% of cases develop a solid fusion with medical therapy alone.

Chronic pain is the most likely complication associated with vertebral column infections, with 64% of patients treated conservatively reporting residual back pain, versus 26% of patients treated operatively.[103] In a systematic review of pyogenic vertebral osteomyelitis case series, over a quarter of patients had a complication that significantly worsened their quality of life, including 28% with chronic pain, 16% with persistent weakness, and 7% with bowel or bladder dysfunction.[5] Postoperative vertebral column infections significantly increase the cost of spine surgery, the length of hospitalization, and the number of complications, including neurologic deficits.[11,20,104]

Worse outcomes are associated with motor weakness or complete paralysis at presentation, delay of diagnosis beyond 2 months, and hospital-acquired infections.[8] Mortality for spontaneous pyogenic spondylodiskitis is approximately 6% (range, 2 to 12%).[1,5] Mortality is usually related to sepsis, endocarditis, or an underlying medical condition.[2,63] In a series of patients undergoing surgical decompression and fusion, postoperative infection increased the mortality rate from 0.5 to 1.06%.[104]

## Conclusion

Vertebral column infection should be considered in any patient with back or neck pain and associated fever, elevated inflammatory markers, or bacteremia. Contrasted MR imaging is the most sensitive and specific test to evaluate for vertebral column infection. Obtaining diagnostic cultures is of paramount importance for the proper treatment of both spontaneous and postoperative infections. Antibiotics should be held until cultures are obtained. Postoperative infections are typically treated with a combination of surgery and tailored antibiotics. Spontaneous vertebral column infections can often be treated with antibiotics alone. Surgery is indicated to obtain diagnostic cultures, decompress neural structures, treat spinal instability, and débride infected and necrotic material when infection persists or worsens in the face of appropriate antibiotics.

### References

1. Cottle L, Riordan T. Infectious spondylodiscitis. J Infect 2008;56(6):401–412
2. Hopkinson N, Stevenson J, Benjamin S. A case ascertainment study of septic discitis: clinical, microbiological and radiological features. QJM 2001;94(9):465–470
3. Grammatico L, Baron S, Rusch E, et al. Epidemiology of vertebral osteomyelitis (VO) in France: analysis of hospital-discharge data 2002-2003. Epidemiol Infect 2008;136(5):653–660
4. Legrand E, Flipo RM, Guggenbuhl P, et al; Rheumatology Network Organization. Management of nontuberculous infectious discitis. Treatments used in 110 patients admitted to 12 teaching hospitals in France. Joint Bone Spine 2001; 68(6):504–509
5. Mylona E, Samarkos M, Kakalou E, Fanourgiakis P, Skoutelis A. Pyogenic vertebral osteomyelitis: a systematic review of clinical characteristics. Semin Arthritis Rheum 2009;39(1):10–17
6. Grados F, Lescure FX, Senneville E, Flipo RM, Schmit JL, Fardellone P. Suggestions for managing pyogenic (non-tuberculous) discitis in adults. Joint Bone Spine 2007;74(2):133–139
7. Patzakis MJ, Rao S, Wilkins J, Moore TM, Harvey PJ. Analysis of 61 cases of vertebral osteomyelitis. Clin Orthop Relat Res 1991;(264):178–183
8. McHenry MC, Easley KA, Locker GA. Vertebral osteomyelitis: long-term outcome for 253 pa-

tients from 7 Cleveland-area hospitals. Clin Infect Dis 2002;34(10):1342–1350

9. Kim CW, Perry A, Currier B, Yaszemski M, Garfin SR. Fungal infections of the spine. Clin Orthop Relat Res 2006;444:92–99

10. Skaf GS, Kanafani ZA, Araj GF, Kanj SS. Non-pyogenic infections of the spine. Int J Antimicrob Agents 2010;36(2):99–105

11. Calderone RR, Garland DE, Capen DA, Oster H. Cost of medical care for postoperative spinal infections. Orthop Clin North Am 1996;27(1): 171–182

12. Abbey DM, Turner DM, Warson JS, Wirt TC, Scalley RD. Treatment of postoperative wound infections following spinal fusion with instrumentation. J Spinal Disord 1995;8(4):278–283

13. Glassman SD, Dimar JR, Puno RM, Johnson JR. Salvage of instrumental lumbar fusions complicated by surgical wound infection. Spine 1996;21(18):2163–2169

14. Keller RB, Pappas AM. Infection after spinal fusion using internal fixation instrumentation. Orthop Clin North Am 1972;3(1):99–111

15. Kostuik JP, Israel J, Hall JE. Scoliosis surgery in adults. Clin Orthop Relat Res 1973;(93): 225–234

16. Lonstein J, Winter R, Moe J, Gaines D. Wound infection with Harrington instrumentation and spine fusion for scoliosis. Clin Orthop Relat Res 1973;(96):222–233

17. Roberts FJ, Walsh A, Wing P, Dvorak M, Schweigel J. The influence of surveillance methods on surgical wound infection rates in a tertiary care spinal surgery service. Spine 1998;23(3):366–370

18. West JL III, Ogilvie JW, Bradford DS. Complications of the variable screw plate pedicle screw fixation. Spine 1991;16(5):576–579

19. Balderston RA, Blumberg KD, eds. Infection in spine surgery. In Balderston RA, An HS, eds. Complications in Spinal Surgery. Philadelphia, PA: Saunders; 1991:157–168

20. Olsen MA, Mayfield J, Lauryssen C, et al. Risk factors for surgical site infection in spinal surgery. J Neurosurg 2003;98(2, Suppl):149–155

21. Bongartz EB, Ulrich P, Fidler M, Bernucci C. Reoperation in the management of post-operative disc space infection. Zentralbl Neurochir 1994;55(2):120–124

22. Weinstein MA, McCabe JP, Cammisa FP Jr. Postoperative spinal wound infection: a review of 2,391 consecutive index procedures. J Spinal Disord 2000;13(5):422–426

23. Massie JB, Heller JG, Abitbol JJ, McPherson D, Garfin SR. Postoperative posterior spinal wound infections. Clin Orthop Relat Res 1992;(284): 99–108

24. Wimmer C, Gluch H, Franzreb M, Ogon M. Predisposing factors for infection in spine surgery: a survey of 850 spinal procedures. J Spinal Disord 1998;11(2):124–128

25. Sasso RC, Garrido BJ. Postoperative spinal wound infections. J Am Acad Orthop Surg 2008; 16(6):330–337

26. Blam OG, Vaccaro AR, Vanichkachorn JS, et al. Risk factors for surgical site infection in the patient with spinal injury. Spine 2003;28(13): 1475–1480

27. Klein JD, Hey LA, Yu CS, et al. Perioperative nutrition and postoperative complications in patients undergoing spinal surgery. Spine 1996;21(22): 2676–2682

28. Tenney JH, Vlahov D, Salcman M, Ducker TB. Wide variation in risk of wound infection following clean neurosurgery. Implications for perioperative antibiotic prophylaxis. J Neurosurg 1985;62(2):243–247

29. Andreshak TG, An HS, Hall J, Stein B. Lumbar spine surgery in the obese patient. J Spinal Disord 1997;10(5):376–379

30. Capen DA, Calderone RR, Green A. Perioperative risk factors for wound infections after lower back fusions. Orthop Clin North Am 1996;27(1): 83–86

31. Patel N, Bagan B, Vadera S, et al. Obesity and spine surgery: relation to perioperative complications. J Neurosurg Spine 2007;6(4):291–297

32. Ho C, Sucato DJ, Richards BS. Risk factors for the development of delayed infections following posterior spinal fusion and instrumentation in adolescent idiopathic scoliosis patients. Spine 2007;32(20):2272–2277

33. Simpson JM, Silveri CP, Balderston RA, Simeone FA, An HS. The results of operations on the lumbar spine in patients who have diabetes mellitus. J Bone Joint Surg Am 1993;75(12):1823–1829

34. Rechtine GR, Bono PL, Cahill D, Bolesta MJ, Chrin AM. Postoperative wound infection after instrumentation of thoracic and lumbar fractures. J Orthop Trauma 2001;15(8):566–569

35. Sponseller PD, LaPorte DM, Hungerford MW, Eck K, Bridwell KH, Lenke LG. Deep wound infections after neuromuscular scoliosis surgery: a multicenter study of risk factors and treatment outcomes. Spine 2000;25(19):2461–2466

36. Hales DD, Duffy K, Dawson EG, Delamarter R. Lumbar osteomyelitis and epidural and paraspinous abscesses. Case report of an unusual source of contamination from a gunshot wound to the abdomen. Spine 1991;16(3):380–383

37. Schulze CJ, Mayer HM. Exogenous lumbar spondylodiscitis following a stabwound injury and vertebral fracture. A case report and review of the literature. Eur Spine J 1995;4(6):357–359

38. Batson OV. The function of the vertebral veins and their role in the spread of metastases. Ann Surg 1940;112(1):138–149

39. Fernandez M, Carrol CL, Baker CJ. Discitis and vertebral osteomyelitis in children: an 18-year review. Pediatrics 2000;105(6):1299–1304

40. Chia SL, Tan BH, Tan CT, Tan SB. *Candida* spondylodiscitis and epidural abscess: management with shorter courses of anti-fungal therapy in combination with surgical debridement. J Infect 2005;51(1):17–23

41. Babinchak TJ, Riley DK, Rotheram EB Jr. Pyogenic vertebral osteomyelitis of the posterior elements. Clin Infect Dis 1997;25(2):221–224

42. Katonis P, Tzermiadianos M, Gikas A, Papagelopoulos P, Hadjipavlou A. Surgical treatment of spinal brucellosis. Clin Orthop Relat Res 2006;444: 66–72

43. Schnepper GD, Johnson WD. Recurrent spinal hydatidosis in North America. Case report and

review of the literature. Neurosurg Focus 2004; 17(6):E8

44. Haidar R, Najjar M, Der Boghossian A, Tabbarah Z. *Propionibacterium acnes* causing delayed postoperative spine infection: review. Scand J Infect Dis 2010;42(6-7):405–411

45. Darouiche RO, Wall MJ Jr, Itani KMF, et al. Chlorhexidine-alcohol versus povidone-iodine for surgical-site antisepsis. N Engl J Med 2010; 362(1):18–26

46. Tanner J, Swarbrook S, Stuart J. Surgical hand antisepsis to reduce surgical site infection. Cochrane Database Syst Rev 2008;(1):CD004288

47. Tanner J, Parkinson H. Double gloving to reduce surgical cross-infection. Cochrane Database Syst Rev 2006;3(3):CD003087

48. Gruenberg MF, Campaner GL, Sola CA, Ortolan EG. Ultraclean air for prevention of postoperative infection after posterior spinal fusion with instrumentation: a comparison between surgeries performed with and without a vertical exponential filtered air-flow system. Spine 2004;29(20):2330–2334

49. Wimmer C, Gluch H. Management of postoperative wound infection in posterior spinal fusion with instrumentation. J Spinal Disord 1996;9(6):505–508

50. Picada R, Winter RB, Lonstein JE, et al. Postoperative deep wound infection in adults after posterior lumbosacral spine fusion with instrumentation: incidence and management. J Spinal Disord 2000;13(1):42–45

51. Levi AD, Dickman CA, Sonntag VK. Management of postoperative infections after spinal instrumentation. J Neurosurg 1997;86(6):975–980

52. Brown EM, Pople IK, de Louvois J, et al; British Society for Antimicrobial Chemotherapy Working Party on Neurosurgical Infections. Spine update: prevention of postoperative infection in patients undergoing spinal surgery. Spine 2004;29(8): 938–945

53. Watters WC III, Baisden J, Bono CM, et al; North American Spine Society. Antibiotic prophylaxis in spine surgery: an evidence-based clinical guideline for the use of prophylactic antibiotics in spine surgery. Spine J 2009;9(2):142–146

54. Barker FG II. Efficacy of prophylactic antibiotic therapy in spinal surgery: a meta-analysis. Neurosurgery 2002;51(2):391–400, discussion 400–401

55. Rohde V, Meyer B, Schaller C, Hassler WE. Spondylodiscitis after lumbar discectomy. Incidence and a proposal for prophylaxis. Spine 1998;23(5):615–620

56. O'Neill KR, Smith JG, Abtahi AM, et al. Reduced surgical site infections in patients undergoing posterior spinal stabilization of traumatic injuries using vancomycin powder. Spine J 2011;11(7): 641–646

57. Sweet FA, Roh M, Sliva C. Intrawound application of vancomycin for prophylaxis in instrumented thoracolumbar fusions: efficacy, drug levels, and patient outcomes. Spine 2011;36(24):2084–2088

58. Haines SJ. Topical antibiotic prophylaxis in neurosurgery. Neurosurgery 1982;11(2):250–253

59. Priest DH, Peacock JE Jr. Hematogenous vertebral osteomyelitis due to *Staphylococcus aureus* in the adult: clinical features and therapeutic outcomes. South Med J 2005;98(9):854–862

60. Zimmerli W. Clinical practice. Vertebral osteomyelitis. N Engl J Med 2010;362(11):1022–1029

61. Rigamonti D, Liem L, Sampath P, et al. Spinal epidural abscess: contemporary trends in etiology, evaluation, and management. Surg Neurol 1999;52(2):189–196, discussion 197

62. Jensen AG, Espersen F, Skinhøj P, Frimodt-Møller N. Bacteremic *Staphylococcus aureus* spondylitis. Arch Intern Med 1998;158(5):509–517

63. Friedman JA, Maher CO, Quast LM, McClelland RL, Ebersold MJ. Spontaneous disc space infections in adults. Surg Neurol 2002;57(2):81–86

64. Khan MH, Smith PN, Rao N, Donaldson WF. Serum C-reactive protein levels correlate with clinical response in patients treated with antibiotics for wound infections after spinal surgery. Spine J 2006;6(3):311–315

65. Thelander U, Larsson S. Quantitation of C-reactive protein levels and erythrocyte sedimentation rate after spinal surgery. Spine 1992;17(4): 400–404

66. Le Moal G, Roblot F, Paccalin M, et al. Clinical and laboratory characteristics of infective endocarditis when associated with spondylodiscitis. Eur J Clin Microbiol Infect Dis 2002;21(9):671–675

67. Graveleau J, Grossi O, Lefebvre M, et al. Vertebral osteomyelitis: an unusual presentation of *Bartonella henselae* infection. Semin Arthritis Rheum 2011;41(3):511–516

68. Kothari NA, Pelchovitz DJ, Meyer JS. Imaging of musculoskeletal infections. Radiol Clin North Am 2001;39(4):653–671

69. Boden SD, Davis DO, Dina TS, Sunner JL, Wiesel SW. Postoperative diskitis: distinguishing early MR imaging findings from normal postoperative disk space changes. Radiology 1992;184(3): 765–771

70. Palestro CJ, Love C, Miller TT. Infection and musculoskeletal conditions: imaging of musculoskeletal infections. Best Pract Res Clin Rheumatol 2006;20(6):1197–1218

71. Shousha M, Boehm H. Surgical treatment of cervical spondylodiscitis: a review of 30 consecutive patients. Spine 2012;37(1):E30–E36

72. Carragee E, Iezza A. Does acute placement of instrumentation in the treatment of vertebral osteomyelitis predispose to recurrent infection: long-term follow-up in immune-suppressed patients. Spine 2008;33(19):2089–2093

73. Ross JS, Zepp R, Modic MT. The postoperative lumbar spine: enhanced MR evaluation of the intervertebral disk. AJNR Am J Neuroradiol 1996;17(2):323–331

74. Beiner JM, Grauer J, Kwon BK, Vaccaro AR. Postoperative wound infections of the spine. Neurosurg Focus 2003;15(3):E14

75. Khoo LT, Mikawa K, Fessler RG. A surgical revisitation of Pott distemper of the spine. Spine J 2003;3(2):130–145

76. Butler JS, Shelly MJ, Timlin M, Powderly WG, O'Byrne JM. Nontuberculous pyogenic spinal infection in adults: a 12-year experience from

a tertiary referral center. Spine 2006;31(23): 2695–2700

77. Rajasekaran S, Soundarapandian S. Progression of kyphosis in tuberculosis of the spine treated by anterior arthrodesis. J Bone Joint Surg Am 1989;71(9):1314–1323

78. Przybylski GJ, Sharan AD. Single-stage autogenous bone grafting and internal fixation in the surgical management of pyogenic discitis and vertebral osteomyelitis. J Neurosurg 2001;94(1, Suppl): 1–7

79. Schuster JM, Avellino AM, Mann FA, et al. Use of structural allografts in spinal osteomyelitis: a review of 47 cases. J Neurosurg 2000;93(1, Suppl): 8–14

80. Rath SA, Neff U, Schneider O, Richter HP. Neurosurgical management of thoracic and lumbar vertebral osteomyelitis and discitis in adults: a review of 43 consecutive surgically treated patients. Neurosurgery 1996;38(5):926–933

81. Stone JL, Cybulski GR, Rodriguez J, Gryfinski ME, Kant R. Anterior cervical debridement and strut-grafting for osteomyelitis of the cervical spine. J Neurosurg 1989;70(6):879–883

82. Karikari IO, Powers CJ, Isaacs RE. Simple method for determining the need for sternotomy/manubriotomy with the anterior approach to the cervicothoracic junction. Neurosurgery 2009;65(6, Suppl):E165–E166, discussion E166

83. Benzel EC. The lateral extracavitary approach to the spine using the three-quarter prone position. J Neurosurg 1989;71(6):837–841

84. Larson SJ, Holst RA, Hemmy DC, Sances A Jr. Lateral extracavitary approach to traumatic lesions of the thoracic and lumbar spine. J Neurosurg 1976;45(6):628–637

85. Fessler RG, Dietze DD Jr, Millan MM, Peace D. Lateral parascapular extrapleural approach to the upper thoracic spine. J Neurosurg 1991;75(3): 349–355

86. Arnold PM, Baek PN, Bernardi RJ, Luck EA, Larson SJ. Surgical management of nontuberculous thoracic and lumbar vertebral osteomyelitis: report of 33 cases. Surg Neurol 1997;47(6):551–561

87. McCormick PC. Retropleural approach to the thoracic and thoracolumbar spine. Neurosurgery 1995;37(5):908–914

88. Anderson TM, Mansour KA, Miller JI Jr. Thoracic approaches to anterior spinal operations: anterior thoracic approaches. Ann Thorac Surg 1993;55(6): 1447–1451, discussion 1451–1452

89. Mok JM, Guillaume TJ, Talu U, et al. Clinical outcome of deep wound infection after instrumented posterior spinal fusion: a matched cohort analysis. Spine 2009;34(6):578–583

90. Stambough JL, Beringer D. Postoperative wound infections complicating adult spine surgery. J Spinal Disord 1992;5(3):277–285

91. Kowalski TJ, Berbari EF, Huddleston PM, Steckelberg JM, Mandrekar JN, Osmon DR. The management and outcome of spinal implant infections: contemporary retrospective cohort study. Clin Infect Dis 2007;44(7):913–920

92. Ploumis A, Mehbod AA, Dressel TD, Dykes DC, Transfeldt EE, Lonstein JE. Therapy of spinal wound infections using vacuum-assisted wound closure: risk factors leading to resistance to treatment. J Spinal Disord Tech 2008;21(5):320–323

93. Yuan-Innes MJ, Temple CL, Lacey MS. Vacuum-assisted wound closure: a new approach to spinal wounds with exposed hardware. Spine 2001;26(3):E30–E33

94. Ubbink DT, Westerbos SJ, Evans D, Land L, Vermeulen H. Topical negative pressure for treating chronic wounds. Cochrane Database Syst Rev 2008;(3):CD001898

95. Viola RW, King HA, Adler SM, Wilson CB. Delayed infection after elective spinal instrumentation and fusion. A retrospective analysis of eight cases. Spine 1997;22(20):2444–2450, discussion 2450–2451

96. Clark CE, Shufflebarger HL. Late-developing infection in instrumented idiopathic scoliosis. Spine 1999;24(18):1909–1912

97. Roblot F, Besnier JM, Juhel L, et al. Optimal duration of antibiotic therapy in vertebral osteomyelitis. Semin Arthritis Rheum 2007;36(5): 269–277

98. Sapico FL, Montgomerie JZ. Pyogenic vertebral osteomyelitis: report of nine cases and review of the literature. Rev Infect Dis 1979;1(5): 754–776

99. Schrenzel J, Harbarth S, Schockmel G, et al; Swiss Staphylococcal Study Group. A randomized clinical trial to compare fleroxacin-rifampicin with flucloxacillin or vancomycin for the treatment of staphylococcal infection. Clin Infect Dis 2004;39(9):1285–1292

100. Gouliouris T, Aliyu SH, Brown NM. Spondylodiscitis: update on diagnosis and management. J Antimicrob Chemother 2010;65(Suppl 3): iii11–iii24

101. American Thoracic Society; CDC; Infectious Diseases Society of America. Treatment of tuberculosis. MMWR Recomm Rep 2003;52(RR-11): 1–77

102. An HS, Seldomridge JA. Spinal infections: diagnostic tests and imaging studies. Clin Orthop Relat Res 2006;444:27–33

103. Hadjipavlou AG, Mader JT, Necessary JT, Muffoletto AJ. Hematogenous pyogenic spinal infections and their surgical management. Spine 2000;25(13):1668–1679

104. Veeravagu A, Patil CG, Lad SP, Boakye M. Risk factors for postoperative spinal wound infections after spinal decompression and fusion surgeries. Spine 2009;34(17):1869–1872

# 13

# Spinal Canal Infections

Ian E. McCutcheon

Although uncommon, infections of the spinal canal have profound clinical implications and pose a risk for paralysis. Their early diagnosis and prompt, effective treatment are therefore very important in maintaining neurologic function and quality of life. Improvements in radiographic imaging, most notably the widespread availability of magnetic resonance (MR) imaging, allow such conditions to be localized because they typically cause the gross structural abnormality of an abscess rather than the more subtle microscopic findings of meningitis. These infections have actually become more common in recent decades as a consequence of the increasing number of patients with chronic or immunosuppressive illness whose life expectancy modern medicine has extended.

The spectrum of such disorders falls into three categories: (1) spinal epidural abscess (SEA), typically bacterial in origin and the most common of the three; (2) spinal subdural abscess, which is much less common; and (3) intramedullary abscess of the spinal cord, which is also rare, although more often reported than subdural abscess in the spinal compartment. Each of these infections is generally pyogenic (i.e., producing a purulent and mainly neutrophilic infiltrate), but infections caused by mycobacteria, fungi, and *Nocardia* species are also occasionally seen. This chapter specifically excludes discussion of focal infection of the vertebrae, known as vertebral osteomyelitis, which is addressed in a separate chapter.

## ■ Spinal Epidural Abscess

Infections in the epidural space can be isolated but are often associated with infection in the vertebral body, disk space, or both. Thus, an anatomic distinction is somewhat artificial and not the principal factor in determining therapy, although an important distinction is that the medical cure of osteomyelitis requires a longer duration of antibiotic administration than does infection of the disk or epidural space. The first pathologic description of a bacterial vertebral osteomyelitis was published in 1820 by Bergamaschi. By the 1890s, surgery had been reported for pyogenic vertebral infections by Ollier and Chipault; in 1896, Makins and Abbott associated vertebral infection with epidural suppuration and advocated both removal of the infected bone and evacuation of the epidural pus.[1] This concept was also promoted by Ramsay Hunt in 1904 in the first paper devoted to establishing epidural abscess as a separate entity.[2] The first attempt at surgical drainage of an isolated SEA without vertebral involvement was performed by Delorme in 1892; the patient succumbed to bacterial endocarditis quickly thereafter, and functional recovery after successful drainage was first reported in 1901 by Barth.[3] These early papers promoted SEA as a distinct condition and began the trend toward surgical drainage of such abscesses, which continues to this day. Because such abscesses are now frequently diagnosed in immunocompromised and elderly patients, many of whom are medically fragile, there has been a reassessment of the need for surgery in all cases and a reconsideration of medical treatment in selected patients, which is now performed with some success (**Table 13.1**).

## Anatomy

The spinal epidural space under normal conditions is filled with fat, a loose areolar connective tissue network, and an exuberant venous plexus. This space sits between the spinal dura and the bony ring that forms the vertebral canal. The dura is relatively adherent to the posterior longitudinal ligament in the anterior aspect of the canal, and thus the dorsal and lateral components of the epidural space are more prominent and are the typical sites for abscess. Because of the larger diameter of the spinal cord in the cervical spine, the space is minimal in the neck; however, it enlarges in the midthoracic region (T4–T8), where it has a depth of 5 to 7 mm, then narrows gradually to accommodate the lumbar cord enlargement, with progressive widening caudal to L2 until the dura ends at S2. It has been suggested that this anatomic variation promotes the formation of SEAs in the thoracolumbar area. However, the distribution of SEAs is relatively even along the spine. Epidural abscesses found in the anterior epidural space are almost always associated with diskitis or vertebral osteomyelitis extending past the posterior longitudinal ligament into the epidural compartment. Because the anterior dural attachments are stronger, epidural abscesses in the anterior space tend to be more limited in extent, whereas those in the posterior aspect of the canal extend over more segments. A typical SEA covers three to five segments, but many more can be involved.

## Epidemiology

The incidence of SEA has risen in recent years, likely through a combination of increased detection, increased life expectancy for immunocompromised patients, and aging of the population. The incidence is variously reported as between 0.2 and 2 cases per 10,000 hospital admissions.[4,5] The elderly are prone to such infections, with the peak incidence in the sixth and seventh decades; SEAs are also relatively uncommon in the pediatric age range. The two most common correlates are frequent bacteremia and significant impairment of immune function. Both acquired immunodeficiency syndrome (AIDS) and intravenous drug use are thus very significant risk factors for SEA, as are diabetes mellitus, end-stage renal disease, and hepatic cirrhosis. In addition, any medical treatment that uses immunosuppression to a therapeutic end or provokes it as a side effect (including long-term steroid therapy, chemotherapy, and suppression of the antigraft response in transplant recipients) can promote SEA.[6,7] In such patients, the spontaneous bacteremia that all people harbor from time to time (and that is cleared by competent immune mechanisms) is more likely to progress unchecked, resulting in SEA.

**Table 13.1** Risk factors for spinal epidural abscess in a general hospital

| Risk Factor[a] | Percentage |
| --- | --- |
| Intravenous drug use | 37 |
| Diabetes mellitus | 29 |
| Multiple medical illnesses | 23 |
| Trauma | 17 |
| Prior spinal surgery | 15 |
| Morbid obesity | 9 |
| HIV infection | 9 |
| End-stage renal disease | 8 |
| Spinal nerve block | 7 |

*Abbreviation*: HIV, human immunodeficiency virus
[a] Risk factors add up to more than 100% because of overlapping conditions in many patients.

## Microbiology

The most common causative organism is *Staphylococcus aureus*,[8] which in conjunction with other gram-positive microbes (e.g., *Staphylococcus epidermidis*, *Streptococcus pneumoniae*, *Streptococcus viridans*, *Enterococcus*, and *Propionibacterium acnes*) causes most epidural abscesses. Gram-negative species are less often cultured from SEAs, but abscesses containing *Escherichia coli*, *Pseudomonas aeruginosa*, *Salmonella*, *Klebsiella*, and other species are sometimes found after infection of the urinary or gastrointestinal tract. Anaerobes rarely cause spinal epidural infections in the general population but sometimes cause infection in intravenous drug abusers. Unfortunately, 10 to 20% of patients show no growth on culture of the abscess material, even in the absence of prior antibiotic therapy.[6,7]

*Streptococcus* species are the second most common bacteria (after *Staphylococcus* species) to cause SEA and are often seen in association with recent pneumonia or after dental procedures. The gram-negative species dominate in intravenous drug abusers, while *Mycobacterium tuberculosis* is quite common in Asia and Africa, and such cases are starting to seep into North America as well. Fungal infections are also becoming slightly more common.

## Mechanisms of Pathogenesis

The venous route of infection from pelvis to vertebral column, proposed by Batson in 1957, has had much traction over the years but is now largely discredited. Hematogenous dissemination of bacteria likely occurs most often through arterial transfer, particularly to the metaphyseal area near the anterior longitudinal ligament. Abscesses in the epidural space can arise through bacterial embolization to this part of the vertebral body with secondary propagation into the adjacent epidural space, or through direct spread to the epidural space posteriorly. Adjacent foci of infection, such as pulmonary, retropharyngeal, or intra-abdominal abscess, are also occasional sources of SEA.[9] Infection and thrombosis of the nutrient metaphyseal artery produce avascular necrosis of bone and thus create a nidus for infection. Ischemia of the disk occurs through the same mechanism, rendering it more susceptible to infection.

Both bone and disk can act as sources of infection in the neighboring epidural space. Some infections may emanate from the epidural veins alone, thus allowing involvement of several spinal segments without concomitant infection of bone or disk.

Bacterial contamination can occur directly in patients undergoing open surgery with exposure of the epidural space. The dead space left after instrumentation is a particularly suitable environment for the growth of bacteria implanted at the time of surgery. Foreign bodies placed in the disk space (e.g., epidural stimulators or catheters) can also carry bacteria into this compartment, as can penetrating injuries or direct breakdown, as occurs in a decubitus ulcer.

The development of neurologic deficits follows the onset of SEA in 5 to 50% of patients. Such deficits occur through direct compression caused by an expanding abscess; this is further exacerbated when spinal deformity occurs as a consequence of biomechanical impairment of the spine as infected bone leads to vertebral wedging. It has long been noted, however, that cord dysfunction on a clinical level is often significantly more evident than the degree of compression alone should cause. Some patients acquire a central cord syndrome that is hard to explain as a result of mass effect.[4] In addition, the rapidity and occasional irreversibility of the neurologic deterioration associated with the onset of SEA suggests that a vascular mechanism underlies these clinical phenomena.

Autopsy studies by Russell et al showed thrombosis of the epidural arteries and veins as well as venous infarction and edema within the cord in patients with SEA.[10] However, experimental model systems (as exemplified by the rabbit model of Feldenzer et al) show an explicit lack of microangiopathy in the cord except in animals with severely compressive lesions, and they found no thrombosis or venous occlusion.[11–13] Such findings argue in favor of the compressive theory, yet the clinical course of the disease in humans does not fully support it. This contradiction may simply reflect the limits of the experimental rabbit model in mimicking the human clinical situation, as well as the heterogeneity of such infections in their microbial pathogenesis and the underlying clinical conditions that predispose patients to SEA. Unfortunately, this ambiguity of etiology and of substrate has prevented a consensus on the appropriate method of therapy across all groups.

## Clinical Features

A broad range of symptoms can signify an SEA, and classic features are not always present. The diagnosis can be missed unless the index of suspicion is high.[14] Although a very small fraction of patients with back pain harbor a spinal infection, a pattern can be gleaned that should point to the diagnosis of epidural abscess and drive the performance of studies to determine whether one is present. The first symptom of an SEA is isolated back pain, and more generalized infection is often absent. Because the symptoms are clarified over time, it is typical for patients to seek medical attention repeatedly before the diagnosis is made. Symptoms usually progress through four stages: (1) an aching pain in the spine, (2) root pain or radiculopathy, (3) weakness, and (4) paralysis.[11] Usually, a patient's symptoms do not follow this pattern perfectly and may consist either of local pain manifestations or systemic signs of infection (fever, malaise, night sweats). The interval between the onset of pain and the onset of neurologic deficit also varies.[4,15,16] The combination of fever and back pain in a patient with immunocompromise or a history of drug abuse should lead to the suspicion of SEA. The back pain is not always associated with local tenderness of the spine, and the pain is usually severe. Fever is often slight and may be masked by the patient's use of analgesics for the back pain or through the prior use of antibiotics. In some, septicemia occurs, and this can be the primary presentation. One-third of patients are neurologically intact at presentation. The rate of progression of the neurologic deficits varies greatly, with some advancing slowly and others causing paralysis within hours.

About 75% of patients have signs of spinal cord or nerve root dysfunction when the diagnosis is made. Monoparesis is common, and paraparesis or quadriparesis is occasionally seen. Patients with severe back pain or encephalopathy may be more difficult to examine, and confusion is noted in 15 to 35% of patients. Loss of bowel or bladder control and sensory deficit can also occur, but a complete loss of sensation below a sensory level is usually seen only with profound and often irreversible loss of motor function. In patients with urinary retention or incontinence, measuring post-void residual volumes with subsequent Foley catheter placement provides clarity as to bladder function.[17]

The presence of fever and back pain, particularly in immunocompromised patients or in those with a history of intravenous drug abuse, should prompt testing for SEA, especially when recent bacteremia is documented.

Secondary extraspinal infection is occasionally seen in people with SEA. Infection in a vertebra can seep into the adjacent fascial layers to cause abscess in the psoas or paraspinal muscles, can cause retropharyngeal abscess, and sometimes provokes a sympathetic pleural effusion.

## Diagnosis

### Laboratory Studies

Serum markers of acute inflammation are helpful in screening patients for SEA. It is important to remember, however, that at least 10% of patients later proven to have an epidural abscess show no inflammatory markers. The three markers generally used are the white blood cell count, the erythrocyte sedimentation rate (ESR), and the C-reactive protein (CRP) level. Most sensitive is the ESR, elevated in 90% of patients with spinal infection, often dramatically so.[18] This readily available test can be used to monitor response to therapy, and it should always be measured during initial evaluation. However, it is not particularly specific, and some patients have an elevated basal ESR from other causes even before onset of the infection. One such example would be a patient with hepatic cirrhosis. Such patients are prone to acquiring SEA; however, their ESR elevations do not correct even when treatment of the infection is successful. The CRP level is less sensitive but somewhat better in the detection of early infections because serum levels rise within hours after the initiation of a bacterial infection. It is also useful in the postoperative setting in patients suspected of having an SEA after spinal surgery. Both the ESR and the CRP level rise after spine surgery, but the CRP level returns to normal more quickly and thus may have more utility in the work-up of patients in the postoperative period. The ESR can take 2 to 3 months to normalize after successful treatment (**Fig. 13.1**). Lumbar puncture is not usually performed when an epidural infection is suspected because it may inoculate infected material into the subarachnoid space and because the cerebrospinal fluid (CSF) from most patients with SEA demonstrates evidence of a nonspecific parameningeal process, with a high protein level and a mild leukocytosis.

## Imaging

Confirmation of the presence of infection and determination of its site in the spine are usually achieved by MR imaging. The multiplanar capacity of MR imaging and its ability to distinguish infection from other pathology make it the imaging method of choice. Many patients will have had preceding plain X-rays or computed tomography (CT) scans. CT is most useful when it includes three-dimensional reconstructions of the spinal anatomy. The main findings of SEA on plain films are indirectly associated anomalies of the bone or disk, including narrowing of the disk space, erosion of the vertebral end plate, and lytic erosion of the vertebral bodies. Plain films can also show spinal alignment and thus may be useful to establish a baseline status. Bone scans (radionuclide scintigraphy) are not very specific and have a sensitivity of only 70%,[15] although they sometimes show early foci of osteomyelitis before plain films do. Gallium 67 and technetium 99 tracers both have reasonable sensitivity, with gallium slightly more specific than technetium as a tracer, but neither has high specificity over all. Sensitivity can be raised by performing a tagged white blood cell scan, but even this shows a lack of sensitivity that impairs its utility. Other markers, including biotin labeled with indium-111, are now being investigated as more specific indicators of infection.[19] Plain films and CT show no change during the earliest stages of infection. It takes several weeks for a disk to lose height and for trabecular erosion to occur on either side of a disk from which infection will ultimately spread to the epidural space. Vertebral collapse and loss of lordosis occur only when infection is advanced.

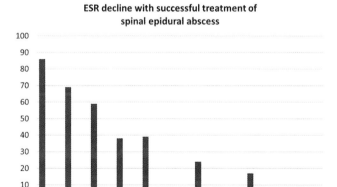

**ESR decline with successful treatment of spinal epidural abscess**

**Fig. 13.1** Restoration of a normal erythrocyte sedimentation rate (ESR) occurs gradually after surgical evacuation of spinal epidural abscess. In this patient, the ESR took 3½ months to normalize. The y-axis shows the ESR, and the x-axis shows time in weeks after surgery. Antibiotics were given for 10 weeks after surgery.

CT is most often used in guiding the percutaneous aspiration of disk spaces, vertebral bodies, or paraspinal fluid collections to provide microbiological identification of infection. CT myelography is still occasionally needed for patients in whom metallic implants degrade the quality of MR images. With the advent of open MR imaging, the previous contraindication of obesity is no longer as important in driving patients toward CT. The absence of ionizing radiation in MR imaging is another advantage of this modality compared with CT.

Contrast-enhanced MR imaging should thus be performed in all patients suspected of having an SEA unless contraindications exist. Imaging before and after the infusion of gadolinium will provide images that are sufficient to distinguish between different pathologies and to determine their location. T1-weighted images before contrast show bone infection as a hypointense signal, with particular focus on the end plates, as well as loss of the normal hyperintensity caused by fat in the vertebral marrow. On T2-weighted images, hyperintensity represents edema in the disk space, which is sometimes found in the vertebra and paravertebral region as well. In post-contrast studies, T1-weighted images show enhancement of the vertebral body, its end plates, the paravertebral soft tissues, and the epidural space[20] (**Fig. 13.2**). Because spinal infections are sometimes multifocal, the entire spine should be imaged.

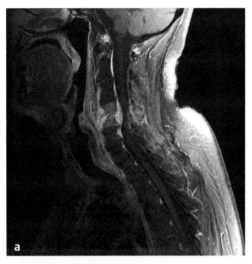

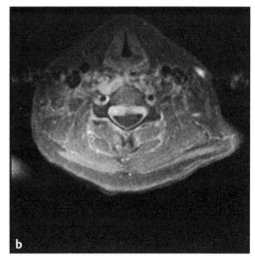

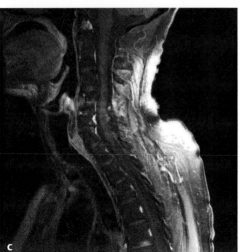

**Fig. 13.2a–c** Epidural abscess. This 51-year-old man in remission from prior acute myelogenous leukemia developed severe neck pain 1 year later. The pain radiated into both shoulders and was associated with dysphagia. Post-contrast magnetic resonance imaging showed osteomyelitis of C4 and C5 with involvement of the intervening disk space and a contiguous enhancing epidural mass anterior to the thecal sac, consistent with epidural abscess. Both sagittal **(a)** and axial **(b)** images reveal the lesion. The patient underwent biopsy and culture of the C5 vertebral body and the C4–5 disk, which confirmed osteomyelitis due to *Staphylococcus epidermidis*. He was treated with intravenous antibiotics for 10 days and then oral antibiotics. Because of persistent elevation of the erythrocyte sedimentation rate, he continued oral therapy for 9 months. He ultimately experienced complete resolution of the infection and likely fusion of C4 and C5 with this prolonged medical therapy **(c)**.

## Identifying the Pathogen

Once imaging has suggested an epidural abscess, the causative agent(s) must be identified to direct the antibiotic choices. Because hematogenous spread from other infected sites is the usual cause of SEA, cultures of urine and septum should be obtained, as should blood cultures in multiple sets. Ideally, blood cultures should be done during a septicemic phase or when temperature spikes occur. Blood cultures identify the organism in only half of cases, however, so needle biopsy of the involved vertebral body or disk space should be carried out under radiographic control. Once this is done, broad-spectrum antibiotic coverage of the usual pathogens (*Staphylococcus* species and *Streptococcus* species) should be initiated. Percutaneous biopsy yields material for successful culture in 60 to 80% of cases. When percutaneous attempts fail to yield a positive specimen, open biopsy is the next step and has a similar rate of success. Withholding antibiotics until all necessary material has been taken for culture will maximize the success of such cultures. If cultures are negative in the face of obvious clinical infection, broad-range polymerase chain reaction (PCR) techniques can be used to enhance the sensitivity of detection.[20] When no bacterial organism can be identified after several attempts, mycobacterial and fungal infections should also be considered, particularly in at-risk patients.

## Treatment

### Surgery

The mainstay of treatment for SEA has traditionally been surgery, and it remains so despite inroads that have been made by medical therapy in recent years.[6,7] Factors to be considered in the choice of treatment (surgical versus medical) include degree of sepsis, neurologic status, extent of cord compression, degree of vertebral destruction, and presence of spinal instability. Most epidural abscesses require urgent although not emergent care; however, any patient with significant myelopathy should receive prompt surgical treatment.

The heterogeneity of the clinical course in SEA makes it difficult to standardize treatment decisions. Delay in treatment can be entertained only when neurologic deficits are minimal or when comorbidities such as sepsis and coagulopathy require correction before surgery. Careful and frequent monitoring should be used for any patient undergoing medical management alone because deficits can progress rapidly and so may require a surgical strategy instead.

Planning surgery requires consideration of the level or levels of spinal involvement, the degree of cord compression, the location of the abscess within the spinal canal (anterior versus posterior), and the physical nature of the material compressing the cord. The strategies for dealing with pus and retropulsed bone are quite different. In addition, simple laminectomy may be effective for washing out a posteriorly or posterolaterally situated phlegmon and for providing cord decompression, but it may also worsen spinal instability when vertebral involvement is profound at the same level. The goals of surgery are decompression of neural structures, including cord and roots; removal of purulent material from the epidural space; removal of any granulation tissue present; and, when necessary, correction of deformity and instability caused by disruption of the vertebral column.

The great majority of patients are still treated primarily with surgery, with antibiotic therapy to follow for a period of several weeks.[21] In general, the probability of success is maximized by the removal of as much infectious material as possible. Doing this may induce or worsen instability; therefore, the surgeon must be prepared to restabilize the spine at the same sitting. Tissue adherent to the dura should not be removed too vigorously because breaching the dura may allow the infected material to be introduced into the subarachnoid space, resulting in meningitis. Once the solid material has been removed from the epidural compartment, copious irrigation with antibiotic solutions is performed. With anterior decompression, a fusion will typically be required, which is commonly done with an interposition autograft or allograft.

When necessary, reconstruction and stabilization can be delayed to a second-stage procedure. It is also important to remember that in patients with only a slight loss of lordosis or slight kyphosis, fusion may occur over time during antibiotic therapy without instrumentation. Therefore, when it is not certain that instrumentation is necessary, delaying a decision on its placement (and using an external brace in the meantime) is reasonable.

Further treatment difficulties arise when the abscess is largely ventral. In the cervical spine, a ventrally placed abscess without adjacent bony involvement can usually be treated safely by laminectomy with maintenance of the facet joints. When vertebral body involvement is more extensive, the best option is generally a formal diskectomy and vertebrectomy via an anterior approach, followed by bone grafting or cage placement with anterior plating. Trough corpectomies can be used to limit bone removal and preserve the biomechanical stability in cases of ventral SEA.[22] In the thoracic spine, a transpedicular or lateral extracavitary approach to an anterior phlegmon may be preferable, often with posterior instrumentation being necessary. Anterior infections within the midthoracic or low thoracic spine respond well to transthoracic approaches performed through a thoracotomy, but the lateral extracavitary approach can be utilized in these cases as well. A laminectomy alone for ventral thoracic disease is not advisable.

Ventral abscesses of the lower thoracic and upper lumbar spine generally require débridement by a thoracoabdominal approach, which allows bone or cage reconstruction with plating as well as removal of the phlegmon. Those patients with infection in the midlumbar or low lumbar spine can undergo decompression via a retroperitoneal approach when the infection is anteriorly placed, with the reconstruction similar to that used at higher levels. Below L2, a posterior approach is generally used.

When infection persists despite antibiotics or when it recurs, reoperation may be necessary. In this scenario, a search for sequestered and devascularized bone is needed, and thus a full corpectomy is commonly performed with reconstruction thereafter.

When patients have significant compression of the cord and thus a clinical myelopathy, steroid administration is considered both safe and useful at high doses.

Current studies suggest that the spine can be reconstructed and stabilized with safety and effectiveness even within a surgical wound contaminated by an epidural infection. As long as necrotic bone and infectious material are removed to the maximum degree, bone grafts can be used as either autografts or allografts and can fuse to native bone. By putting the fusion construct under compression, the placement of plates, rods, and screws as needed promotes bone fusion in this circumstance. As long as the infectious material is well removed and a sufficiently long course of antibiotics is given, it is rarely necessary to reoperate to remove infected or colonized instrumentation or bone graft.[17,23–26]

## Medical Therapy

Some patients can be managed with medical therapy alone and can thus avoid surgical intervention.[6,7,27,28] This choice must be made carefully and with due consideration given to the MR imaging characteristics of the epidural lesion and the neurologic status of the patient. Collections that are fluid and thus easily drained tend to be hyperintense on T2-weighted images and to enhance only peripherally around a central core of hypointensity. More solid, organized lesions (granulation tissue) tend to enhance throughout and to appear iso- or hypointense on T2-weighted images. When such a phlegmon is present and the patient is neurologically intact, medical therapy can be considered. When a patient has radiographic signs of a fluid collection but lacks any neurologic compromise, the decision is more controversial. Certainly abscesses below the conus are less surgically compelling, whereas those in the cervical and thoracic spine pose more danger for a sudden neurologic decline and thus are better managed with an operative strategy. Neurologic recovery can occur after surgery even in patients with abscesses extending over many segments, and even in those presenting with several days of complete paralysis.[29,30] Any patient treated conservatively must be frequently reassessed, and a low threshold for surgical intervention must be maintained.

The risk for deterioration while a patient is on medical therapy is not trivial. Khanna et al showed that 19% of patients who had been selected for medical therapy alone because of their relatively intact neurologic status and identifiable organism eventually required surgery because of neurologic decline while they were on medical therapy.[16] A similar rate of neurologic progression was cited by Darouiche et al and other authors.[6,15] Nevertheless, not all patients with SEA are good candidates for surgery, and the absence of spinal instability in neurologically intact patients may make medical therapy attractive.

Medical therapy requires both the administration of intravenous antibiotics (as determined by bacterial sensitivity profiling) and immobilization of the affected portion of the spine, which helps control pain and may promote fusion. The duration of therapy has not been standardized, but in general, the SEAs of patients with lesser degrees of bone infection and who are immunocompetent can clear with 6 to 8 weeks of antibiotic therapy. When osteomyelitis is present or when the patient is immunocompromised, 8 weeks of antibiotic therapy or longer is the recommended duration.[31] The route of administration is generally intravenous, with supplemental oral antibiotics used in some cases. Relapses generally occur within 6 months after the conclusion of therapy and affect up to 15% of patients.[32] The route of administration is generally intravenous. Supplemental oral antibiotics are used in some cases; however, there is no evidence that oral antibiotics are helpful, and they may be suppressive rather than curative.

The effectiveness of such therapy is gauged by reductions in pain and fever and by a decrease in the ESR. However, the ESR is not entirely reliable as a marker for infection, and some patients show sustained elevations in the face of clinical improvement.[18] In such cases, it is reasonable to extend the length of antibiotic treatment and, if the ESR elevation persists, to repeat imaging and perform a biopsy to clarify the clinical situation.

Because the most common bacterial species causing SEA are staphylococcal and streptococcal species, the most commonly used antibiotics are cephalosporins, vancomycin, and β-lactams. Vancomycin and cephalosporins penetrate infected bone and disk inefficiently, and when bone disease is extensive, a second agent (rifampin or a fluoroquinolone) may be valuable. When cultures are negative and no sensitivity typing can be meaningful, empiric therapy must be used. If treatment fails, then reimaging and repeat culturing are indicated and should include a search for less common causative agents, such as fungi and mycobacteria. Usually, those receiving intravenous antibiotics are restricted to bed for 2 weeks and thereafter are mobilized with a fitted orthosis to prevent spinal deformity and pain.

## ■ Outcome

The best predictor of outcome is the clinical and neurologic condition of the patient at the time of surgery. Neurologic deficits can decrease after decompression and washout of the abscess, and indeed patients do better after surgery for SEA than after surgery for other extrinsic compressive causes of myelopathy. In one series, surgical intervention within 24 hours of the onset of paralysis resulted in neurologic improvements in 6 of 14 patients (42%).[15] The prognosis for recovery is worse in patients who present with established and extensive deficits due to delays in treatment, or in those in whom sudden and profound decline from spinal vascular occlusion has occurred. In addition, those who present with overt sepsis do poorly.

Factors influencing outcome as determined by Khanna et al are discussed below.[16] Those who do better are neurologically intact at presentation, younger than 60 years of age, have less than 50% spinal canal compromise, have a lumbosacral location of the abscess, and undergo surgery within 72 hours. Those in whom the SEA comprises pus rather than phlegmon also have better prognosis. It is likely that multiple comorbidities and a complete sensory or motor deficit predispose to a poorer outcome. Significant recovery from a profound neurologic deficit does occur, with one study of the effectiveness of rehabilitation in SEA after surgery showing 5 of 11 patients recovering from plegia to full function over time.[33] With medical management, the prognosis depends on the patient's age, on the rate of decrease in the ESR, and on the presence of immunocompromise. Although the elderly have a poor outcome in general, when they are managed with aggressive surgery, they can do well.[7,34]

Other measures of outcome include mortality, which ranges from 3 to 23% in several series of SEA.[6,7] When it occurs, death usually stems from a missed diagnosis or from a severe coexisting illness outside the nervous system. Another important measure of outcome is maintenance of sagittal balance in the spine over time. Thus, spontaneous fusion of contiguous affected levels is a positive outcome, as is radiographic incorporation of the bone graft after surgical treatment. The best predictors of a successful outcome relate to clinical status of the patient, and in particular the disappearance of fever and pretreatment laboratory abnormalities as well as the relief of spinal and radicular pain. MR imaging findings in SEA take months to resolve, and serial imaging correlates poorly with clinical improvement.[35]

## ■ Unusual Bacteria Causing Epidural Abscess

Very occasionally, bacterial pathogens other than the usual species (*Staphylococcus*, *Streptococcus*, and *Enterococcus* species, *E. coli*, *Pseudomonas aeruginosa*, and *Proteus* species) act as the causative agents for epidural abscess. Most notable of these are *Nocardia*, *Brucella*, and *Actinomyces* species.

*Nocardia asteroides* is a gram-positive aerobe with a filamentous structure. This organism typically produces pulmonary infection in patients with immunocompromise and only rarely involves the spine. The mechanism of spread to the spine is thought to be either through direct extension from a thoracic infection or by hematogenous routes. Treatment usually includes some combination of penicillin, cephalosporin, and aminoglycoside, and treatment may be prolonged. Surgical treatment is similar to that used in SEA caused by other pathogens.[36,37]

*Actinomyces israelii* is a gram-positive bacterium that also has a filamentous structure. It typically results in a chronic draining infection containing "sulfur granules," which are not sulfur but clumps of the actual organism. This microbe commonly affects the oral cavity and paranasal sinuses and thus may extend into the soft tissues of the neck. Involvement of the spine usually is the result of contiguous spread from either the retropharyngeal area or the lungs. This bacterium usually causes vertebral destruction or deformity. Surgical intervention is used only in patients with neurologic compromise. Medical treatment includes intravenous penicillin G, ciprofloxacin, or rifampin.[38,39]

Brucellosis is uncommon in the United States but remains epidemic in countries bordering the Mediterranean Sea and in Central and South America. Human infection comes through contact with livestock or from consumption of unpasteurized milk. In 25% of cases, osteoarticular complications arise, half of which involve the spine. Thus, vertebral infections occur in 10 to 12% of cases and produce a subacute clinical scenario similar to that seen in spinal infections caused by other microbes. Spinal deformity is rarely seen, and cure occurs with antibiotic therapy in 90% of patients. Antibiotics used include tetracycline, aminoglycosides, and trimethoprim-sulfamethoxazole. Surgery is not typically necessary but occasionally is required for decompression or correction of deformity.[40–42]

Tuberculosis remains an important public health hazard throughout the world, particularly in less developed countries. The causative organism is highly prevalent in Russia, the Indian subcontinent, and eastern and central Africa because of the high incidence of human immunodeficiency virus (HIV) infection in those regions. Poor nutrition and crowded living conditions also predispose to cultivation of the disease, as does inappropriate antibiotic treatment leading to resistant strains of mycobacterial species. Involvement of the bones and joints occurs in 3 to 5% of patients with tuberculosis and rises to 60% in those with coexisting HIV infection. Half of the cases affecting bone occur in the spine and have a propensity to create deformity and thus paraplegia. Although involvement at the thoracolumbar junction is most common, any level can be affected. As with actinomycosis, tubercular involvement of the spine occurs both from hematogenous spread and by direct extension from an infected lung. Tuberculosis tends to be more indolent than other infections of the spine, more commonly involves the posterior elements of the vertebral body, and produces deformity more often. Paraspinal phlegmon or abscess is frequent. Although initial inflammation leads to abscess formation with liquid pus, in later stages caseous material forms, and both bony necrosis and ligamentous disruption contribute to spinal deformity. As the acute infection fades, a chronic infection with a fibrous reaction improves but does not typically restore complete spinal stability. Tuberculosis of the spine may be associated with calcification and even ossification, which when exuberant produces a chronic compression of the cord.

The standard treatment of spinal tuberculosis is by medical therapy with multiple agents for a prolonged period of time. The most common regimen includes isoniazid, rifampin, and pyrazinamide for 12 months or more. Although some authors recommend bed rest in the initial management of spinal tuberculosis, this is impractical in many of the countries where the disease is most prevalent. As with other forms of SEA, surgical treatment is valuable in patients with instability of the spine or in those in whom progressive neurologic symptoms stem from cord compression. The role of surgical drainage of extraspinal collections or of débridement of involved bone in helping to clear infection remains unclear. However, the confirmed indications of spinal instability, pronounced deformity, and neurologic deficit still apply as reasons to perform surgery.[43–47]

## Fungal Pathogens

Fungal infection of the spine is rarely seen and is generally associated with immunosuppression resulting from lengthy steroid use, diabetes mellitus, HIV infection, or intravenous drug abuse or occurring in conjunction with severe systemic illnesses. The most common fungal infection is candidiasis, which presents in immunocompromised patients as an opportunistic infection but in which vertebral involvement is not common. SEA occurs typically in the setting of disseminated candidiasis, and its clinical features are not particularly different from those seen with classic bacterial SEA. Treatment is also similar, and amphotericin B is the standard medical therapy. Osteomyelitis responds in 85% of the patients thus treated, but mortality is high because of the comorbid conditions usually present in other organ systems.[48,49]

Other fungal infections include coccidioidomycosis, aspergillosis, and blastomycosis. Although infection with *Coccidioides immitis* is relatively benign and usually occurs in the respiratory tract, it can disseminate. Rarely, infections within the spine occur, usually within the vertebral body and commonly extending into the epidural space. In the United States, such cases are seen mainly in the southwestern quadrant. They are treated surgically in the fashion usual for other forms of SEA and then with lifelong antifungal therapy.[50,51] Aspergillosis occurs in patients similar to those affected by *Candida* species and has a very similar treatment profile. *Aspergillus* species involve the spine more commonly than coccidioidomycosis does and rarely afflict immunocompetent patients.[52,53] Blastomycosis, which is epidemic in the southeastern United States and the Midwest, produces a granuloma presenting as a cutaneous or respiratory infection. Dissemination may produce bony involvement, particularly within the spine. The typical situation involves a destructive vertebral lesion associated with a paraspinal mass that is treated with amphotericin B or newer drugs, such as itraconazole. Epidural involvement is exceptionally unusual but has been reported.[54]

### Parasitic Infection

Occasional reports in the literature describe epidural involvement with parasitic infections of the spine. Parasitic infestation of the spinal canal is very rare in developed countries and is usually treated surgically. Examples include cases of *Echinococcus granulosus* (hydatid disease),[55] *Schistosoma mansonii* (bilharziasis),[56] and dracunculiasis (guinea worm).[57] Like schistosomiasis, cysticercosis is usually a parenchymal disease of the spinal cord or occurs in the subarachnoid space, yet cysticercosis can also form masses or collections that occupy the epidural space, producing neural compromise.[58] In general, patients with parasitic involvement of the epidural space still require systemic therapy because of the disseminated nature of such infections.

### Epidural Abscess after Therapeutic Intervention

Postoperative infections in spinal operative wounds typically do provoke an epidural abscess as well as an overlying cellulitis. Because most spinal procedures involve a laminectomy with dural exposure, any collection of purulent material within the surgical site tends to track down to the dura. The incidence of wound infection after spinal surgery averages 2%, but more infections occur in reoperative procedures or in those patients in whom prior irradiation, chemotherapy, or steroid therapy has been used. In addition, patients with poor nutrition, impaired mobility, diabetes mellitus, or a history of smoking are all at increased risk for SEA. The duration of surgery also appears to correlate positive-

ly with the risk for wound infection. We routinely give intravenous antibiotics for prophylaxis within the 60 minutes before surgery and continue them at scheduled intervals throughout the case and for 24 hours afterward. We also routinely irrigate copiously with antibiotic-containing saline to prevent intraoperative contamination.

The causative organisms in postoperative infections are typically skin flora, usually *S. aureus* or *S. epidermidis*. The diagnosis is largely a clinical one, prompted by finding drainage from a wound between 2 days and 2 weeks after surgery. Interpretation of the ESR or CRP level can be problematic because each is elevated by surgery in general; the CRP level returns to normal more quickly, but without a baseline value (often not previously obtained), a trend cannot be ascertained. CT or MR imaging usually shows a shaggy subincisional space, and although strong peripheral enhancement of this cavity may denote infection, false-positive results are common. If it appears that infection is only superficial, we treat with antibiotics alone. With frank drainage and particularly if purulent material extrudes from the wound, reexploration is indicated. This involves washout of the wound with large amounts of antibiotic solution and débridement of the depths of the wound to remove any necrotic tissue or granulation tissue. The epidural component of these abscesses may require gentle scraping of granulation tissue from the dural surface. As this may provoke a CSF leak, care must be exercised while such material is physically removed from the epidural space. After wound washout, antibiotics are continued intravenously for several days, and conversion to oral administration takes place when and if sensitivities allow. The total duration of antibiotic therapy depends on the severity of the infection but may extend for 3 to 4 weeks.

When instrumentation has been placed, a larger dead space is created that promotes infection through the buildup of epidural hematoma, an increase in necrosis of the overlying paraspinal muscles, and tissue ischemia caused by prolonged retraction. The presence of a large hematoma around the instrumentation also provides a good culture medium for the growth of microorganisms. Usually, infections after spinal instrumentation surgery take 2 to 6 weeks to become clinically apparent. A scenario of wound breakdown within this time frame does suggest an infection within the wound, as does more focal drainage. The principles of treatment are the same as those described above for simpler spinal operations, and it is generally not necessary to remove the instrumentation. If methylmethacrylate has been used, it should be removed; however, metallic implants resist infection well, and as long as isolated soft tissue has been removed from within the various crevices of the instrumentation system, a good resolution of the infection usually occurs. When necessary to relieve tension on the overlying skin and subcutaneous tissue, plastic surgical flaps can be rotated to offer better coverage of the wound and promote its ultimate healing. When loose bone graft is present within an infected area, it too should be removed because it is devitalized tissue and can provide a nidus for recurrence of the infection. Delayed infections occurring several months after surgery are usually caused by more indolent microorganisms, including *Propionibacterium acnes*, *Corynebacterium* species, and *S. epidermidis*. We do not recommend hardware removal as some authors have done.[59] Rather, we strip the glycocalyx polysaccharide shell that usually coats the instrumentation, and we do so in meticulous manner with a copious washout with antibiotic solution. If such a procedure fails to eliminate the infection, then only do we consider hardware removal. This allows as much time as possible for bony fusion to occur and thus permits removal of the instrumentation without reintroducing spinal instability.

### Infections after Other Spinal Procedures

Diskography is not done now as commonly as it once was. Infections do occur after diskography, and these include diskitis, epidural abscess, and subdural abscess if the dura has been penetrated. Severe local pain occurs a few days after the procedure with elevation of the ESR and CRP level, and a local inflammatory process can be visible on MR imaging, particularly on the post-contrast images. Treatment is medical, and the patient may also require external bracing with a period of immobilization if the pain is severe. The use of needles with a stylet helps prevent this complication but does not completely eliminate it.[60,61]

Epidural catheter placement can also provide a route of access for bacteria into the epidural space. Here again, the usual causative bacteria are staphylococcal species, reflecting skin flora. The incidence of such infections rises with the length of time the catheter is in place, with an overall incidence of 0.2 to 0.77 per 1,000 catheter-days.[62,63] Thus, patients receiving longer-term epidural catheters for control of cancer pain face a higher infectious risk. In such cases, therefore, the practice is to implant an indwelling subcutaneous system including a refillable pump attached to a completely internalized epidural catheter after a percutaneous trial to ensure effectiveness. The early signs of infection in this scenario include pain around the catheter insertion site, superficial infection at that site, and in some cases blockage of the catheter. The formation of an epidural abscess around the catheter within the nonlaminectomized portion of the spine eventually leads to a neurologic deficit. MR imaging can provide a fairly certain diagnosis.[63] When infection is mild, catheter removal with subsequent antibiotic therapy will usually clear the infection. Successful clearance of infection with medical therapy alone (and without catheter removal) has been reported but is not recommended for most patients.[28] When a neurologic deficit has developed, surgical intervention is necessary. The catheter tip should be cultured immediately on removal to allow identification of the organism and the determination of its antibiotic sensitivities. Occasional cases of sepsis with serious consequences have been reported after catheter-related epidural abscess. We recommend tunneling the catheter whenever possible as a way of preventing infection.

With the advent of percutaneous vertebroplasty and kyphoplasty as methods of treating pain caused by spinal compression fractures, a new source of epidural abscess has joined the list of those associated with foreign body placement in and around the spine. The technique involves the injection of methylmethacrylate into the cancellous center of a collapsed vertebral body. Although infection is uncommon, occasional reports are now appearing as a consequence of the widespread use of this technique in the elderly, in patients with osteoporosis, and in those with metastatic cancer.[64,65] Because methylmethacrylate is a porous, avascular substance, it is a very retentive harbor for microorganisms once they are introduced. Therefore, simple antibiotic therapy is usually unsuccessful in clearing infections associated with such vertebral augmentation. The recommended treatment for an infected vertebroplasty or kyphoplasty site, particularly when it involves an epidural abscess, is removal of the involved vertebral segment with its methylmethacrylate, copious washout with antibiotic solution, and appropriate reconstruction and instrumentation.

## Spinal Subdural Abscess

A subdural empyema contained focally within the intradural extramedullary space of the spinal canal is exceptionally rare. The literature contains approximately 65 reports, with *S. aureus* the most common bacterial source and the thoracolumbar spine the most commonly affected region. As with other spinal infections, MR imaging is the diagnostic procedure of choice. The first spinal subdural empyema was reported in 1927.[66] There is no clear pattern for gender or age. Whereas the epidural space has anatomic barriers, described previously, that limit the spread of an abscess from its point of origin, no such constraints apply within the subdural space, and thus the infectious process can extend along multiple segments of the spinal canal. The incidence of spinal subdural infection is much lower than that of cranial subdural empyema; the reasons for this are speculative but likely relate to the absence of air sinuses in the spine and to the more voluminous epidural space located there. Half of the cases involve *S. aureus*, and the others are due to the same diverse species found from time to time in SEA (*E. coli*, *M. tuberculosis*, others). Most patients with a spinal subdural abscess carry at least one factor predisposing them to infection. These include diabetes mellitus, alcoholism, and HIV infection. Many patients who develop such abscesses have had recent spinal surgery, and many have concurrent or recent infections elsewhere. In 20% of cases, the abscess occurs because of a spinal tap or a diskogram gone awry.[67] Another quarter of the cases emanate from cutaneous infections or defects, such as cellulitis, congenital dermal sinuses, and furuncles[68,69] (**Fig. 13.3**). Only 15% of these abscesses occur outside the thoracic and lumbar spine.

The symptoms usually include back pain at the affected level, fever, and neurologic deficits appropriate to the site and degree of compression exerted by the phlegmon.

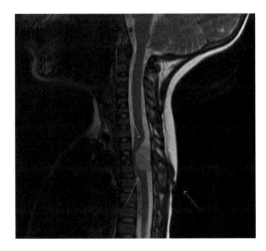

**Fig. 13.3** Epidural abscess developing in association with a congenital dermal sinus tract in an infant. This T2-weighted sagittal magnetic resonance image shows significant cord compression from a well-defined abscess. The arrows show both the dorsally placed globular lesion and the immediately adjacent sinus tract coursing cephalad from its origin on the skin. The abscess was surgically drained and the sinus tract excised, with normal development thereafter.

Disturbance of consciousness can occur if the abscess generalizes into a diffuse spinal meningitis leading to meningoencephalitis. Spinal tenderness is present in only 20 to 30% of patients, so it cannot be used as a feature to differentiate a subdural infection from an epidural abscess. Meningitis is common in these cases, and more of the patients are ill at presentation than those with SEA; the progression of the disease is usually quite rapid. Diagnosis is generally made by reviewing the MR images. If lumbar puncture is done because of meningeal signs and fever and pus is demonstrated, then spinal subdural empyema should be suspected. Intraspinal gas on imaging should lead to inclusion in the differential diagnosis of spinal subdural empyema caused by a gas-forming microorganism. Both aerobic and anaerobic microbes can produce gases, including hydrogen, nitrogen, hydrogen sulfide, and methane, which accumulate because of their low degree of aqueous solubility.[70]

The treatment of choice for spinal subdural abscess is surgical drainage of the abscess. The mortality rate is much higher in patients treated with medical therapy alone (80%) than in those treated with surgery (18%).[71] Like intracranial subdural empyemas, spinal cases should be considered as surgical emergencies because patients can become paralyzed within hours after the onset of the deficit due to vascular thrombosis induced by the infection. Because of the intradural location of the abscess, dural opening is required, and closure in such cases should be done with monofilament suture, such as polypropylene (Prolene; Ethicon 360), rather than braided suture, such as nylon (Nurolon; Ethicon 360) or silk. In cases extending over multiple levels, it may be possible to do a more limited laminectomy and use a lavage system within the subdural space.[72] During drainage of the intradural pus, preservation of the arachnoid is ideal but usually not possible. After surgery, intravenous antibiotics appropriately chosen from culture results are given for 4 to 6 weeks. The role of dexamethasone in preventing or moderating occlusive thrombolysis remains controversial.

Because the subdural space is the central compartment sandwiched between the epidural space and the spinal cord, it is possible for a subdural spinal abscess also to involve either of the two contiguous compartments by crossing the dural or pial barrier.[73,74] Involvement of all three has not as yet been reported.

## Spinal Intramedullary Abscess

Spinal intramedullary abscess is rare but somewhat more common than a subdural abscess of the spine. Cases tend to arise either in young people (younger than 25 years of age) or in older adults (older than 50 years of age). The usual route of dissemination is hematogenous in adults, and occasional correlation with patent foramen ovale has been reported.[75,76] In children, spinal intramedullary abscess may be associated with a dermal sinus tract.[77]

*Staphylococcus* species, *Streptococcus* species, and gram-negative bacilli are responsible for most intramedullary abscesses from which bacteria can be cultured. The most common finding, however, is a sterile culture, seen in 25 to 40% of cases. Polymicrobial infections account for up to 21% of cases.[78,79] Less common pathogens can also cause intramedullary infection and include *Listeria*, *Brucella*, *Actinomyces*, *Nocardia*, *Candida*, and *Toxoplasma*. In the work-up before surgery, post-contrast MRI is the diagnostic test of choice. This study may show a nodular pattern of enhancement rather than ring enhancement, which with a lack of pleocytosis in any CSF sampled helps to distinguish an abscess from a metastatic tumor in the cord. A typical example is shown in **Fig. 13.4**. Cord edema with variable and heterogeneous enhancement may signify early myelitis as a precursor to an abscess, which takes 7 to 15 days to form after local bacterial inoculation. It has been suggested that enhancement at the poles of the lesion and a peri-ependymal pattern should raise the suspicion for an intramedullary abscess.[80] The same authors report that pial and arachnoidal enhancement can reflect perimedullary venous dilatation representing thrombosed veins and may offer

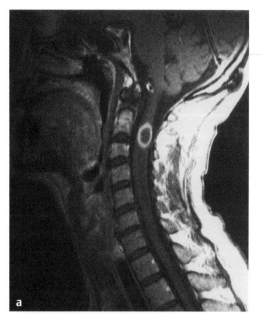

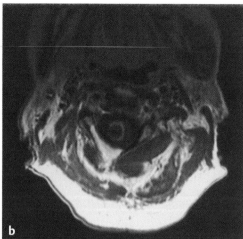

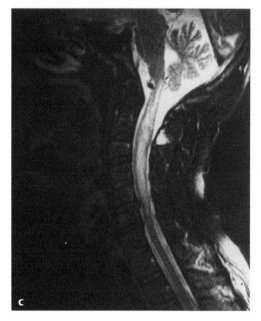

**Fig. 13.4a–c** Intramedullary abscess. A 54-year-old man with the onset of hemiparesis 8 months after removal of an adenocarcinoma of the gastroesophageal junction. In the interim, he had had two episodes of empyema at a chest tube site; the first occurred 5 weeks after surgery and the second 5 months after the first. With the earlier episode of empyema, he had generalized sepsis. Six weeks after the later episode, neurologic decline began. He was afebrile with leukocytosis to 13,200/mm³ and a left shift. Post-contrast magnetic resonance imaging showed an intramedullary ring-enhancing lesion at C2–3 **(a)** that was eccentric within the cord **(b)** and associated with significant edema extending from the cervicomedullary junction to C6 on T2-weighted images **(c)**. The bacterium cultured from the abscess at surgery was *Streptococcus milleri*, and the patient regained significant neurologic function while completing 4 weeks of intravenous antibiotics. He died of pulmonary embolism 7 weeks after surgery.

evidence of an infectious etiology for any ring-enhancing lesion in the cord.

A high index of suspicion, early diagnosis, and prompt surgical evacuation in conjunction with appropriate intravenous antibiotics given for up to 8 weeks constitute the best strategy for treating an intramedullary abscess. The initial antibiotic coverage should be broad enough to treat gram-positive and gram-negative organisms as well as anaerobes, but coverage should be tailored to the causative pathogens once they have been identified. Although no data exist on antibiotic penetration into the spinal cord (as opposed to the brain, where much evidence has been gathered), it seems logical to choose drugs that penetrate the blood–brain and blood–CSF barriers. We tend to use a combination of vancomycin, ceftazidime, and metronidazole as initial therapy for this disorder. Penicillin should be added or substituted to cover *Listeria* if the patient is immunocompromised or has a history of alcohol abuse, hepatic cirrhosis, or diabetes mellitus.[81] Antibiotic treatment alone is occasionally successful if the infection is chronic, the pathogen known, the abscess small, and neurologic deficits absent, and myelitis without defined abscess formation is usually treated with antibiotics alone.[75,79,80] The use of perioperative steroids must be carefully individualized, with the benefits of reducing cord edema balanced against the immunosuppressive and other potentially harmful properties of such medications.

Early recognition optimizes the chances for functional recovery, with the best results occurring when treatment begins within 3 days after the onset of symptoms. Once treatment concludes, the overall rate of residual neurologic impairment is 70%, and prolonged antibiotic therapy is recommended because these lesions have a propensity to recur.[79,82]

The pathogenesis of spinal intramedullary abscess recapitulates that of an intracerebral abscess. The bacterial nidus is first infiltrated by polymorphonuclear leukocytes. Suppurative myelitis follows, then the development of a necrotic center with liquefaction.[83] Spreading along the white matter tracts, the average lesion extends over three to six spinal segments. Ultimately, the central pus is circumscribed by the development of fibrous granulation tissues. All levels of the cord are equally affected. The lesions can be acute, subacute, or chronic in nature. An acute intramedullary abscess presents with back pain, fever, and neurologic deficits in a fashion similar to that of an acute transverse myelitis. A chronic abscess more closely mimics an intramedullary tumor, with the absence of fever, a gradually developing back pain, and the slow onset of neurologic deficit. Most patients have motor impairment and bladder impairment, pain, and often sensory loss. Interestingly, only half are febrile.[75]

Surgical treatment generally involves laminectomy with a midline myelotomy to gain access to the abscess cavity, which tends to be relatively central within the cord. After gentle irrigation, the patient's wound is closed with monofilament sutures, and then he or she is placed on antibiotics for 6 to 8 weeks. Although the mortality rate (unlike that in epidural or subdural abscesses) is quite low, the neurologic recovery tends to be incomplete. As in any spinal cord procedure, neurologic outcome depends mainly on the preoperative level of function of the patient.

## References

1. Makins GH, Abbott FC. II. On acute primary osteomyelitis of the vertebrae. Ann Surg 1896; 23(5):510–539

2. Ramsay Hunt J. Acute infectious osteomyelitis of the spine and acute suppurative perimeningitis. Med Record 1904;65:641–650

3. Walker AE. A History of Neurological Surgery. Baltimore, MD: Williams & Wilkins; 1951

4. Hlavin ML, Kaminski HJ, Ross JS, Ganz E. Spinal epidural abscess: a ten-year perspective. Neurosurgery 1990;27(2):177–184

5. Rigamonti D, Liem L, Sampath P, et al. Spinal epidural abscess: contemporary trends in etiology, evaluation, and management. Surg Neurol 1999;52(2):189–196, discussion 197

6. Darouiche RO. Spinal epidural abscess. N Engl J Med 2006;355(19):2012–2020

7. Pradilla G, Nagahama Y, Spivak AM, Bydon A, Rigamonti D. Spinal epidural abscess: current diagnosis and management. Curr Infect Dis Rep 2010;12(6):484–491

8. Chen SH, Chang WN, Lu CH, et al. The clinical characteristics, therapeutic outcome, and prognostic factors of non-tuberculous bacterial spinal epidural abscess in adults: a hospital-based study. Acta Neurol Taiwan 2011;20(2):107–113

9. Smith C, Kavar B. Extensive spinal epidural abscess as a complication of Crohn's disease. J Clin Neurosci 2010;17(1):144–146

10. Russell NA, Vaughan R, Morley TP. Spinal epidural infection. Can J Neurol Sci 1979;6(3): 325–328

11. Rankin RM, Flothow PG. Pyogenic infection of the spinal epidural space. West J Surg Obstet Gynecol 1946;54:320–323

12. Feldenzer JA, McKeever PE, Schaberg DR, Campbell JA, Hoff JT. Experimental spinal epidural abscess: a pathophysiological model in the rabbit. Neurosurgery 1987;20(6):859–867

13. Feldenzer JA, McKeever PE, Schaberg DR, Campbell JA, Hoff JT. The pathogenesis of spinal epidural abscess: microangiographic studies in an experimental model. J Neurosurg 1988;69(1):110–114

14. Davis DP, Salazar A, Chan TC, Vilke GM. Prospective evaluation of a clinical decision guideline to diagnose spinal epidural abscess in patients who present to the emergency department with spine pain. J Neurosurg Spine 2011;14(6):765–770

15. Darouiche RO, Hamill RJ, Greenberg SB, Weathers SW, Musher DM. Bacterial spinal epidural abscess. Review of 43 cases and literature survey. Medicine (Baltimore) 1992;71(6):369–385

16. Khanna RK, Malik GM, Rock JP, Rosenblum ML. Spinal epidural abscess: evaluation of factors

influencing outcome. Neurosurgery 1996;39(5): 958–964

17. Lifeso RM. Pyogenic spinal sepsis in adults. Spine 1990;15(12):1265–1271

18. Carragee EJ, Kim D, van der Vlugt T, Vittum D. The clinical use of erythrocyte sedimentation rate in pyogenic vertebral osteomyelitis. Spine 1997; 22(18):2089–2093

19. Lazzeri E, Erba P, Perri M, et al. Scintigraphic imaging of vertebral osteomyelitis with 111in-biotin. Spine 2008;33(7):E198–E204

20. Fuursted K, Arpi M, Lindblad BE, Pedersen LN. Broad-range PCR as a supplement to culture for detection of bacterial pathogens in patients with a clinically diagnosed spinal infection. Scand J Infect Dis 2008;40(10):772–777

21. Boström A, Oertel M, Ryang Y, et al. Treatment strategies and outcome in patients with non-tuberculous spinal epidural abscess—a review of 46 cases. Minim Invasive Neurosurg 2008;51(1):36–42

22. Deshmukh VR. Midline trough corpectomies for the evacuation of an extensive ventral cervical and upper thoracic spinal epidural abscess. J Neurosurg Spine 2010;13(2):229–233

23. Przybylski GJ, Sharan AD. Single-stage autogenous bone grafting and internal fixation in the surgical management of pyogenic discitis and vertebral osteomyelitis. J Neurosurg 2001;94(1, Suppl): 1–7

24. Ruf M, Stoltze D, Merk HR, Ames M, Harms J. Treatment of vertebral osteomyelitis by radical debridement and stabilization using titanium mesh cages. Spine 2007;32(9):E275–E280

25. Carragee E, Iezza A. Does acute placement of instrumentation in the treatment of vertebral osteomyelitis predispose to recurrent infection: long-term follow-up in immune-suppressed patients. Spine 2008;33(19):2089–2093

26. Robinson Y, Tschoeke SK, Kayser R, Boehm H, Heyde CE. Reconstruction of large defects in vertebral osteomyelitis with expandable titanium cages. Int Orthop 2009;33(3):745–749

27. Lyu RK, Chen CJ, Tang LM, Chen ST. Spinal epidural abscess successfully treated with percutaneous, computed tomography-guided, needle aspiration and parenteral antibiotic therapy: case report and review of the literature. Neurosurgery 2002;51(2):509–512, discussion 512

28. Perez-Toro MR, Burton AW, Hamid B, Koyyalagunta D. Two-Tuohy needle and catheter technique for fluoroscopically guided percutaneous drainage of spinal epidural abscess: a case report. Pain Med 2009;10(3):501–505

29. Grieve JP, Ashwood N, O'Neill KS, Moore AJ. A retrospective study of surgical and conservative treatment for spinal extradural abscess. Eur Spine J 2000;9(1):67–71

30. Katonis P, Souvatzis X, Tsavalas N, Alpantaki K. Reversal of tetraplegia in a patient with haematogenous cervical epidural abscess. Acta Orthop Belg 2011;77(4):543–547

31. Jensen AG, Espersen F, Skinhøj P, Frimodt-Møller N. Bacteremic *Staphylococcus aureus* spondylitis. Arch Intern Med 1998;158(5):509–517

32. Roblot F, Besnier JM, Juhel L, et al. Optimal duration of antibiotic therapy in vertebral osteo-

myelitis. Semin Arthritis Rheum 2007;36(5): 269–277

33. Koo DW, Townson AF, Dvorak MF, Fisher CG. Spinal epidural abscess: a 5-year case-controlled review of neurologic outcomes after rehabilitation. Arch Phys Med Rehabil 2009;90(3):512–516

34. Cahill DW, Love LC, Rechtine GR. Pyogenic osteomyelitis of the spine in the elderly. J Neurosurg 1991;74(6):878–886

35. Kowalski TJ, Layton KF, Berbari EF, et al. Follow-up MR imaging in patients with pyogenic spine infections: lack of correlation with clinical features. AJNR Am J Neuroradiol 2007;28(4):693–699

36. Atalay B, Azap O, Cekinmez M, Caner H, Haberal M. Nocardial epidural abscess of the thoracic spinal cord and review of the literature. J Infect Chemother 2005;11(3):169–171

37. West KR, Mason RC, Sun M. *Nocardia* spinal epidural abscess: 14-year follow-up. Orthopedics 2012;35(1):e128–e131

38. Yung BC, Cheng JC, Chan TT, Loke TK, Lo J, Lau PY. Aggressive thoracic actinomycosis complicated by vertebral osteomyelitis and epidural abscess leading to spinal cord compression. Spine 2000;25(6):745–748

39. Eftekhar B, Ketabchi E, Ghodsi M, Ahmadi A. Cervical epidural actinomycosis. Case report. J Neurosurg 2001;95(1, Suppl):132–134

40. Pina MA, Modrego PJ, Uroz JJ, Cobeta JC, Lerin FJ, Baiges JJ. Brucellar spinal epidural abscess of cervical location: report of four cases. Eur Neurol 2001; 45(4):249–253

41. Ugarriza LF, Porras LF, Lorenzana LM, Rodríguez-Sánchez JA, García-Yagüe LM, Cabezudo JM. Brucellar spinal epidural abscesses. Analysis of eleven cases. Br J Neurosurg 2005;19(3):235–240

42. Gerberding JL, Romero JM, Ferraro MJ. Case records of the Massachusetts General Hospital. Case 34-2008. A 58-year-old woman with neck pain and fever. N Engl J Med 2008;359(18):1942–1949

43. Rezai AR, Lee M, Cooper PR, Errico TJ, Koslow M. Modern management of spinal tuberculosis. Neurosurgery 1995;36(1):87–97, discussion 97–98

44. Lindahl S, Nyman RS, Brismar J, Hugosson C, Lundstedt C. Imaging of tuberculosis. IV. Spinal manifestations in 63 patients. Acta Radiol 1996;37(4):506–511

45. Metta H, Corti M, Redini L, Yampolsky C, Schtirbu R. Spinal epidural abscess due to *Mycobacterium tuberculosis* in a patient with AIDS: case report and review of the literature. Braz J Infect Dis 2006; 10(2):146–148

46. Muzii VF, Mariottini A, Zalaffi A, Carangelo BR, Palma L. Cervical spine epidural abscess: experience with microsurgical treatment in eight cases. J Neurosurg Spine 2006;5(5):392–397

47. Mathew J, Tripathy P, Grewal S. Epidural tuberculosis involving the entire spine. Neurol Neurochir Pol 2009;43(5):470–474

48. Chia SL, Tan BH, Tan CT, Tan SB. *Candida* spondylodiscitis and epidural abscess: management with shorter courses of anti-fungal therapy in combination with surgical debridement. J Infect 2005; 51(1):17–23

49. Metcalfe S, Morgan-Hough C. Cervical epidural abscess and vertebral osteomyelitis following non-traumatic oesophageal rupture: a case report and discussion. Eur Spine J 2009;18(Suppl 2): 224–227

50. Herron LD, Kissel P, Smilovitz D. Treatment of coccidioidal spinal infection: experience in 16 cases. J Spinal Disord 1997;10(3):215–222

51. Kakarla UK, Kalani MY, Sharma GK, Sonntag VK, Theodore N. Surgical management of coccidioidomycosis of the spine: clinical article. J Neurosurg Spine 2011;15(4):441–446

52. Dubbeld P, van Oostenbrugge RJ, Twinjstra A, Schouten HC. Spinal epidural abscess due to *Aspergillus* infection of the vertebrae: report of 3 cases. Neth J Med 1996;48(1):18–23

53. Tew CW, Han FC, Jureen R, Tey BH. *Aspergillus* vertebral osteomyelitis and epidural abscess. Singapore Med J 2009;50(4):e151–e154

54. Hardjasudarma M, Willis B, Black-Payne C, Edwards R. Pediatric spinal blastomycosis: case report. Neurosurgery 1995;37(3):534–536

55. Karadereler S, Orakdögen M, Kiliç K, Ozdogan C. Primary spinal extradural hydatid cyst in a child: case report and review of the literature. Eur Spine J 2002;11(5):500–503

56. Ruberti RF, Saio M. Epidural *Bilharzioma mansoni* compressing the spinal cord: case report. East Afr Med J 1999;76(7):414–416

57. Legmann P, Chiras J, Launay M, Philippon J, Bories J. Epidural dracunculiasis: a rare cause of spinal cord compression. Neuroradiology 1980;20(1): 43–45

58. Delobel P, Signate A, El Guedj M, et al. Unusual form of neurocysticercosis associated with HIV infection. Eur J Neurol 2004;11(1):55–58

59. Richards BR, Emara KM. Delayed infections after posterior TSRH spinal instrumentation for idiopathic scoliosis: revisited. Spine 2001;26(18): 1990–1996

60. Connor PM, Darden BV II. Cervical discography complications and clinical efficacy. Spine 1993;18(14):2035–2038

61. Junila J, Niinimäki T, Tervonen O. Epidural abscess after lumbar discography. A case report. Spine 1997;22(18):2191–2193

62. Byers K, Axelrod P, Michael S, Rosen S. Infections complicating tunneled intraspinal catheter systems used to treat chronic pain. Clin Infect Dis 1995;21(2):403–408

63. Sillevis Smitt P, Tsafka A, van den Bent M, et al. Spinal epidural abscess complicating chronic epidural analgesia in 11 cancer patients: clinical findings and magnetic resonance imaging. J Neurol 1999;246(9):815–820

64. Vats HS, McKiernan FE. Infected vertebroplasty: case report and review of literature. Spine 2006;31(22):E859–E862

65. Cosar M, Sasani M, Oktenoglu T, et al. The major complications of transpedicular vertebroplasty. J Neurosurg Spine 2009;11(5):607–613

66. Velissaris D, Aretha D, Fligou F, Filos KS. Spinal subdural *Staphylococcus aureus* abscess: case report and review of the literature. World J Emerg Surg 2009;4:31

67. Lownie SP, Ferguson GG. Spinal subdural empyema complicating cervical discography. Spine 1989;14(12):1415–1417

68. Levy ML, Wieder BH, Schneider J, Zee CS, Weiss MH. Subdural empyema of the cervical spine: clinicopathological correlates and magnetic resonance imaging. Report of three cases. J Neurosurg 1993;79(6):929–935

69. Park SW, Yoon SH, Cho KH, Shin YS, Ahn YH. Infantile lumbosacral spinal subdural abscess with sacral dermal sinus tract. Spine 2007;32(1): E52–E55

70. Nadkarni T, Shah A, Kansal R, Goel A. An intradural-extramedullary gas-forming spinal abscess in a patient with diabetes mellitus. J Clin Neurosci 2010;17(2):263–265

71. Bartels RH, de Jong TR, Grotenhuis JA. Spinal subdural abscess. Case report. J Neurosurg 1992; 76(2):307–311

72. Kim SH, Lee JK, Jang JW, Seo BR, Kim TS, Kim SH. Laminotomy with continuous irrigation in patients with pyogenic spondylitis in thoracic and lumbar spine. J Korean Neurosurg Soc 2011; 50(4):332–340

73. Hershkowitz S, Link R, Ravden M, Lipow K. Spinal empyema in Crohn's disease. J Clin Gastroenterol 1990;12(1):67–69

74. Alessi G, Lemmerling M, Nathoo N. Combined spinal subdural tuberculous empyema and intramedullary tuberculoma in an HIV-positive patient. Eur Radiol 2003;13(8):1899–1901

75. Byrne RW, von Roenn KA, Whisler WW. Intramedullary abscess: a report of two cases and a review of the literature. Neurosurgery 1994;35(2): 321–326, discussion 326

76. David C, Brasme L, Peruzzi P, Bertault R, Vinsonneau M, Ingrand D. Intramedullary abscess of the spinal cord in a patient with a right-to-left shunt: case report. Clin Infect Dis 1997;24(1):89–90

77. Tufan K, Cekinmez M, Sener L, Erdogan B. Infected lumbar dermoid cyst presenting with tetraparesis secondary to holocord central lesion. J Child Neurol 2008;23(8):934–937

78. Candon E, Frerebeau P. Bacterial abscesses of the spinal cord. Review of the literature (73 cases) [in French]. Rev Neurol (Paris) 1994;150(5): 370–376

79. Chan CT, Gold WL. Intramedullary abscess of the spinal cord in the antibiotic era: clinical features, microbial etiologies, trends in pathogenesis, and outcomes. Clin Infect Dis 1998;27(3):619–626

80. Condette-Auliac S, Lacour JC, Anxionnat R, et al. MRI aspects of spinal cord abscesses. Report of 5 cases and review of the literature [in French]. J Neuroradiol 1998;25(3):189–200

81. Pfadenhauer K, Rossmanith T. Spinal manifestation of neurolisteriosis. J Neurol 1995;242(3): 153–156

82. Morandi X, Mercier P, Fournier HD, Brassier G. Dermal sinus and intramedullary spinal cord abscess. Report of two cases and review of the literature. Childs Nerv Syst 1999;15(4):202–206, discussion 207–208

83. DiTullio MV Jr. Intramedullary spinal abscess: a case report with a review of 53 previously described cases. Surg Neurol 1977;7(6):351–354

# IV

# Neurosurgical Issues

# 14

# Neurosurgical Antibiotic Prophylaxis

Daraspreet Singh Kainth, Dino Terzic, and Stephen J. Haines

## ◼ General Principles of Antibiotic Prophylaxis

Effective antibiotics for use in neurosurgical procedures provide adequate coverage of the organisms commonly associated with neurosurgical infections, such as staphylococci. An ideal antibiotic will have minimal adverse effects and be low in cost.[1] In addition, it should reach adequate concentrations in the tissues of the operative site, have the least potential for adverse side effects, have a half-life that permits single-dose injections, and not interact with other drugs given perioperatively.[2]

The Centers for Disease Control and Prevention (CDC) has provided recommendations in regard to the administration of prophylactic antibiotics. The CDC recommendations are based on a thorough review of the literature and are categorized

based on the level of evidence to support them. These recommendations are outlined in **Tables 14.1** and **14.2**.[3] The CDC recommends that a prophylactic antibiotic be administered intravenously at the appropriate time before an incision is made such that the bactericidal concentration of the drug has been established when the incision is made.[3] Prophylactic antibiotics should not be extended significantly into the postoperative period.

The administration of prophylactic antibiotics is not without risks. Before administration, the clinical history should be examined to prevent the administration of antibiotics to which the patient may have an allergic reaction. Other risks associated with antibiotic use include thrombophlebitis and the suppression of natural flora, which can lead to urinary or gastrointestinal infections.[4] Allergic reactions to

**Table 14.1** Classification of Centers for Disease Control and Prevention recommendations for the prevention of surgical site infections[3]

| Rankings | Recommendations |
|---|---|
| Category 1A | Strongly recommended for implementation and supported by well-designed experimental, clinical, or epidemiologic studies |
| Category 1B | Strongly recommended for implementation and supported by some experimental, clinical, or epidemiologic studies and strong theoretical rationale |
| Category II | Suggested for implementation and supported by suggestive clinical or epidemiologic studies or theoretical rationale |
| No recommendation; unresolved issue | Practices for which insufficient evidence or no consensus regarding efficacy exists |

**Table 14.2** Antimicrobial prophylaxis recommendations[3]

| Category IA |
|---|
| • Select an antimicrobial agent with efficacy against expected pathogens. For neurosurgical patients, the antibiotic regimen should cover gram-positive organisms such as *Staphylococcus* species. |
| • The intravenous route should be used to obtain adequate serum levels during the operation and for at most a few hours after the incision is closed. |

| Category IB |
|---|
| • Vancomycin should not be routinely used for antimicrobial prophylaxis. |
| • Additional intraoperative doses of prophylactic antibiotics should be considered in cases in which operative length exceeds the half-life of the drug, in operations with significant blood loss, and in operations on morbidly obese patients. |

penicillin derivatives are quite common. Cephalosporins cause fewer allergic reactions; however, they demonstrate cross reactivity in roughly 10% of patients with penicillin allergy.[2] In addition, prophylactic antibiotics have been found to be associated with the risk for developing *Clostridium difficile* colitis, although *C. difficile* colonization is more commonly associated with prolonged antibiotic treatment.[5,6]

Antibiotics for surgical prophylaxis should be chosen to have as narrow a spectrum as possible while still covering relevant pathogens. The widespread use of broad-spectrum antibiotics leads to the development of resistant organisms.[2] For example, the increasing prevalence of methicillin-resistant *Staphylococcus aureus* (MRSA) is concerning.[4] Antibiotics that are typically used to treat resistant organisms should not routinely be used for prophylaxis unless no alternative is available.[2]

Even with the use of prophylactic antibiotics, infections are not completely preventable. Inherent factors may exist that increase the risk for developing a postoperative infection, such as malnutrition, immunosuppression, diabetes mellitus, and steroid use. Intraoperative conditions that increase the risk for infection include longer duration of the operation, placement of drains in the wound, blood transfusions, cerebrospinal fluid (CSF) fistulas, and tissue injury.[2]

## ■ Clinical Data Regarding Systemic Antimicrobial Prophylaxis in Neurosurgical Procedures

The incidence of infection after clean neurosurgical procedures ranges from 1 to 3%.[1] Although the incidence of infection is low, such infections carry the risk for potentially devastating complications in neurosurgical procedures. Currently, prophylactic antibiotics in clean neurosurgical procedures are used routinely and have become the standard of care.[7] Randomized controlled trials have demonstrated that the use of prophylactic antibiotics reduces the incidence of surgical site infections. Randomized studies from the 1970s, 1980s, and early 1990s have concluded that systemic antibiotic prophylaxis is effective at reducing the infection rate in clean neurosurgical procedures.[8–16]

In 1994, Barker conducted a meta-analysis of randomized studies published prior to 1992, comparing antibiotics with placebo in clean neurosurgical procedures.[17] Pooled data from eight eligible randomized studies showed 19 infections in 1,014 craniotomies with prophylactic antibiotics and 93 infections in 1,061 craniotomies without prophylactic antibiotics. The difference was statistically significant, and the author estimated that the odds of infection without the use of antibiotics are 4.2 times higher than the odds of infection with the use of antibiotic prophylaxis. Over all, the estimated incidence of infection was 2% with antibiotics and 8% without antibiotics ($p < 0.001$).[17] These results confirmed that systemic antibiotic prophylaxis is effective in reducing the infection rate after clean neurosurgical procedures. After the establishment that systemic antibiotic prophylaxis is superior to placebo, subsequent trials have focused on comparing different antibiotic regimens.

When the blood–CSF barrier is intact, the cephalosporins commonly used for prophylaxis in neurosurgical procedures do not penetrate the CSF.[18–20] In 1979, Friedrich et al demonstrated that cephacetril, a first-generation cephalosporin, is not detectable in the CSF when the blood–CSF barrier is intact.[19] Similarly, Knoop et al demonstrated that cefotiam, a second-generation cephalosporin, does not penetrate the CSF during surgery.[20] On the other hand, cephalosporins do demonstrate good penetration of the CSF when the blood–brain barrier is disrupted, as in the case of meningeal inflammation. For example, Cherubin et al in 1989 and Cadoz et al in 1981 described the excellent penetration of ceftriaxone into the CSF and the quick clearance of bacteria in children with meningitis.[21,22] Case series and randomized controlled trials have shown that ceftriaxone used as prophylaxis in neurosurgical procedures is effective at reducing surgical site infections.[14,23,24]

Even though cephalosporins do not effectively penetrate the CSF in the absence of meningeal inflammation, they are able to reach effective concentrations in the tissue to prevent surgical site infections.[25] However, after a neurosurgical procedure, damage may occur to the blood–brain barrier that enables the CSF penetration of antibiotics.[26,27] Other prophylactic systemic antibiotic regimens that have been used in neurosurgical procedures include piperacillin, vancomycin, vancomycin with gentamicin, cloxacillin, and oxacillin.[9–12,14–16,28]

At present, no regimen has been shown to be superior to others in terms of reducing the infection rate. The attempt to demonstrate different degrees of effectiveness for different antibiotics is constrained by the sample sizes required for definitive studies. When the clean neurosurgical procedure infection rate with the use of antibiotic prophylaxis approximates 1%, trials with an 80% chance of demonstrating an infection rate decrease to 0.5% need to have approximately 2,000 patients. Decisions regarding the appropriate prophylactic antibiotic to administer will depend on local microorganism sensitivity profiles and external factors, such as cost.

In 2001, Zhu et al conducted a prospective randomized trial comparing the use of prophylactic ceftriaxone and ampicillin-sulbactam in clean neurosurgical operations. Surgical site infections occurred in 3.3% of patients in the ceftriaxone group and 2.3% of patients in the ampicillin-sulbactam group. There was no statistically significant difference in the infection rates.[1] However, because the trial was not designed as an equivalence trial, the absence of a significant difference must be interpreted with caution. We cannot reliably conclude whether differences actually exist in various antibiotic regimens unless such trials are designed as equivalence trials or unless they are adequately powered to detect differences in infection rates.

Similarly, Whitby et al[29] compared infection rates in neurosurgical procedures that used either cefotaxime or trimethoprim-sulfamethoxazole as systemic antibiotic prophylaxis. The infection rate in the cefotaxime group was 2.5%, and the infection rate was 2.3% in the trimethoprim-sulfamethoxazole group. The authors concluded that both regimens are equally effective at controlling neurosurgical infection rates.[29] The sample size was calculated to achieve a power of 0.8 or greater, assuming an infection rate of 4% in the absence of prophylaxis and a reduction in the rate to 2% with prophylaxis.

The neurosurgical literature discussing the use of prophylactic antibiotics in clean–contaminated procedures is limited. Clean–contaminated procedures are defined by entry into the respiratory, gastrointestinal, or genitourinary tract under controlled conditions. This circumstance is encountered during transnasal trans-sphenoidal approaches, transoral approaches, or other complex cranial base approaches. The general surgery literature has demonstrated the beneficial role of prophylactic antibiotics in this group, such as in cases in which the bowel or biliary tract is entered.[30,31]

Dirty and contaminated wounds are frequently encountered in the trauma setting. The use of antibiotics in this situation is of therapeutic value and no longer prophylactic. Factors such as the level of contamination, the patient's immune status, violation of the dura mater, and the extent of débridement required will play a role in determining the administration of antibiotics.

## ■ Timing and Duration of Prophylaxis

Early animal model experiments by Burke and by Miles et al established the importance of the timing of antibiotic administration in preventing incision infections.[32,33] Burke established that systemic antibiotics have no effect on primary staphylococcal infections if the bacteria have been present in the tissue longer than 3 hours before the administration of antibiotics. In order for the antibiotic to suppress an infection, the antibiotic has to be present before the bacteria have time to gain access to the tissue.

With regard to the timing of the administration of prophylactic antibiotics, the antibiotic should be given at the appropriate time before the operation begins such that the bactericidal concentration of the drug has been established when the incision is made.[3] The exact timing will depend on the pharmacokinetics of the drug. In general, prophylactic antibiotics are suggested to be given within 1 hour before the incision is made.[2] A study by Galandiuk et al showed that the infection rate is higher in general surgery patients who receive prophylactic antibiotics more than 1 hour before the incision is made.[34]

Similarly, Classen et al[35] showed that the timing of prophylactic antibiotic administration has an impact on the rate of developing an infection. They prospectively monitored the infection rate in 2,847 patients undergoing elective clean or clean–contaminated surgical procedures. The patients were divided into four groups according to the time of prophylactic antibiotic administration. The groups included patients who received antibiotics between 24 and 2 hours before incision time (early), within 2 hours before incision (preoperative), within 3 hours after incision (perioperative), and between 3 and 24 hours after incision (postoperative). The patients who received the antibiotic within 2 hours before incision had the lowest infection rate (0.6%), which suggested that appropriate timing of administration should fall within this window.

In terms of the duration of prophylactic antibiotic, there is no evidence to support multiple-dose versus single-dose administration. No neurosurgical trials exist on this topic, although it has been examined in the surgery literature. DiPiro et al have reported on eight studies that compared a single-dose prophylactic regimen versus multiple-dose regimens of the same drug. In all of these studies, no difference in the infection rates was witnessed.[36] Such results fit with pioneering experimental animal data, which showed that antimicrobials administered as soon as within 3 hours after bacterial contamination of the wound do not influence the size of the skin lesion measured at 24 hours.[32,33,36]

Similarly, in a prospective randomized trial by Nooyen et al, no statistically significant difference in infection rates was seen in patients undergoing coronary artery bypass grafting who were randomized to receive either a single dose of cefuroxime at the induction of anesthesia or the same dose for an additional 3 days consecutively.[37] A total of 844 patients were randomized, and the sternal site infection rate was 14% in the single-dose group compared with 13% in the 3-day-course group.

These trials demonstrate that there is no significant benefit to extending the administration of prophylactic antibiotics. Given the risks and complications that can occur with antibiotic administration, without any definitive evidence for extended use, such a practice is not recommended. However, antibiotics may need to be redosed in lengthy operations and in cases in which there is significant blood loss.[2]

## Antimicrobial Prophylaxis in Special Circumstances

### External Cerebrospinal Fluid Drains

The rate of infection with placement of an external ventricular drain varies in the literature based on the criteria and methodology used to determine the presence of infection. External ventricular drain infection rates have been reported to range from 4% to more than 20% per procedure per patient.[38–42]

Reported risk factors for infection include longer duration of catheter placement,[41] CSF leakage,[38] presence of intraventricular blood, and trauma.[39] The most common pathogens involved in external ventricular drain infections are gram-positive microorganisms of the skin flora, most often coagulase-negative staphylococci.[39,41]

A study by Mayhall et al in 1984 suggested that ventricular catheters be changed and inserted in a different site if monitoring is required more than 5 days to reduce the risk for ventriculostomy-related infections.[42] This remains a debated topic. In 2002, Wong et al published a randomized prospective trial that was powered to detect a statistically significant difference between the infection rates of patients randomized to external ventricular drainage with the drain changed at 5-day intervals and the infection rates of those randomized to external ventricular drainage with the drain not changed. This study demonstrated that there was no statistically significant difference between the infection rates of the two groups: 7.8% versus 3.8% ($p = 0.50$).[43] However, when designing this study, the authors used a historical infection rate of 30% in patients whose ventricular catheter remained unchanged after 5 days versus an infection rate of 8% in patients whose ventricular catheter was changed at 5-day intervals to calculate the power for the study. The finding of a difference of almost 50% in the infection rates raises the question of whether the use of the historical infection rates led to this study being underpowered.

Advances in technology have led to the availability of antibiotic-impregnated ventricular catheters. Catheters can be impregnated with more than one antibiotic to prevent the development of antibiotic resistance. In vitro studies have shown that impregnated catheters can decrease colonization by *Staphylococcus epidermidis* for at least 1 year and prevent the spread of bacteria along the catheter surface. Studies demonstrate that antibiotic-impregnated catheters decrease the incidence of catheter-related infections.[44,45] Rivero-Garvía et al reported a decrease in the catheter infection rate from 17% to 2.4% with the use of antibiotic-impregnated catheters.[45] In a prospective randomized trial by Wong et al, it was demonstrated that antibiotic-impregnated catheters were as effective as systemic antibiotics in preventing CSF infections. Patients were randomized to receive an antibiotic-impregnated catheter with no systemic antibiotics versus systemic antibiotics without an antibiotic-impregnated catheter. The difference between the infection rates, 1% versus 3%, was not statistically significant.[46]

Higher infection rates have been observed when the catheter has been tunneled in the subcutaneous tissue for a distance of less than 5 cm. Sandalcioglu et al found that the ventricular catheter was tunneled less than 5 cm in 83% of their patients with CSF infections.[47] The authors hypothesize that this disproportion was related to the observation that CSF leakage was more common when the catheter was not tunneled an adequate distance, increasing the chance for colonization and infection.

The use of antibiotic treatment during external ventricular drainage remains an issue of debate.[40,48,49] The practice of using prophylactic antibiotics is variable. In a survey of the members of the Neurocritical

Care Society, of whom 77% (599 individuals) were neurosurgeons, 56% recommended the use of antibiotics while the catheter was in place.[49] In 1985, Blomstedt conducted a prospective randomized trial in which one group of patients was randomized to be given trimethoprim-sulfamethoxazole as prophylaxis during ventricular drainage and a second group to be given no antibiotic prophylaxis. The study contained 52 patients and did not show a difference in the infection rates, but the study was not powered adequately. A retrospective study by Alleyne et al in 2000 did not show a difference between the rates of ventriculitis in patients who received continued antibiotics while their ventricular drain remained in place and the rates of those who did not receive continued antibiotics.[48] Currently, practices vary based on limited evidence. However, the routine use of antibiotics is not without risks and has the potential to lead to the development of drug-resistant organisms and *C. difficile* colitis.[49,51] We would benefit from a prospective randomized trial of adequate power to answer this question.

In patients who received antibiotics through the duration of ventricular drainage, Wong et al in 2006 reported that a single broad-spectrum antibiotic such as cefepime was as effective in preventing ventriculitis as alternative regimens that contained dual antibiotics, such as ampicillin-sulbactam with aztreonam. In this prospective randomized controlled trial, the infection rate was 6.6% in the single-antibiotic group and 2.3% in the dual-antibiotic group ($p = 0.17$).[52]

Protocols for the placement of ventricular drains, surveillance, and treatment of catheter-related infections vary between institutions. Over all, recommendations for the placement of an external ventricular drain include antibiotic prophylaxis at the time of catheter insertion, placement of an antibiotic-impregnated catheter under sterile conditions, catheter exchange in the event of positive CSF culture demonstrating CSF infection, and minimization of catheter manipulation.

Similar principles apply to the insertion and maintenance of lumbar drains. Lumbar drains similarly can lead to the development of CSF infections. The risks for infection increase with drain leakage or blockage, hemorrhagic CSF, and the length of time the drain remains in place.[53] In a cohort study by Schade et al in 2005, the authors compared the rates of infection in ventricular and lumbar drainage. After correcting for duration of drainage, they did not find a significant difference between the infection rates for these two drainage techniques.[52]

## Cerebrospinal Fluid Shunts and Other Foreign Bodies

The placement of CSF shunts is one the most frequent neurosurgical procedures performed. Other neurosurgical procedures that require the implantation of a foreign body include synthetic cranioplasties, placement of intrathecal catheters for drug delivery, and implantation of deep brain and epidural spinal cord electrodes. Shunt infection can complicate the placement of a CSF shunt, and the infection rate ranges from 5 to 10%.[54] The common organisms responsible for shunt infections include those that are part of the skin flora: *S. epidermidis, S. aureus*, and *Propionibacterium acnes*. The clustering of 70% of shunt infections within 2 months after shunt placement suggests that initial colonization during shunt placement contributes significantly to resulting shunt infections.[53] Many studies have examined the role that prophylactic systemic antibiotics can play in reducing the shunt infection rate.

Before the meta-analysis performed by Haines and Walters in 1994, attempts to confirm the efficacy of antibiotic prophylaxis for CSF shunt operations had yielded inconclusive results.[55-58] Haines and Walters combined the results of seven high-quality controlled trials into a meta-analysis. A reduction of approximately 50% ($p = 0.001$) in infection risk was demonstrated when antibiotic prophylaxis was used. The infection rate in the prophylactic antibiotic group was 7%, compared with 13% in the control group ($p = 0.003$). The study also showed a correlation between the efficacy of prophylactic antibiotics in reducing the infection rate and the baseline infection rate. Through the use of a regression equation, it was demonstrated that once the baseline infection rate fell below 5.5%, the efficacy of prophylactic antibiotics on the infection rate was negligible. It is interesting to note that prophylactic antibiotics have been found to reduce the infection rate in clean neurosurgical procedures even with baseline infection rates as low as 3%.[58] The difference may relate to the ability of foreign body implants to harbor microorganisms and provide an environment that makes the microorganisms less accessible to the antibiotic effect.[58,59]

Similarly, Langley et al performed a meta-analysis of 12 randomized controlled trials in patients who had undergone CSF shunt placement with random allocation either to perioperative systemic antibiotics or to no perioperative antibiotics. One study achieved statistical significance on its own, and the other 11 studies had relative risks in the same direction as the combined analysis. In total, 1,359 patients had been randomized, and the pooled results demonstrated a 50% ($p = 0.0002$) reduction in risk for subsequent CSF shunt infections with the use of perioperative systemic antibiotics.[59] In the groups treated with prophylactic antibiotics, the shunt infection rate averaged 6.8% (range, 1.9 to 17%).[60]

Ratilal et al also performed a meta-analysis that included 17 trials and a total number of 2,134 patients.[61] Their results confirmed that the use of systemic antibiotic prophylaxis decreased the shunt infection rate by approximately 50%. The results of these studies show that antibiotic prophylaxis is useful in reducing shunt infection rates; however, the impact appears to be marginal in conditions in which a low baseline infection rate exists.

In terms of choosing the appropriate perioperative prophylactic antibiotic, local resistance rates should guide decision making. For example, the current prevalence of MRSA among *S. aureus* isolates is roughly 20 to 25%, but this varies among institutions and communities.[62] A randomized controlled trial by Tacconelli et al demonstrated the shunt infection rate

could be reduced at their hospital, where MRSA was prevalent, with the use of perioperative vancomycin instead of cefazolin.[28] They categorized their institution as having a high prevalence of MRSA based on published consensus guidelines suggesting that a high rate of MRSA transmission is indicated by a threshold of 0.5 new nosocomial cases of MRSA per 100 admissions in a hospital that has more than 500 beds.[62] The shunt infection rate was 4% in the patients treated with vancomycin, compared with 14% in the patients who received cefazolin ($p = 0.03$).[28]

In regard to the efficacy of prophylactic antibiotics in the implantation of other foreign bodies in neurosurgical procedures (e.g., synthetic cranioplasties, intrathecal catheters for drug delivery, deep brain and epidural spinal cord electrodes), a paucity of trials exists. Here, we can extrapolate the principles gleaned from studies on antibiotic prophylaxis in CSF shunting and make the argument that theoretically, antibiotic prophylaxis under these circumstances should also play a role in reducing infection rates.

## ■ Spinal Neurosurgery

The vast majority of spinal neurosurgical operations are clean elective operations. Patients in this group have the lowest intrinsic rate of infection to begin with, and some have suggested that the balance between risk and benefit of antibiotic prophylaxis may be swayed toward its harmful and costly side effects. The available data do not support this concern.

Infection of the operated spine can undermine its mechanical stability and extend to involve neural structures, leading to debilitating deformity and compromise of neurologic function. The potential of such devastating consequences has secured widespread acceptance of antibiotic prophylaxis before spinal surgeries in the past three decades. Multiple studies have examined this question, but all have significant shortcomings. Taken together, they indicate a trend toward a benefit of antibiotic prophylaxis for clean spine surgery. The evidence supporting this policy is reviewed below.

Among the most important of the studies is that of Pavel et al,[63] who demonstrated reduced infection rates after preoperative antibiotics for a variety of orthopedic procedures. The spinal surgery subgroup was too small for the difference to reach statistical significance.

Rubinstein et al reported a double-blind randomized controlled trial comparing cefazolin with placebo in 141 patients undergoing clean spine surgery.[64] They showed a 12.7% infection rate in the placebo group versus 4.3% in the cefazolin group.

The strongest evidence has been derived from a meta-analysis of multiple trials that individually failed to show benefit.[65] The results of six randomized controlled trials with 843 patients were pooled. There was a 2.2% infection rate if antibiotics were given (10/451) and 5.9% (23/392) without prophylaxis ($p < 0.01$). Barker's review also showed that additional coverage of gram-negative organisms, as well as multiple dosing, did not show superiority over a single agent.

The specific antibiotic, repetitive dosing, instrumented versus noninstrumented surgery, and the effect of additional risk factors have not been sufficiently studied to allow firm conclusions to be drawn. Watters et al summarized the current evidence in 2009 and put forward recommendations regarding prophylaxis in spine surgery[66]: A single dose of a broad-spectrum antibiotic, covering gram-positive organisms and taking into account the spectrum of infectious agents at the local institution, given before incision in time sufficient to reach adequate serum concentration, is the accepted practice for this type of surgery.

## Cerebrospinal Fluid Fistulas

The role of antibiotics in preventing meningitis due to open communication between the CSF and the nonsterile world remains a controversial subject. Leakage of CSF following neurosurgical procedures has long been recognized as a risk factor for postsurgical infection. The evidence for or against prophylactic antibiotics in such cases, as well as in cases of traumatic or spontaneous CSF leakage, is slim. When Brodie conducted a meta-analysis of trials, each individually failing to show a benefit of antibiotic prophylaxis in posttraumatic CSF fistulas, the results suggested a significant reduction in infection from 2.5 to 10% ($p = 0.006$).[67] This study, however, included nonrandomized case series, and 73% of the patients received antibiotic prophylaxis. Villalobos et al conducted a meta-analysis in 1998, examining antibiotic prophylaxis in the setting of basilar skull fractures, and concluded that there was no benefit to antibiotic prophylaxis against meningitis.[68]

Following those studies, several randomized controlled trials were conducted. A Cochrane review by Ratilal et al analyzed the utility of antibiotics in preventing meningitis following basilar skull fractures. His group was able to combine four randomized controlled trials with a total of 208 patients, 109 in the treatment group and 99 in the control group, but not all of them had a CSF leak. Given the data at hand, they were unable to demonstrate a benefit of prophylactic antibiotics in patients with basilar skull fractures. Nevertheless, they concluded that there is insufficient evidence to support or refute such practice.[69]

## Topical Antibiotic Prophylaxis

Topical antiseptic prophylaxis is a well-accepted procedure. The application of alcohol and turpentine to wounds, in an attempt to prevent wound infections, was described by 1700 BC in the Edwin-Smith Papyrus. Antiseptic preparation of the skin before incision is a standard practice in modern surgery.

After the advent of antibiotics in the second half of the previous century, the practice of powdering or spraying them into wounds developed. It was Malis, however, who by 1979 established the practice of continuous antibiotic solution irrigation together with parenteral administration.[70] He proceeded to demonstrate the benefit of that practice but never separated the analysis of topical and parenteral approaches.

Although it has become a widely accepted practice since then, it remains poorly studied, and solid evidence supporting or refuting it is lacking. Miller et al performed a retrospective analysis demonstrating a reduction of stereotactic and functional hardware infections after the injection of antibiotics into wounds before closure, in addition to systemic prophylaxis and local irrigation.[71] Alves and Godoy[72] performed a review of the literature on this subject in 2010, updating that of Haines,[73] and summarized the few studies looking at this practice in neurosurgery, concluding that they are lacking strength in numbers and design.

Nevertheless, the simplicity, relative lack of toxicity, and superficial reasonableness of the practice make it a common one in modern neurosurgery. When coupled with implant material, such as CSF shunts and other catheters, as well as deep brain stimulation electrodes and batteries, topical antibiosis is almost a universal practice. Several general principles, extrapolated from theory and studies applied in other surgical specialties, should be followed. The antibiotic solution should be bactericidal against the flora present at the institution where it is applied, and antibiotics with minimal potential for toxicity should be chosen. Penicillins should be avoided when the cerebrum is exposed because of their epileptogenic potential. Bacitracin and metronidazole, conversely, have been shown to be the least likely to produce epileptiform activity.

## Conclusion

Antibiotic prophylaxis before surgery has been demonstrated to play a major role in the avoidance of operative site infections and has become the standard of practice. Because the rate of postoperative infections in most neurosurgical procedures is low, there is a paucity of evidence regarding several aspects of perioperative antibiotic prophylaxis, including the ideal prophylactic antibiotic regimen and certain aspects of the timing of administration.

## References

1. Zhu XL, Wong WK, Yeung WM, et al. A randomized, double-blind comparison of ampicillin/sulbactam and ceftriaxone in the prevention of surgical-site infections after neurosurgery. Clin Ther 2001;23(8):1281–1291
2. Gyssens IC. Preventing postoperative infections: current treatment recommendations. Drugs 1999;57(2):175–185
3. Mangram AJ, Horan TC, Pearson ML, Silver LC, Jarvis WR; Centers for Disease Control and Prevention (CDC) Hospital Infection Control Practices Advisory Committee. Guideline for Prevention of Surgical Site Infection, 1999. Am J Infect Control 1999;27(2):97–132, quiz 133–134, discussion 96
4. Tadiparthi S. Prophylactic antibiotics for clean, non-implant plastic surgery: what is the evidence? J Wound Care 2008;17(9):392–394, 396–398
5. Spencer RC. The role of antimicrobial agents in the aetiology of *Clostridium difficile*-associated disease. J Antimicrob Chemother 1998;41(Suppl C):21–27
6. Mukhtar S, Shaker H, Basarab A, Byrne JP. Prophylactic antibiotics and *Clostridium difficile* infection. J Hosp Infect 2006;64(1):93–94
7. Malis LI, Ruberti RF, Kaufman AB, et al. Intraoperative antibiotic prophylaxis. Surg Neurol 1997;47(5):481–483
8. Savitz MH, Malis LI. Prophylactic clindamycin for neurosurgical patients. NY State J Med 1976;76(1):64–67
9. Bullock R, van Dellen JR, Ketelbey W, Reinach SG. A double-blind placebo-controlled trial of perioperative prophylactic antibiotics for elective neurosurgery. J Neurosurg 1988;69(5):687–691
10. Blomstedt GC, Kyttä J. Results of a randomized trial of vancomycin prophylaxis in craniotomy. J Neurosurg 1988;69(2):216–220
11. Geraghty J, Feely M. Antibiotic prophylaxis in neurosurgery. A randomized controlled trial. J Neurosurg 1984;60(4):724–726
12. Shapiro M, Wald U, Simchen E, et al. Randomized clinical trial of intra-operative antimicrobial prophylaxis of infection after neurosurgical procedures. J Hosp Infect 1986;8(3):283–295
13. van Ek B, Dijkmans BA, van Dulken H, van Furth R. Antibiotic prophylaxis in craniotomy: a prospective double-blind placebo-controlled study. Scand J Infect Dis 1988;20(6):633–639
14. Winkler D, Rehn H, Freckmann N, Nowak G, Herrmann HD. Clinical efficacy of perioperative antimicrobial prophylaxis in neurosurgery—a prospective randomized study involving 159 patients. Chemotherapy 1989;35(4):304–312
15. Young RF, Lawner PM. Perioperative antibiotic prophylaxis for prevention of postoperative neurosurgical infections. A randomized clinical trial. J Neurosurg 1987;66(5):701–705
16. Djindjian M, Lepresle E, Homs JB. Antibiotic prophylaxis during prolonged clean neurosurgery. Results of a randomized double-blind study using oxacillin. J Neurosurg 1990;73(3):383–386
17. Barker FG II. Efficacy of prophylactic antibiotics for craniotomy: a meta-analysis. Neurosurgery 1994;35(3):484–490, discussion 491–492

18. Walstad RA, Hellum KB, Blika S, et al. Pharmaco-kinetics and tissue penetration of ceftazidime: studies on lymph, aqueous humour, skin blister, cerebrospinal and pleural fluid. J Antimicrob Chemother 1983;12(Suppl A):275–282

19. Friedrich H, Pelz K, Hänsel-Friedrich G. Lack of penetration of cephacetril into the cerebro-spinal fluid of patients without meningitis. Infection 1979;7(1):41–44

20. Knoop M, Schütze M, Piek J, Drewelow B, Mundkowski R. Antibiotic prophylaxis in cerebrospinal fluid shunting: reassessment of Cefotiam penetration into human CSF. Zentralbl Neurochir 2007; 68(1):14–18

21. Cherubin CE, Eng RH, Norrby R, Modai J, Humbert G, Overturf G. Penetration of newer cephalosporins into cerebrospinal fluid. Rev Infect Dis 1989;11(4):526–548

22. Cadoz M, Denis F, Félix H, Diop Mar I. Treatment of purulent meningitis with a new cephalosporin–Rocephin (Ro 13-9904). Clinical, bacteriological and pharmacological observations in 24 cases. Chemotherapy 1981;27(Suppl 1):57–61

23. Rehn H, Winkler D, Freckmann N, Nowak G, Herrmann H. Perioperative prophylaxis in neurosurgery with ceftriaxone. Chemioterapia 1987;6(2, Suppl):566–568

24. Zhao JZ, Wang S, Li JS, et al. The perioperative use of ceftriaxone as infection prophylaxis in neurosurgery. Clin Neurol Neurosurg 1995;97(4): 285–289

25. White RR IV, Pitzer KD, Fader RC, Rajab MH, Song J. Pharmacokinetics of topical and intravenous cefazolin in patients with clean surgical wounds. Plast Reconstr Surg 2008;122(6):1773–1779

26. Wang Q, Shi Z, Wang J, Shi G, Wang S, Zhou J. Postoperatively administered vancomycin reaches therapeutic concentration in the cerebral spinal fluid of neurosurgical patients. Surg Neurol 2008;69(2): 126–129, discussion 129

27. Wang JF, Wang Q, Zhao LH, Shi GZ, Zhou JX. Blood-brain barrier penetration of cefepime after neurosurgery. Chin Med J (Engl) 2007;120(13): 1176–1178

28. Tacconelli E, Cataldo MA, Albanese A, et al. Vancomycin versus cefazolin prophylaxis for cerebrospinal shunt placement in a hospital with a high prevalence of methicillin-resistant *Staphylococcus aureus*. J Hosp Infect 2008;69(4):337–344

29. Whitby M, Johnson BC, Atkinson RL, Stuart G; Brisbane Neurosurgical Infection Group. The comparative efficacy of intravenous cefotaxime and trimethoprim/sulfamethoxazole in preventing infection after neurosurgery: a prospective, randomized study. Br J Neurosurg 2000;14(1): 13–18

30. Stone HH, Hooper CA, Kolb LD, Geheber CE, Dawkins EJ. Antibiotic prophylaxis in gastric, biliary and colonic surgery. Ann Surg 1976;184(4): 443–452

31. Polk HC Jr, Lopez-Mayor JF. Postoperative wound infection: a prospective study of determinant factors and prevention. Surgery 1969;66(1): 97–103

32. Burke JF. The effective period of preventive antibiotic action in experimental incisions and dermal lesions. Surgery 1961;50:161–168

33. Miles AA, Miles EM, Burke J. The value and duration of defence reactions of the skin to the primary lodgement of bacteria. Br J Exp Pathol 1957;38(1): 79–96

34. Galandiuk S, Polk HC Jr, Jagelman DG, Fazio VW. Re-emphasis of priorities in surgical antibiotic prophylaxis. Surg Gynecol Obstet 1989;169(3): 219–222

35. Classen DC, Evans RS, Pestotnik SL, Horn SD, Menlove RL, Burke JP. The timing of prophylactic administration of antibiotics and the risk of surgical-wound infection. N Engl J Med 1992;326(5): 281–286

36. DiPiro JT, Cheung RP, Bowden TA Jr, Mansberger JA. Single dose systemic antibiotic prophylaxis of surgical wound infections. Am J Surg 1986;152(5): 552–559

37. Nooyen SM, Overbeek BP, Brutel de la Rivière A, Storm AJ, Langemeyer JJ. Prospective randomised comparison of single-dose versus multiple-dose cefuroxime for prophylaxis in coronary artery bypass grafting. Eur J Clin Microbiol Infect Dis 1994;13(12):1033–1037

38. Korinek AM, Reina M, Boch AL, Rivera AO, De Bels D, Puybasset L. Prevention of external ventricular drain–related ventriculitis. Acta Neurochir (Wien) 2005;147(1):39–45, discussion 45–46

39. Scheithauer S, Bürgel U, Ryang YM, et al. Prospective surveillance of drain associated meningitis/ventriculitis in a neurosurgery and neurological intensive care unit. J Neurol Neurosurg Psychiatry 2009;80(12):1381–1385

40. Aucoin PJ, Kotilainen HR, Gantz NM, Davidson R, Kellogg P, Stone B. Intracranial pressure monitors. Epidemiologic study of risk factors and infections. Am J Med 1986;80(3):369–376

41. Camacho EF, Boszczowski I, Basso M, et al. Infection rate and risk factors associated with infections related to external ventricular drain. Infection 2011;39(1):47–51

42. Mayhall CG, Archer NH, Lamb VA, et al. Ventriculostomy-related infections. A prospective epidemiologic study. N Engl J Med 1984;310(9): 553–559

43. Wong GK, Poon WS, Wai S, Yu LM, Lyon D, Lam JM. Failure of regular external ventricular drain exchange to reduce cerebrospinal fluid infection: result of a randomised controlled trial. J Neurol Neurosurg Psychiatry 2002;73(6):759–761

44. Muttaiyah S, Ritchie S, John S, Mee E, Roberts S. Efficacy of antibiotic-impregnated external ventricular drain catheters. J Clin Neurosci 2010;17(3):296–298

45. Rivero-Garvía M, Márquez-Rivas J, Jiménez-Mejías ME, Neth O, Rueda-Torres AB. Reduction in external ventricular drain infection rate. Impact of a minimal handling protocol and antibiotic-impregnated catheters. Acta Neurochir (Wien) 2011;153(3):647–651

46. Wong GK, Ip M, Poon WS, Mak CW, Ng RY. Antibiotics-impregnated ventricular catheter versus systemic antibiotics for prevention of nosocomial CSF and non-CSF infections: a prospective randomised clinical trial. J Neurol Neurosurg Psychiatry 2010;81(10):1064–1067

47. Sandalcioglu IE, Stolke D. Failure of regular external ventricular drain exchange to reduce CSF infection.

J Neurol Neurosurg Psychiatry 2003;74(11):1598–1599, author reply 1599

48. Alleyne CH Jr, Hassan M, Zabramski JM. The efficacy and cost of prophylactic and periprocedural antibiotics in patients with external ventricular drains. Neurosurgery 2000;47(5):1124–1127, discussion 1127–1129

49. McCarthy PJ, Patil S, Conrad SA, Scott LK. International and specialty trends in the use of prophylactic antibiotics to prevent infectious complications after insertion of external ventricular drainage devices. Neurocrit Care 2010;12(2):220–224

50. Blomstedt GC. Results of trimethoprimsulfamethoxazole prophylaxis in ventriculostomy and shunting procedures. A double-blind randomized trial. J Neurosurg 1985;62(5):694–697

51. Ortiz R, Lee K. Nosocomial infections in neurocritical care. Curr Neurol Neurosci Rep 2006;6(6):525–530

52. Wong GK, Poon WS, Lyon D, Wai S. Cefepime vs. ampicillin/sulbactam and aztreonam as antibiotic prophylaxis in neurosurgical patients with external ventricular drain: result of a prospective randomized controlled clinical trial. J Clin Pharm Ther 2006;31(3):231–235

53. Schade RP, Schinkel J, Visser LG, Van Dijk JM, Voormolen JH, Kuijper EJ. Bacterial meningitis caused by the use of ventricular or lumbar cerebrospinal fluid catheters. J Neurosurg 2005;102(2):229–234

54. Gardner P, Leipzig TJ, Sadigh M. Infections of mechanical cerebrospinal fluid shunts. Curr Clin Top Infect Dis 1988;9:185–214

55. Zentner J, Gilsbach J, Felder T. Antibiotic prophylaxis in cerebrospinal fluid shunting: a prospective randomized trial in 129 patients. Neurosurg Rev 1995;18(3):169–172

56. Schmidt K, Gjerris F, Osgaard O, et al. Antibiotic prophylaxis in cerebrospinal fluid shunting: a prospective randomized trial in 152 hydrocephalic patients. Neurosurgery 1985;17(1):1–5

57. Wang EE, Prober CG, Hendrick BE, Hoffman HJ, Humphreys RP. Prophylactic sulfamethoxazole and trimethoprim in ventriculoperitoneal shunt surgery. A double-blind, randomized, placebo-controlled trial. JAMA 1984;251(9):1174–1177

58. Haines SJ, Walters BC. Antibiotic prophylaxis for cerebrospinal fluid shunts: a metanalysis. Neurosurgery 1994;34(1):87–92

59. Borges LF. Cerebrospinal fluid shunts interfere with host defenses. Neurosurgery 1982;10(1):55–60

60. Ratial B, Costa J, Sampaio C. Antibiotic prophylaxis for surgical introduction of intracranial ventricular shunts. Cochrane Database Syst Rev 2006 July 19;(3):CD005365

61. Langley JM, LeBlanc JC, Drake J, Milner R. Efficacy of antimicrobial prophylaxis in placement of cerebrospinal fluid shunts: meta-analysis. Clin Infect Dis 1993;17(1):98–103

62. Wenzel RP, Reagan DR, Bertino JS Jr, Baron EJ, Arias K. Methicillin-resistant *Staphylococcus aureus* outbreak: a consensus panel's definition and management guidelines. Am J Infect Control 1998;26(2):102–110

63. Pavel A, Smith RL, Ballard A, Larson IJ. Prophylactic antibiotics in elective orthopedic surgery: a prospective study of 1,591 cases. South Med J 1977;70(Suppl 1):50–55

64. Rubenstein E, Findler G, Amit P, Shaked I. Perioperative prophylactic cephazolin in spinal surgery. A double-blind placebo-controlled trial. J Bone Joint Surg Br 1994;76(1):99–102

65. Barker FG II. Efficacy of prophylactic antibiotic therapy in spinal surgery: a meta-analysis. Neurosurgery 2002;51(2):391–400, discussion 400–401

66. Watters WC III, Baisden J, Bono CM, et al; North American Spine Society. Antibiotic prophylaxis in spine surgery: an evidence-based clinical guideline for the use of prophylactic antibiotics in spine surgery. Spine J 2009;9(2):142–146

67. Brodie HA. Prophylactic antibiotics for posttraumatic cerebrospinal fluid fistulae. A meta-analysis. Arch Otolaryngol Head Neck Surg 1997;123(7):749–752

68. Villalobos T, Arango C, Kubilis P, Rathore M. Antibiotic prophylaxis after basilar skull fractures: a meta-analysis. Clin Infect Dis 1998;27(2):364–369

69. Ratial B, Costa J, Sampaio C. Antibiotic prophylaxis for preventing meningitis in patients with basilar skull fractures. Cochrane Database Syst Rev 2006;(1):CD004884

70. Malis LI. Prevention of neurosurgical infection by intraoperative antibiotics. Neurosurgery 1979;5(3):339–343

71. Miller JP, Acar F, Burchiel KJ. Significant reduction in stereotactic and functional neurosurgical hardware infection after local neomycin/polymyxin application. J Neurosurg 2009;110(2):247–250

72. Alves RV, Godoy R. Topical antibiotics and neurosurgery: have we forgotten to study it? Surg Neurol Int 2010;1(1):22

73. Haines SJ. Topical antibiotic prophylaxis in neurosurgery. Neurosurgery 1982;11(2):250–253

# 15

# Postoperative Intracranial Infections

Arya Nabavi, Frederike Knerlich-Lukoschus, and Andreas M. Stark

Postoperative infections in cranial neurosurgery are reported within a range of 0.5 to 6.6%.[1–3] An analysis of predisposing conditions and risk factors, in addition to sufficient preventative measures, should provide a solid basis for further evaluation of this problem. However, closer scrutiny of the literature before 1992[4–6] and the contemporary literature, which provides the basis for this chapter, raises concern.

The rarity of this complication demands high case numbers to permit conclusive analysis beyond anecdotal case reports. As such, some studies combine the results of spinal and cranial (burr holes and open craniotomies) cases to generate a single neurosurgical infection rate.[3,7,8] When these subdivisions are accounted for, only a few contemporary studies remain with sufficient case numbers for a meaningful analysis of cranial postoperative infections. As a consequence, McClelland could find only two recent neurosurgical studies to include in a meta-analysis.[9] Furthermore, basic inconsistencies in adherence to an antibiotic prophylaxis protocol (e.g., incorrect timing, wrong or no prophylaxis, continuation at the surgeon's discretion, regionally adapted unconventional combinations[8,10,11]) and in reporting of infections (wound or general infections,[11] only infections that were reoperated,[12,13] classification of wound infections) prevent comparison. In addition to these issues, potential detection error,[14] referral bias, and unrecorded treatment at different institutions[12] may result in miscalculation of the "true" infection rate.

Besides open questions in epidemiology, the rarity of postoperative infections combined with the irregularities encountered in reporting represents a challenge in evaluating and a still greater challenge in comparing prevention techniques with sufficient statistical power.

To obtain such information, examination of the literature for other surgical specialties is useful.[1,15–18] The Centers for Disease Control and Prevention (CDC) has provided a working definition of surgical wound infections, more precisely labeled as surgical site infections (SSIs), as a basis for structured reporting.[1,15,19,20] Risk factors for infection have been corroborated in various series.[1–3,7,8,10,17,21–24]

Only a few neurosurgical reports that address wound infections are structured accordingly.[2,7] Most publications report infection rates indiscriminately, precluding further analysis, or consider only those complications that required reoperation,[12,13] obscuring the true dimension of the problem. Information with regard to risk factors, follow-up, and true infection rate remains vague. Larger studies that enable a more thorough investigation are infrequent.

McClelland and Hall[3] analyzed 1,587 elective cranial cases performed by the senior author as a "single-surgeon" series. For the 562 elective craniotomies, five infections were reported, resulting in an infection rate of 0.89%. Korinek et al[2] reported an overall infection rate of 6.6% in a single-center, "multiple-surgeon" study with 4,578 craniotomies (emergency and elective). While the former study shows how under the best possible circumstances infection rates can be lowered and almost eradicated, the latter most likely reflects the challenge that confronts most neurosurgical units.[2]

In this chapter, we review the contemporary literature with respect to risk factors, the classification of postoperative wound infections (SSIs), and potential methods for future analysis. The specific postoperative infections in cranial neurosurgery are discussed within this framework.

# Risk Factors for Surgical Site Infections

A multitude of factors have been identified that result in SSI. Although information remains contradictory on their respective validity, risk factors can be categorized as patient- or procedure-related.[17]

## Patient-Related Risk Factors

Patient-related risk factors include vulnerability due to metabolic states[21] (e.g., diabetes mellitus); unbalanced nutritional states (obesity, malnutrition manifested by weight loss and a low preoperative albumin level); tobacco use; specific exposure risks (infection at another site at the time of surgery, prolonged preoperative hospital stay, colonization with *Staphylococcus aureus*); reduced defensive capacity (impaired immune response, corticosteroid use, irradiation to the surgical field); and age.

Although these factors may be interrelated and thus not valid as independent risk factors, they warrant heightened attention. Furthermore, a closer investigation of these risk factors may yield potential approaches to reduce or prevent their impact.[17] For instance, diabetes is not in itself a risk factor[3] for infection in the absence of preoperative hyperglycemia.[17] Therefore, metabolic correction to normoglycemia reduces the infection risk in every patient, irrespective of the underlying disorder. Advanced age has also been considered a risk factor. Various

hypotheses on decreased wound healing and a defective immune system have been discussed. However, Kaye et al[23] showed that longitudinally, the risk for SSI increases up to the age of 65, after which there is a decrease in a linear fashion at a rate of 1.1% per year.[17,23]

Various patient-related characteristics can reasonably be identified as risk factors. Careful reevaluation may provide new insights[17] that will enable us to influence preoperative states to reduce the hazard of infections.

## Procedure-Related Risk Factors

Procedure-related risk factors can be broadly categorized as local (related to the surgical site) or general (related to systemic issues).[18,25] Most of the local factors pertain to site preparation: lack of preoperative cleansing (antiseptic shower); hair removal[26–28] (type and timing, improper skin preparation); and surgical techniques[25] (excessive tissue damage, intraoperative placement of chemotherapeutic wafers[22,29]). General issues include inappropriate antibiotic prophylaxis with regard to timing, reapplication, and choice[2]; hypothermia and hypoxia; perioperative blood transfusion; and postoperative anemia.[17] Special risks in the neurosurgical population are implantation of foreign material (i.e., ventriculoperitoneal shunts, dural substitutes); local radiation (causing subsequent decreased vascularity of the skin) and chemotherapy (prior treatment[24] or intracavitary wafers[22]); and early reoperation.[2]

The single most important procedure-related risk factor for a postoperative infection in neurosurgery is cerebrospinal fluid (CSF) leakage.[2,7,8,13,30–33] A multicenter study by Korinek et al[10] identified emergency surgery, clean–contaminated class of surgery, length of surgery of more than 4 hours, and reoperation as additional risk factors for infection. In the subsequent single-center study,[2] CSF leakage remained the most important risk factor (odds ratio, 11.48), whereas neither emergency surgery nor contamination class was found to be statistically significant. However, surgical diagnosis, surgeon, early reoperation, and surgery lasting more than 4 hours were identified as independent risk factors. Meningiomas (76/729, or 10%) and metastases (29/183, or 15%) accounted for 34.7% of 303 infections in 4,578 surgeries, making the surgical diagnosis an independent risk factor. The reason for the high incidence of infection in metastases remains unclear, but it has been attributed to altered immune defenses. Although in meningiomas[2,13] the individual circumstances are not specified, the most likely explanation is the potential for CSF leakage after dural reconstruction.

Because surgery is the required event for SSI, it is not surprising that the surgeon plays an important role. Although it is misleading to describe the surgeon as a general risk factor,[2] there are interesting implications. In the available reports, single-surgeon studies[3] provide the lower end of the infection range, and multicenter studies[2] determine the upper end. Cushing (1915) pointed out the surgeon's pivotal role in postoperative infections: "Certainly infections cannot be attributed to the intervention of the devil but must be laid at the surgeon's door." It is important to interpret this statement properly; it is neither accusatory nor placing blame, but rather represents a challenge to the individual surgeon to live up to this essential obligation.

Two other aspects of the surgical site that warrant a more elaborate discussion are classification of the wound and shaving of the operative field.

## Wound Categories

The National Academy of Sciences has proposed the widely accepted classification of the contamination status of sites of surgery as clean, clean–contaminated, contaminated, and dirty.[15] With the correct administration of antibiotic prophylaxis and appropriate aseptic technique, the infection rates are lowered in all categories.[1,15,20,21] In neurosurgery, most cases are considered clean; however, reported infection rates for shunt implantations, which are considered clean surgeries, are higher

than those for other cranial procedures. To account for this discrepancy, the cases in the clean subdivision have been separated into those with and those without foreign body implantation.[34] Although the question remains of how much material constitutes the difference between clean and clean with foreign body, this seems like a reasonable subdivision, in particular with regard to shunt procedures, cranioplasty, and surgeries involving dural substitutes.[34]

The term *clean–contaminated* describes procedures in which the respiratory or alimentary membranes are entered under controlled conditions, as in trans-sphenoidal or endoscopic approaches[30,33] to the skull base. With proper attention to antiseptic techniques, these cases can have similar infection rates (1.8%),[33] as can clean elective craniotomies. Contaminated and dirty procedures are rarely performed in neurosurgery and are mostly associated with emergency situations, which in themselves represent a risk factor.

## Shaving of the Surgical Site

Hair has previously been considered a risk factor for wound infections. However, evidence exists that shaving itself poses a risk. A clear association between the manner of hair removal and SSI has been found in that the use of a razor results in a higher risk for SSI than do clippers or a depilation cream.[26] A razor produces microscopic abrasions of the skin, which are subsequently colonized by bacteria. Shaving the surgical site the evening before surgery poses the greatest risk for SSI because of the extended period in which bacterial colonization can occur, and this practice has largely been abandoned.

A comprehensive article by Winston[26] offers an enjoyable analysis of this issue of hair removal. Hair can be rendered void of infecting organisms by using proper local preparation and surgical scrubbing. The infecting flora is found in the deeper layers of the skin, which are not affected by shaving. There is no increase in infection rates if the hair is not removed. Subsequently, various groups have published their data on surgery without shaving.[26–28] A prerequisite to prevent infection is thorough preparation of the site before surgery with shampooing and antiseptic cleansing. Furthermore, in closing the wound, the surgeon must ensure that no hair remains in the wound, thus making the final part of the procedure more involved. Staples and interrupted sutures[26–28] are used to close the skin. The studies were carefully designed and should be read attentively before a "no-shave" policy is adopted. Bekar et al[27] administered antibiotics for 3 days after surgery. This practice may have resulted in a skewed representation of the true infection risk posed by not shaving. Tokimura et al[28] administered antibiotics for 24 hours and had the patients' hair washed on the second, fourth, and sixth postoperative days. Accordingly, all studies that pertain to "no-shaving" routines instituted additional safety measures. Thus, "not shaving" poses no additional risk for infection if proper precautions are taken.

## ▪ Estimating the Risk for Surgical Site Infection: NNIS Risk Index

In an effort to identify patients with a susceptibility to postoperative infection, the CDC (National Nosocomial Infections Surveillance [NNIS] system) developed a risk index, which has been validated and found to correlate well with infection rates.[15] The risk index is based on an ASA (American Society of Anesthesiologists) preoperative assessment, the wound category, and the duration of surgery (75th percentile of the NNIS data for craniotomies rounded to the nearest whole number of hours: 4 hours). The index is divided into four categories (0 to 3), which correlate with increasing risk for postoperative wound infections. The categories are calculated by adding one point for each of the following when present: an ASA score of 3, 4, or 5; contaminated or dirty wounds; and a duration of surgery exceeding 4 hours. This NNIS risk score allows an estimate of the risk for developing an SSI.[1,10,20]

## ▪ Surgical Site Infections in Postoperative Cranial Surgery

To distinguish general postoperative from wound infections, the latter are appropriately termed SSIs.[19] The neurosurgical site is divided into extra- and intradural parts. Extradural infections involve every level from the skin to the dura mater, including the bone flap. Intradural infections can be localized to the subdural space (empyema) or to an intracerebral location (abscess), or they can be generalized (meningitis and ventriculitis). To allow a more thorough analysis of SSIs, the CDC introduced a classification[19] that differentiates between incisional (superficial and deep) and organ-related SSIs. In neurosurgery, incisional SSIs represent extradural infections. Organ-related SSIs include every intradural infection (subdural empyema, intracerebral abscess, meningitis, and ventriculitis). In the CDC definition, organ SSIs are specified as "all infections . . . [which] . . . involve any part of the anatomy other than the incision opened or manipulated during the operative procedure,"[19] which includes the cranial opening. Thus, epidural abscess and bone flap infection are considered deep wound infections, whereas osteomyelitis as a CDC organ/space SSI refers to orthopedic surgery.

Although this clear categorization of location can facilitate appropriate reporting, a gray zone exists for potential underreporting. In the neurosurgical literature, a particularly pragmatic approach is taken whereby only those SSIs that required reoperation are considered. This practice covers only those complications with immediate serious consequences, whereas "near-complications" such as superficial SSIs treated on the ward (e.g., additional stitches, lumbar drainage for CSF collections without leakage) may be incompletely reported. However, these near-complications or incidents allow us to understand and address the issue of SSI more comprehensively. In risk management and prevention, special emphasis is given to near-incidents, which are more frequent than actual events and therefore represent a larger database. This more extensive pool of information facilitates the analysis of potential risk factors and the assessment of surgical and preventive techniques.

Additional concern exists that SSIs may be underreported because of cases that are not detected by the surgeon,[14] as well as infections that occur after discharge[7,10,16,35] and are handled either on an outpatient basis or at other institutions. This is particularly relevant for infection of the bone flap, which may manifest months after surgery.[6] With shorter hospital stays and increased patient transfer to specialized centers,[12] referral and admission patterns may indeed result in problems with accurately reporting SSIs. Patient transfer, which is less developed in Europe, has to be considered when infection rates[9] are compared by countries or continents.

The CDC criteria for wound infection include "purulent discharge" and the "surgeon's impression" of the wound as key features. Infections present mostly with local signs of inflammation. Fever is an explicit symptom, but in milder courses of infection, temperature elevation can be either absent or slight. Neurologic symptoms in intracranial infections range from headaches to altered mental status and focal deficits.

Currently, the most useful postoperative laboratory parameter is the C-reactive protein (CRP) level.[36-38] Although elevated levels are not surprising after surgery (correlating with tissue damage), sustained elevation beyond the fourth day or renewed elevation after normalization should raise suspicion for infection. In the presence of neurologic symptoms, imaging is indicated to assess for the presence of intracranial suppuration. Computed tomography (CT) is the most readily available imaging modality. Contrast-enhanced CT provides a firm basis for the diagnosis of intracranial and epidural infectious complications. Although nonspecific contrast enhancement may appear a few days postoperatively, when considered together with clinical suspicion and laboratory findings, the results rarely remain ambiguous. Generally, infections present as fluid collections with pronounced ring enhancement. To plan the surgical procedure, the extent of the infection must be defined. The increased availability of magnetic resonance (MR) imaging provides further structural and pathophysiologic (perfusion) information.

Most often, the offending organisms are gram-positive skin flora (i.e., coagulase-negative staphylococci, *S. aureus*, and *Propionibacterium acnes*). Various reports on rare and resistant bacterial strains emphasize the importance of adhering to the general principles of antibiotic prophylaxis and of coordinating treatment closely with microbiologists. Fungal SSIs are rare but should not be disregarded.

Although incisional and organ SSIs manifest at different time intervals after surgery, the range is too wide to provide a solid basis for differential diagnosis. In a population of 2,944 patients in a multicenter study,[10] scalp infections (5 ± 9 days; median, 13 days) and meningitis/ventriculitis (10 ± 8 days; median, 7 days) occurred earlier than intradural infections (empyema and abscess, 25 ± 31 days; median, 15 days), with the longest latency seen for bone flap infection (42 ± 56 days; median, 27 days). In a single-institution[2] follow-up study with a larger population of 4,578 patients, the authors corroborated the order with time to manifestation—with, however, an even larger range (mean time between surgery and onset of infection in days: meningitis, 12 ± 14; scalp infection, 23 ± 51; brain abscess or empyema, 25 ± 27; bone flap, 118 ± 157), reemphasizing the long latency period for bone flap infection.

## ■ Incisional Surgical Site Infections

Incisional SSIs are subdivided into superficial and deep infections.[19]

### Superficial Incisional Surgical Site Infections

The CDC defines superficial incisional wound infections as ". . . infection . . . [which] . . . occurs within 30 days after the operative procedure and involves only skin and subcutaneous tissue of the incision and at least one . . . [of the following] . . .: purulent discharge from the superficial incision/organisms isolated/signs of infection/diagnosis by the surgeon or attending physician. (Stitch abscess is not an SSI)." Korinek et al[2] reported 191 scalp infections in 4,578 patients. Because multiple infection sites per patient could be recorded, it remains unclear how many scalp infections were isolated or associated with deeper infections. Generally, if not associated with deeper infections, incisional SSIs can be managed by local measures. Awareness, prevention, and immediate treatment of these infections can prevent progression. Most patients with an epidural abscess had a previous superficial wound infection.[5,39,40] Although bacteriologic samples are mandatory, these usually represent noncausative skin flora.

### Deep Incisional Surgical Site Infections

Deep incisional wound infections are ". . . infections within 30 days after the operative procedure if no implant is left in place or within 1 year, if implant is in place and infection involves the deep soft tissue and one of the following: purulent discharge/ spontaneously dehisces or opened because of fever, local pain, or tenderness/pathological, radiological, or intraoperative proof/ diagnosis by physician."

Deep incisional infections should be inspected in the operating room with cleaning, débridement, local antiseptic techniques, and readaptation. In our practice, we apply a specially constructed ball tip ultrasonic aspirator for wound débridement and local antibacterial effect through the cavitation (unpublished data).

### ■ Bone Flap Infection with Epidural Abscess

Bone flap infections and epidural abscesses are deep incisional infections. Hlavin et al reported on 23 patients over a period of 11 years with postoperative epidural abscess and bone flap infection.[39,41] Korinek et al[2]

identified 77 of 4,578 patients (1.68%) as having bone flap infection. Dashti et al[12] reoperated on 22 patients for this diagnosis among 16,540 craniotomies over 10 years. Considering that bone flaps are devascularized and that 50% of flaps lifted for craniotomy are contaminated[29] (albeit with few colony-forming units), this low rate is remarkable.

The clinical symptoms are limited, usually without headache and neurologic signs; local symptoms of wound infection are often present. An epidural abscess can develop local mass effect, causing focal neurologic deficit. Fever can occur but is not obligatory for the diagnosis. Manifestation of bone flap infection can be delayed. The reported mean presentation time lies beyond 30 to 40 days and up to 180 days after surgery.[2,5,6,29,40,42]

Surgical débridement with removal of foreign material is mandatory, as is obtaining a specimen for microbiological analysis. Subsequently, antibiotic irrigation and a "ball pen" ultrasonic aspirator (personal experience) are employed to clean the surgical site. Intradural inspection should be avoided unless the dura appears tense. [6] With prior surgery, however, deeper extension of the epidural infection should be suspected. Preoperative MR imaging is helpful in planning the extent of the operation. Postoperatively, antibiotics are administered according to culture results. In the setting of bone infection, a protracted course of antibiotics is usually administered in accordance with general and local guidelines.

With the surgical evacuation of pus, the standard recommendation is to remove the contaminated bone.[5,6,39,40] Cranioplasty usually is planned 6 months after removal.

Efforts to salvage the bone in position have recently yielded encouraging results. It is evident that antibiotic treatment alone is insufficient, and various surgical methods have been tested. Thorough surgical débridement resulted in the long-term resolution of infection in 11 of 13 uncomplicated cases.[43] In more complex cases, a "wash-in, wash-out indwelling antibiotic irrigation system" was employed, resulting in complete resolution in 11 of 12 patients.[44] However, if the bone flap cannot be salvaged, immediate reconstruction with titanium mesh may be an alternative. After extensive surgical débridement, this approach was successful in 10 of 12 patients.[42] Although these measures may present good alternatives after individual careful consideration, the numbers are too small to permit their general endorsement in the treatment of bone flap infections.

## Organ/Space Surgical Site Infections

The CDC defines organ/space SSI as follows: "An organ/space SSI involves any part of the anatomy other than the incision, opened or manipulated during the operative procedure, with infection within 30 days, if no implant is left in place and . . . [one of the following] . . .: purulent discharge/organisms cultured/an abscess or other evidence of infection on direct reexamination by the surgeon."

The microbiological spectrum of these infections encompasses the most frequent offenders: coagulase-negative staphylococci, *S. aureus*, and *P. acnes*. However, gram-negative and atypical bacteria (documented by a plethora of case reports) are also important. Postoperative subdural suppuration should raise concern with regard to unsuspected sources of bacteremia or communication with air-filled sinuses.[5,6,39–41]

These infections encompass localized subdural empyema and intracerebral abscesses within the resection cavity, as well as generalized infections (i.e., meningitis and ventriculitis). Because the subdural space and post-resection cavity may be interconnected, concomitant empyema and abscess may result.[39] Thus, subdural empyema and intracerebral abscess are often discussed together.[2] However, some studies differentiate between the two clinical entities, permitting a rough estimate[39] of their respective incidence.

## Subdural Empyema

Subdural empyema is infrequently encountered after surgery. In the largest series of subdural empyema, only 4 of 699 cases occurred postoperatively.[45] Hlavin et al identified 11 patients with postoperative suppuration involving the subdural space over 11 years (3 purely subdural empyemas; 1 combined with an intracerebral abscess; 7 patients with subdural empyema and epidural abscess that were regarded as continuous from the epidural to the subdural space).[39] Dashti et al[12] found 7 patients with subdural empyema. However, because multiple sites were affected in their 50 patients with intracranial infections (among a total of 16,540 cases), those were not isolated infections.

Spontaneous subdural empyema (**Fig. 15.1**) generally follows a prodromal infection, most often of the adjacent air-filled

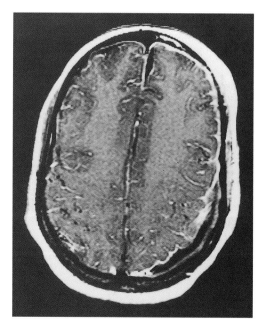

**Fig. 15.1** Contrast-enhanced axial T1-weighted magnetic resonance image demonstrates a subdural empyema located over the left hemisphere in a patient with fever and chronic sinusitis. (Figure courtesy of Walter A. Hall, MD, MBA.)

sinuses. Subsequent spread into the subdural compartment with the rapid accumulation of pus in preformed spaces leads to rapid neurologic deterioration, mandating urgent diagnosis and subsequent surgery. Septa can compartmentalize the subdural space, making the surgical treatment challenging (**Fig. 15.2**). Therefore, a common recommendation in these entities is to remove the pus through a craniotomy because burr holes do not provide access for sufficient drainage.[40,46] Subdural empyema represents a surgical emergency, with a high rate of morbidity (10 to 20% of patients develop purulent meningitis, and 10 to 25% have an associated intraparenchymal abscess) and mortality. Early recognition and treatment are the main factors necessary for a good clinical outcome.[5,39,41,46] Thrombosis of cortical vessels with subsequent venous infarction may accelerate the already rapid clinical decline.[41]

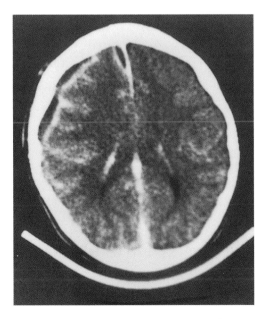

**Fig. 15.2** Axial contrast-enhanced computed tomographic scan of the brain shows a septated subdural empyema over the right frontal lobe. There is also purulence in the interhemispheric fissure. (Figure courtesy of Walter A. Hall, MD, MBA.)

Fortunately, when it occurs as a postoperative complication, the progress and presentation of this entity are often less aggressive.[39] This is attributed to the postoperative formation of membranes that protect the cortex and limit the extension of the empyema.[41] The main symptoms are local pain and tenderness at the surgical site. Recurrent seizures and mild neurologic deficits should draw attention to this possible complication and warrant imaging. Hlavin et al found 30% of their CT scans inconclusive. However, this statement pertains to scans acquired before 1994; moreover, 50% of those imaging studies were done without contrast.[39,41] Contemporary CT with contrast should provide enough information for the diagnosis. Additionally, MR imaging provides structural as well as perfusional information.

Treatment is immediate surgical evacuation by repeat craniotomy. Antibiotics alone are ineffective. One should be prepared to enlarge the cranial opening to reach all potential "pockets" of purulence if imaging suggests a wider extension of the empyema. Where the arachnoid is breached, a resection, which would endanger the underlying cortex and vessels,[39,41] should be avoided. As much pus as is accessible should be removed. Gross total evacuation of the empyema is a prerequisite for successful antibiotic treatment. After treatment is begun with a broad spectrum of antibiotics, targeted treatment should be initiated subsequent to microbiological differentiation.

## ■ Intracerebral Abscess

Postoperative intracerebral abscesses are rare (percentage of abscesses among total number of craniotomies: 0.53% (3/556)[3]; 0.17% (31/18,600)[47]; and 0.05% (8/16,540).[12] This complication occurs primarily in the immediate postoperative period and presents with nonspecific symptoms of meningitis and clinical deterioration. A new neurologic deficit, normal or elevated temperature, and progressively impaired levels of consciousness warrant imaging to obtain a diagnosis. In postoperative abscesses, the frequency of gram-negative and polymicrobial etiologies complicates subsequent antibiotic therapy.[40,47]

The treatment of postoperative abscesses, unlike that of spontaneous cases, requires open surgical reexploration of the surgical site[5,12,13,40,47] to obtain viable specimens, drain the abscess, and inspect and clean the resection cavity. Leaving a drain inside the cavity is not recommended. Antibiotic treatment should be initiated as a broad-spectrum combination and continued according to microbiological differentiation.

An additional noninfectious differential diagnosis for ring-enhancing lesions within the operative cavity has occurred with more aggressive treatment for gliomas. So-called pseudo-progression, with new contrast-enhancing tissue due to concomitant radiation and chemotherapy, may be distinguished by its delayed time course, silent clinical presentation, and patchy appearance on imaging.

Chemotherapy wafer implantation may lead to an enlarging resection cavity that presents with neurologic changes due to the mass lesion.[48] On imaging, homogeneous ring enhancement with perifocal edema may meet the criteria for the diagnosis of an abscess. However, the smooth and linear-appearing contrast ring should raise suspicion that this might be a normal reaction after local chemotherapy. In this case, symptoms resolve with a short course of high-dose dexamethasone. Subsequently, the enhancement decreases and the cavity contracts over the course of several weeks. Occasionally, puncture of the pseudocyst and rarely implantation of a reservoir are needed.

## ■ Meningitis

Postoperative meningitis may be either aseptic or bacterial in origin.[49] This infection manifests within a few days after surgery. Classic signs, such as nuchal rigidity, alteration of consciousness, and fever, oc-

cur. The CRP level rises sharply. Cerebral imaging should be obtained to rule out local causative SSI as well as postoperative mass lesions. After contraindications have been excluded, lumbar puncture should be performed to acquire material for bacteriology. A broad-spectrum antibiotic combination should then be initiated and subsequently changed according to the microbiology culture results.[5,49] If aseptic meningitis is diagnosed, antibiotics should be discontinued. In this condition, corticosteroids relieve the meningeal inflammatory response.[49]

The most common risk factor for bacterial meningitis (organ SSI) is persistent CSF leakage.[2,7,31] CSF cushions without leakage are mostly treated successfully by conservative means. However, fistulas should be addressed surgically when diagnosed to prevent any form of SSI. Under special circumstances, after careful assessment of the intraoperative conditions and an evaluation of the extent of CSF leakage, a short-term conservative treatment with lumbar puncture or drain may be attempted to avoid reopening the surgical site. However, lumbar or ventricular drains are risk factors by themselves.[49,50] In these cases, close clinical and laboratory observation is necessary.[50] There is no consensus with regard to prophylactic antibiotics.

Definitive surgical closure of the CSF leak is preferable in most cases. With persistent CSF leakage, the surrounding inflammation will increase, complicating subsequent wound closure. Foreign material should be removed during revision surgery. Preparations should be made to harvest fascia lata and umbilical fat for dural reconstruction.

## ■ Summary and Conclusion

Postoperative infections in cranial neurosurgery are rare. They encompass bone flap infection, epidural and intracerebral abscesses, subdural empyema, and meningitis. Meningitis can generally be treated with antibiotics, but the other SSIs require surgical treatment.

The single most important risk factor for the development of SSI is CSF leakage.[2,7,8,13]

Further procedural risk factors are the following: absent or inadequate antibiotic prophylaxis, longer duration of surgery, implantation of foreign materials, early re-operation, and irradiated skin.[2,3,7,8,13] Hair removal does not show advantages over unshaven surgical sites.[26] Clean and clean–contaminated wound categories do not have any impact if the surgical site is properly prepared.[2,30,33]

General adherence to CDC wound and SSI definitions[15,19] provides a basis for the structured reporting of postoperative wound infections. Still, because of their scarcity, gathering comprehensive information on the occurrence, causes, and prevention of SSIs remains challenging.

In neurosurgery, there is a considerable variation in reported cranial postoperative infection rates, increasing from single-surgeon series[3] to series with only elective cases[8] to less selective multiple-center[10] and multiple-surgeon studies.[2] However, a comparison of only these rates disregards differences in data accumulation.[9] Regarding postoperative infections in cranial neurosurgery, Bloomsted had already stated in 1992 that "… incidence rates should be read with skepticism." Various reasons for this cautious assessment have been highlighted in this chapter.

For future reporting, adherence to the locations summarized in this chapter would enable a more comprehensive analysis of SSIs across studies in regard to their occurrence, respective risk factors, and prevention. Presently, the surgeon remains the most crucial element in preempting SSIs. Control of the general operating room situation, careful case preparation, adherence to antiseptic principles, minimization of tissue damage, operating in a timely fashion, and meticulous wound closure are all within the surgeon's dominion.

## References

1. Gaynes RP, Culver DH, Horan TC, Edwards JR, Richards C, Tolson JS. Surgical site infection (SSI) rates in the United States, 1992-1998: the National Nosocomial Infections Surveillance System basic SSI risk index. Clin Infect Dis 2001;33(Suppl 2): S69–S77

2. Korinek AM, Golmard JL, Elcheick A, et al. Risk factors for neurosurgical site infections after craniotomy: a critical reappraisal of antibiotic prophylaxis on 4,578 patients. Br J Neurosurg 2005; 19(2):155–162

3. McClelland S III, Hall WA. Postoperative central nervous system infection: incidence and associated factors in 2111 neurosurgical procedures. Clin Infect Dis 2007;45(1):55–59

4. Blomstedt GC. Craniotomy infections. Neurosurg Clin N Am 1992;3(2):375–385

5. Hall WA. Cerebral infectious processes. In: Loftus CM, ed. Neurosurgical Emergencies. Vol 1. Park Ridge, IL: American Association of Neurological Surgeons; 1994:165–182

6. Olsen JJ, Bingaman KD. Cranial bone flap infections and osteomyelitis of the skull. In: Osenbach RK, Zeidman SM, eds. Infections in Neurological Surgery. Philadelphia, PA: Lippincott–Raven Publishers; 1999:65–83

7. Lietard C, Thébaud V, Besson G, Lejeune B. Risk factors for neurosurgical site infections: an 18-month prospective survey. J Neurosurg 2008;109(4):729–734

8. Valentini LG, Casali C, Chatenoud L, Chiaffarino F, Uberti-Foppa C, Broggi G. Surgical site infections after elective neurosurgery: a survey of 1747 patients. Neurosurgery 2008;62(1):88–95, discussion 95–96

9. McClelland S III. Postoperative intracranial neurosurgery infection rates in North America versus Europe: a systematic analysis. Am J Infect Control 2008;36(8):570–573

10. Korinek AM; Service Epidémiologie Hygiène et Prévention. Risk factors for neurosurgical site infections after craniotomy: a prospective multicenter study of 2944 patients. The French Study Group of Neurosurgical Infections, the SEHP, and the C-CLIN Paris-Nord. Neurosurgery 1997;41(5):1073–1079, discussion 1079–1081

11. Sharma MS, Vohra A, Thomas P, et al. Effect of risk-stratified, protocol-based perioperative chemoprophylaxis on nosocomial infection rates in a series of 31,927 consecutive neurosurgical procedures (1994-2006). Neurosurgery 2009;64(6):1123–1130, discussion 1130–1131

12. Dashti SR, Baharvahdat H, Spetzler RF, et al. Operative intracranial infection following craniotomy. Neurosurg Focus 2008;24(6):E10

13. Lassen B, Helseth E, Rønning P, et al. Surgical mortality at 30 days and complications leading to recraniotomy in 2630 consecutive craniotomies for intracranial tumors. Neurosurgery 2011;68(5):1259–1268, discussion 1268–1269

14. Heipel D, Ober JF, Edmond MB, Bearman GM. Surgical site infection surveillance for neurosurgical procedures: a comparison of passive surveillance by surgeons to active surveillance by infection control professionals. Am J Infect Control 2007;35(3):200–202

15. Culver DH, Horan TC, Gaynes RP, et al; National Nosocomial Infections Surveillance System. Surgical wound infection rates by wound class, operative procedure, and patient risk index. Am J Med 1991;91(3B):152S–157S

16. Kasatpibal N, Jamulitrat S, Chongsuvivatwong V. Standardized incidence rates of surgical site infection: a multicenter study in Thailand. Am J Infect Control 2005;33(10):587–594

17. Talbot TR, Schaffner W. Relationship between age and the risk of surgical site infection: a contemporary reexamination of a classic risk factor. J Infect Dis 2005;191(7):1032–1035

18. Owens CD, Stoessel K. Surgical site infections: epidemiology, microbiology and prevention. J Hosp Infect 2008;70(Suppl 2):3–10

19. Horan TC, Gaynes RP, Martone WJ, Jarvis WR, Emori TG. CDC definitions of nosocomial surgical site infections, 1992: a modification of CDC definitions of surgical wound infections. Am J Infect Control 1992;20(5):271–274

20. Mangram AJ, Horan TC, Pearson ML, Silver LC, Jarvis WR; Centers for Disease Control and Prevention (CDC) Hospital Infection Control Practices Advisory Committee. Guideline for prevention of surgical site infection, 1999. Am J Infect Control 1999;27(2):97–132, quiz 133–134, discussion 96

21. Malone DL, Genuit T, Tracy JK, Gannon C, Napolitano LM. Surgical site infections: reanalysis of risk factors. J Surg Res 2002;103(1):89–95

22. McGovern PC, Lautenbach E, Brennan PJ, Lustig RA, Fishman NO. Risk factors for postcraniotomy surgical site infection after 1,3-bis (2-chloroethyl)-1-nitrosourea (Gliadel) wafer placement. Clin Infect Dis 2003;36(6):759–765

23. Kaye KS, Schmit K, Pieper C, et al. The effect of increasing age on the risk of surgical site infection. J Infect Dis 2005;191(7):1056–1062

24. Clark AJ, Butowski NA, Chang SM, et al. Impact of bevacizumab chemotherapy on craniotomy wound healing. J Neurosurg 2011;114(6):1609–1616

25. McHugh SM, Hill AD, Humphreys H. Intraoperative technique as a factor in the prevention of surgical site infection. J Hosp Infect 2011;78(1):1–4

26. Winston KR. Hair and neurosurgery. Neurosurgery 1992;31(2):320–329

27. Bekar A, Korfali E, Doğan S, Yilmazlar S, Başkan Z, Aksoy K. The effect of hair on infection after cranial surgery. Acta Neurochir (Wien) 2001;143(6):533–536, discussion 537

28. Tokimura H, Tajitsu K, Tsuchiya M, et al. Cranial surgery without head shaving. J Craniomaxillofac Surg 2009;37(8):477–480

29. Chiang HY, Steelman VM, Pottinger JM, et al. Clinical significance of positive cranial bone flap cultures and associated risk of surgical site infection after craniotomies or craniectomies. J Neurosurg 2011;114(6):1746–1754

30. Harvey RJ, Smith JE, Wise SK, Patel SJ, Frankel BM, Schlosser RJ. Intracranial complications before and after endoscopic skull base reconstruction. Am J Rhinol 2008;22(5):516–521

31. Korinek AM, Baugnon T, Golmard JL, van Effenterre R, Coriat P, Puybasset L. Risk factors for adult nosocomial meningitis after craniotomy: role of antibiotic prophylaxis. Neurosurgery 2008;62(Suppl 2):532–539

32. Dubey A, Sung WS, Shaya M, et al. Complications of posterior cranial fossa surgery—an institutional experience of 500 patients. Surg Neurol 2009;72(4):369–375

33. Kono Y, Prevedello DM, Snyderman CH, et al. One thousand endoscopic skull base surgical procedures demystifying the infection potential: incidence and description of postoperative meningitis and brain abscesses. Infect Control Hosp Epidemiol 2011;32(1):77–83

34. Narotam PK, van Dellen JR, du Trevou MD, Gouws E. Operative sepsis in neurosurgery: a method of classifying surgical cases. Neurosurgery 1994;34(3):409–415, discussion 415–416

35. Sands K, Vineyard G, Platt R. Surgical site infections occurring after hospital discharge. J Infect Dis 1996;173(4):963–970

36. Bengzon J, Grubb A, Bune A, Hellström K, Lindström V, Brandt L. C-reactive protein levels following standard neurosurgical procedures. Acta Neurochir (Wien) 2003;145(8):667–670, discussion 670–671

37. Mirzayan MJ, Gharabaghi A, Samii M, Tatagiba M, Krauss JK, Rosahl SK. Response of C-reactive protein after craniotomy for microsurgery of intracranial tumors. Neurosurgery 2007;60(4):621–625, discussion 625

38. Al-Jabi Y, El-Shawarby A. Value of C-reactive protein after neurosurgery: a prospective study. Br J Neurosurg 2010;24(6):653–659

39. Hlavin ML, Kaminski HJ, Fenstermaker RA, White RJ. Intracranial suppuration: a modern decade of postoperative subdural empyema and epidural abscess. Neurosurgery 1994;34(6):974–980, discussion 980–981

40. Hall WA, Truwit CL. The surgical management of infections involving the cerebrum. Neurosurgery 2008;62(Suppl 2):519–530, discussion 530–531

41. Hlavin ML, Ratcheson RA. Subdural empyema. In: Kaye AH, Black PM, eds. Operative Neurosurgery. Vol 2. London, England: Churchill Livingstone; 2000:1667–1678

42. Kshettry VR, Hardy S, Weil RJ, Angelov L, Barnett GH. Immediate titanium cranioplasty after debridement and craniectomy for post-craniotomy surgical site infection. Neurosurgery 2011;(Jul):29

43. Bruce JN, Bruce SS. Preservation of bone flaps in patients with postcraniotomy infections. J Neurosurg 2003;98(6):1203–1207

44. Auguste KI, McDermott MW. Salvage of infected craniotomy bone flaps with the wash-in, wash-out indwelling antibiotic irrigation system. Technical note and case series of 12 patients. J Neurosurg 2006;105(4):640–644

45. Nathoo N, Nadvi SS, van Dellen JR, Gouws E. Intracranial subdural empyemas in the era of computed tomography: a review of 699 cases. Neurosurgery 1999;44(3):529–535, discussion 535–536

46. Nathoo N, Nadvi SS, Gouws E, van Dellen JR. Craniotomy improves outcomes for cranial subdural empyemas: computed tomography-era

experience with 699 patients. Neurosurgery 2001;49(4):872–877, discussion 877–878

47. Yang KY, Chang WN, Ho JT, Wang HC, Lu CH. Post-neurosurgical nosocomial bacterial brain abscess in adults. Infection 2006;34(5):247–251

48. Dörner L, Ulmer S, Rohr A, Mehdorn HM, Nabavi A. Space-occupying cyst development in the resection cavity of malignant gliomas following Gliadel® implantation: incidence, therapeutic strategies, and outcome. J Clin Neurosci 2011;18(3):347–351

49. Infection in Neurosurgery Working Party of the British Society for Antimicrobial Chemotherapy. The management of neurosurgical patients with postoperative bacterial or aseptic meningitis or external ventricular drain-associated ventriculitis. Br J Neurosurg 2000;14(1):7–12

50. Scheithauer S, Bürgel U, Bickenbach J, et al. External ventricular and lumbar drainage-associated meningoventriculitis: prospective analysis of time-dependent infection rates and risk factor analysis. Infection 2010;38(3):205–209

# 16

# Implanted Devices and Central Nervous System Infection

**Ramesh Grandhi, Gillian Harrison, and Elizabeth Tyler-Kabara**

The use of implanted devices is commonplace in most neurosurgical practices. Because of the tendency of implanted hardware to harbor microorganisms, the rate of postsurgical infections is generally higher, and the treatment of such infections often necessitates surgical removal of the involved hardware. In this chapter, we review the diagnosis, microbiology, and treatment of these challenging infections by category. We also review current strategies for prevention, which are discussed from other viewpoints in other chapters of this volume.

## ■ Shunt Infections

Hydrocephalus, estimated to affect nearly 1 in every 500 children,[1] is one of the most common pediatric pathologies requiring neurosurgical intervention. This disorder may coexist with a variety of congenital or acquired brain disorders, most commonly myelomeningocele[2] or intraventricular hemorrhage,[3] followed by aqueductal stenosis, tumor, prior central nervous system (CNS) infection, and head injury. In contrast, common forms of hydrocephalus in adults include idiopathic normal-pressure hydrocephalus and obstructive hydrocephalus; it is also caused by cysts, tumors, hemorrhage, head injury, and meningitis.[4] Although a variety of other treatments have been utilized, such as choroid plexectomy, choroid plexus cauterization, and carotid ligation, high morbidity and failure rates have forced these methods to be abandoned. The development of endoscopy has increased the use of third ventriculostomy, but a cerebrospinal fluid (CSF) shunt is the current mainstay of treatment for hydrocephalus.[5]

CSF shunts have three main components—a proximal ventricular catheter, a unidirectional valve, and a distal catheter—that function by diverting fluid from the ventricles to other body cavities, most commonly the peritoneum and rarely the right atrium or pleural space. The first shunts were used in the 1950s,[6] and they currently account for nearly 70,000 hospital discharges and 36,000 surgical procedures in the United States, costing over $100 million annually.[2,7] Although some studies suggest that the incidence of hydrocephalus and corresponding shunt insertion is decreasing,[8,9] others have found that the prevalence has increased because of the improved survival of premature infants and older children with hydrocephalus.[10] Despite nearly 60 years of experience with CSF shunts, their placement remains fraught with complications, and overall failure rates remain high, at nearly 40% in the first year.[11,12] Malfunction due to mechanical obstruction or disconnection remains the most common complication, but infection is arguably the most dangerous, resulting in serious patient morbidity and mortality, long hospital stays, and costly interventions.[5]

## Epidemiology and Risk Factors

The incidence of shunt infection varies greatly, with most modern studies reporting rates ranging from 2.1 to 12% per procedure[4,9,13–27] and from 6.3 to 18% per patient.[15,23,25] Following surgery, the median time to infection ranges from 10 to 72 days,[4,14,21,26] with approximately 60% presenting within the first month[17] and nearly 90% presenting in the first 6 months.[28] Investigators have attempted to identify factors predicting the length of time to the development of infection, such as type of bacteria[28] and whether the shunt is primary insertion or a revision[14]; however, most studies have not identified such a correlation. Although it is difficult to establish significant differences between infection rates in ventriculoperitoneal (VP), ventriculoatrial (VA), and ventriculopleural shunts because of small sample sizes of the latter two, it has been suggested that the infection incidence is lowest for VP shunts.[9]

There is a clear association between age and the incidence of infection, with the highest incidence noted in children. Tulipan and Cleves documented a rate of 15.7% in patients younger than 11.3 years of age, statistically higher than the rate of 6.7% in adults, with the highest incidence of 23% in infants less than 1 month old.[16] These results have been corroborated in multiple studies,[20,27] with a demonstrable inverse relationship between age and the incidence of infection.[21] Most investigators note the highest infection rates in children younger than 1 year of age, many citing early gestational age, preterm birth, hydrocephalus etiology of intraventricular hemorrhage, or younger age at the time of shunt placement as independent risk factors for infection.[15,24,25,28] Although the basis for this trend remains unclear, possible reasons include a relative immunodeficient response to bacterial infection in the first 6 months of life, higher bacterial density on the skin, longer hospital stays, and prior exposure to antibiotics. A multitude of patient, surgeon, and operative factors have been examined to identify risk factors for infection. In addition to age, patient factors found to increase the risk for infection include prior CSF leak, shunt revision, and infection.[3,4,21,28,29] Demographic factors such as race, insurance type, and chronic medical conditions were found to be significant risk factors in one study[15]; however, these results were not widely reproduced. Studies have shown mixed results for the etiology of hydrocephalus as a risk factor for infection. Some suggest that etiologies such as intraventricular hemorrhage or prior shunt infection[15,28] increase risk; however, others have not found any difference between etiologies.[4,30] General risk factors for infection, such as prolonged hospitalization, prolonged steroid treatment, immunosuppressive states, and poor skin condition, may also play a role. Several surgeon and operative factors have also been reported to affect the incidence of infection, such as surgeon experience or case volume,[9,19] time of day and length of surgery,[4,31] use of a neuroendoscope,[21] and the number of times the shunt is handled during surgery.[24]

## Pathogenesis and Microbiology

The bacteria most often responsible for shunt infection are commensal, low-virulence, slowly replicating organisms. By far the most commonly observed pathogens (up to 71.8%)[32] are coagulase-negative staphylococci, with *Staphylococcus epidermidis* the most often reported causative organism (**Table 16.1**). Other gram-positive pathogens observed to cause infection include *Staphylococcus aureus*, particularly in patients with concomitant skin infections,[4] and less frequently viridans-group streptococci, pneumococci, *Enterococcus*, *Propionibacterium acnes*, and *Corynebacterium*. Gram-negative bacteria (e.g., *Escherichia coli*, which accounts for more than 50%[26] of cases, *Klebsiella, Proteus*, and *Pseudomonas*) account for a lower percentage of infections than gram-positive organisms and are usually associated with corresponding abdominal pathology. Although generally considered uncommon, polymicrobial infections account for up to 20% of infections and are often associated with an abdomi-

**Table 16.1** Incidence of specific pathogens in shunt infection

| Pathogen | Incidence, % |
|---|---|
| Gram-positive bacteria | |
| Coagulase-negative staphylococci (*Staphylococcus epidermidis*) | 24–71.8[4,16,17,29,32,37,38] |
| *Staphylococcus aureus* | 9.3–33[3,16,21,22,29,32,37,38] |
| Other (*Propionibacterium acnes*, *Corynebacterium*, viridans-group streptococci, *Streptococcus pneumoniae*, *Enterococcus*) | < 1–21.8[3,21,22,29,32] |
| Gram-negative bacteria (*Escherichia coli*, *Pseudomonas*, *Klebsiella*, *Proteus*) | 6–49[17,22,29] |
| Polymicrobial | 11–20[4,20,32] |

nal origin or contaminated head wounds.[20] Fungal infections, most commonly involving *Candida*, are seen infrequently, usually in premature infants or immunocompromised patients.[28]

Given the frequency with which infection occurs soon after shunt surgery and the predominance of common skin flora as the causative organisms, it is logical to hypothesize that the majority of infections are the result of contamination at the time of surgery; indeed, Conen et al associated 72% of shunt infections with intraoperative sources.[29] Although Bayston and Lari reported wound contamination in 58% of cases at incision closure,[33] the origin of the such organisms was unclear. In a study comparing skin cultures with infection culture results, Shapiro et al noted that 22% of patients were infected with organisms identical to their skin flora, 22% had infections associated with other identifiable causes, and 55% were infected with typical skin flora that were different from the patients' isolates.[27] In addition to intraoperative contamination, other sources of infection include skin

dehiscence over the shunt tract, hematogenous spread, and bowel perforation by the distal catheter tip, resulting in an ascending infection.[29] Although VA shunts are more prone to infection through bacteremia, VP shunts are more susceptible to distal infection by intestinal pathogens.

Once contamination occurs, bacteria colonize the shunt lumen, which is an immune-protected space, and exposure to CSF aids bacterial adherence to the tubing.[34] The prevalence of infection with coagulase-negative staphylococci is particularly important in the pathogenesis of shunt infection because these organisms are able to form an extracellular matrix made of glycoproteins, called a biofilm, that further facilitates adhesion and protects the bacteria from the immune system and antibiotics.[28] Formation of the biofilm and peritoneal inflammation that walls off the distal end of the shunt catheter by forming a pseudocyst are two major contributors to the association between shunt infection and malfunction.[35]

## Diagnosis

### Clinical Presentation

The presentation of a shunt infection may be insidious and nonspecific, with variable clinical features that depend on the site of the infection. The most common manifestation of infection is fever with signs and symptoms indicative of shunt malfunction, such as headache, irritability, nausea and vomiting, and lethargy.[28] Wounds with localized signs and symptoms, such as erythema, pain, swelling, CSF accumulation along the shunt track, and with progression purulent discharge, particularly in children with poor skin quality, may provide a visible source of infection, with at least one of these signs observed in up to half of cases.[29] Less commonly, patients may present with neck stiffness or frank meningismus and, more rarely, seizures[20] or glomerulonephritis.[36] In the case of the VP shunt, abdominal symptoms mimicking common viral syndromes may confound the diagnosis, with signs of intra-abdominal infection being pain, vomiting, food intolerance, and peritonitis.

## Diagnostic Course

In patients presenting with nonspecific signs and symptoms, particularly those with recent shunt surgery, a high level of suspicion for shunt infection should be maintained; however, it is always important, particularly with children, to complete a full history and physical examination to exclude other common infectious sources. Routine blood tests often show a peripheral leukocytosis[22]; positive blood culture in the setting of VP shunt infection is infrequent. Elevated C-reactive protein (CRP) levels may also be observed in nearly three-fourths of cases.[37] Additionally, any apparent sites of infection, such as open wounds, should be cultured.

The most definitive way to diagnose a shunt infection is through the direct sampling of CSF from the shunt, known as a shunt tap, with the observation of organisms on either Gram stain or culture.[39] Culture positivity is highest when sampling is done directly from the valve or reservoir (> 90%) rather than from a lumbar puncture, which yields a positive culture in fewer than half of cases.[29] CSF cultures should be held for a minimum of 7 to 10 days to ensure growth of fastidious organisms.[36,40] Although positive cultures provide a definitive diagnosis, studies have reported negative CSF cultures in infections confirmed by later culture of the shunt tip anywhere from 8%[21] to 55.8%[16] of the time, indicating that a negative culture does not rule out infection but may be due to several factors, such as prior antibiotic use. CSF findings supporting infection include leukocytosis with a predominance of neutrophils, eosinophilia,[22] elevated protein, decreased glucose, and elevated lactate. Although all of these criteria may not be met, CSF analysis is completely normal in fewer than 3% of patients,[29] and the combination of fever and ventricular neutrophils above 10% has a reported specificity of 99% and a positive predictive value of 93% for infection.[22]

Imaging in the diagnosis of shunt infection may include a shunt series to establish continuity of the shunt hardware. Computed tomography (CT) or magnetic resonance (MR) imaging should be used to examine the size of the ventricles, which may be enlarged with concurrent shunt malfunction. CT may show signs of infection in approximately 10% of cases, manifested mainly as meningeal enhancement or the presence of a brain abscess.[29] For suspected cases of distal infection, older studies have suggested the use of ultrasound[35]; however, CT has since been found to be more reliable than ultrasound, demonstrating signs of infection such as inflammation of the fat or muscle around the shunt, thickened intestinal wall, abscess, shunt tip dislocation, or pseudocyst in three-fourths of episodes, in contrast to only half of episodes in which ultrasound was used.[29] In summary, the most important method of diagnosis is a high level of clinical suspicion at the time of presentation, supported by CSF studies and imaging.

## Management

Once the diagnosis of a shunt infection is made, the mainstay of treatment includes antibiotics with or without surgical management. Immediate clinical decisions include the choice of antibiotics, route of administration (systemic with or without intraventricular administration), and the fate of the shunt. Review of the literature reveals three general approaches to the management of an infected shunt[38]:

1. A two-stage surgical procedure with removal of the entire shunt and external drainage of the CSF, either by an external ventricular drain or by periodic tapping of the ventricles, with antibiotics administered systemically, intraventricularly, or both ways, followed by replacement of the shunt when the CSF is sterile

2. A one-stage procedure with removal of the entire shunt and immediate replacement, with antibiotics administered systemically, intraventricularly, or both ways

3. Antibiotic therapy alone, administered systemically, intraventricularly, or both ways

Additional surgical options in combination with antibiotics may include distal externalization of the peritoneal catheter in cases with a mild suspicion for infection or isolated abdominal infection and malfunction,[35,36] complete removal of the shunt without replacement, and complete removal with the later performance of a third ventriculostomy.[23] The majority of patients will continue to require management of their intracranial pressure through CSF drainage, making the latter two options viable in only a small subset of patients.

## Antibiotics

The choice of antibiotics is highly dependent on the presumed etiology of the infection, patterns of susceptibility, and penetration of the blood–brain barrier (BBB). Typical empiric, broad-spectrum antibiotics initiated before culture and sensitivity results are obtained may include vancomycin, a third-generation cephalosporin, and a third agent to cover anaerobes.[36] First-generation cephalosporins should be avoided because of their poor BBB penetration.[39] Because of high rates of resistance to methicillin (> 60%[38]), oxacillin, and penicillin (33%[20]), vancomycin is the drug of choice against staphylococci. Oral or intravenous rifampin may be added in combination with vancomycin because it is able to penetrate the biofilm and attain bactericidal levels at the shunt surface[38]; however, it should not be used alone because of the development of resistance. CSF Gram stain may be of early assistance in choosing an antibiotic regimen, and CSF culture and sensitivity results will allow antibiotic coverage to be tailored to specific pathogens.

All patients should receive systemic antibiotics. Whether or not to add intraventricular antibiotics to the regimen is a point of contention. The logical rationale behind the use of intraventricular antibiotics is to overcome the poor BBB penetration achieved with intravenous administration, especially in shunt infections caused by low-virulence bacteria associated with minimal meningeal inflammation. Intraventricular administration allows maximal drug concentration at the site of infection, with higher peak concentrations and better maintenance of therapeutic levels, as opposed to the observed ratios of CSF concentrations to blood concentrations after systemic antibiotic administration, which can range from 0 to 30%.[41] Reported complications with intraventricular antibiotic administration are infrequent, with the most serious being focal motor seizure.[42]

The appropriate duration of therapy is not well defined in the literature and is predominately based on the observation of clinical improvement combined with sterilization of the CSF. The reported mean duration of antibiotics ranges from 9 to 18 days.[14,29,38,39] Arnell et al reported that clinical improvement paralleled CSF sterilization and suggested performing repeat CSF culture 2 to 3 days after diagnosis, then if the cultures are negative, completing a total of 5 to 10 days of antibiotics, and if they are positive, continuing daily CSF cultures.[40] Anderson and Yogev reported cost and health benefits for shorter periods of antibiotics and recommended as few as 3 days of therapy for the mildest infections and 10 days for persistent cases.[39] The definition of infection "cure" varies; it may be limited to clinical improvement and CSF sterilization or include an extended period of infection-free follow-up. After cure of the immediate infection, if it has been surgically managed with shunt removal and later replacement, antibiotics are typically discontinued on the day of shunt replacement.

## Medical Management

Treatment with antibiotics alone has the benefit of avoiding surgery and its associated morbidity, especially in patients with multiple retained catheters. Simon et al managed 13.3% of patients with antibiotics alone with a statistically significant shorter length of hospital stay, but they also identified a trend toward higher reinfection rates.[14] In contrast to most reported cure rates with antibiotics alone,[40] Brown et al achieved a cure rate of 84% over all and in 93% of patients with *S. epidermidis* infection.[38] Importantly, this study excluded patients with *S. aureus* infection because of a high early failure rate, as well as patients with shunt malfunction, redundant shunts, brain abscess or subdural empyema, external infection, fungal infection, or local abdominal infection, thus making the study population quite specific. Additionally, all patients received intraventricular antibiotics through a ventricular catheter, which was placed if the patient did not have one before presentation. Although likely not the best choice for a majority of patients, this study suggests that antibiotic therapy alone may be efficacious for a carefully selected group of patients.

## Surgical Management

Despite the potential complications associated with undergoing a surgical procedure in view of the adherence of bacteria to shunt material, removal of the hardware is the definitive method of eliminating persistent contamination that could cause recurrent infection.[36] Two primary surgical approaches dominate the treatment of shunt infection: a two-stage and a one-stage procedure. Most institutions report surgical treatment as the standard of care,[3,14,29,39,40] with a majority employing the two-stage method. In the case of a two-stage treatment with placement of an external ventricular drain, the average length of external ventricular drain placement is approximately 1 week; however, reinternalization should not be unnecessarily delayed because reinfection rates correlate with the duration of external ventricular drain placement.[39] Kestle[3] reported a mean time to replacement of 13 days after CSF sterilization; however, in a study of more "aggressive" treatment, James and Bradley reported similar success rates with shunt replacement after antibiotic treatment for less than 12 days and after CSF cultures were negative for 24 compared with 48 hours.[42]

The choice of optimal treatment of shunt infection is hampered by the lack of prospective, randomized clinical trials. An older published trial compared antibiotics alone with one- and two-stage surgical approaches, all patients receiving both systemic and intraventricular antibiotics.[43] This study reported a cure rate of 100% with a two-stage approach, 90% with a one-stage approach, and 30% with antibiotics alone. The antibiotic group also exhibited a higher mortality rate (20% versus 0% in other groups) and longer hospital stays (45, 33, and 24 days for antibiotics, one-stage procedures, and two-stage procedures, respectively). Although this trial was limited by the small sample size, modern reviews of published studies have corroborated the results. In 1985, Yogev reviewed 18 studies and documented cure rates of 96%, 65%, and 36% for two-stage procedures, one-stage procedures, and antibiotics alone, respectively.[44] Similarly, in 2002, Schreffler et al performed a decision analysis and reviewed 17 studies with corroborating cure rates of 87.7%, 64.4%, and 33.5% for each approach.[45]

With respect to morbidity and mortality, historical studies have shown that morbidity, measured as average number of subsequent hospital admissions and average number of days in the hospital for each infection, is lowest for surgical treatment, as is mortality.[23] In a more recent study of treatment approaches, a trend toward lower mortality was documented for a two-stage approach,[37] and reviews have documented 5.7%, 11.1%, and 20.4% mortality rates for two-stage procedures, one-stage procedures, and antibiotic treatments, respectively.[45] The decision analysis for this same study assigned utility values to each approach based on cure, morbidity, and mortality and concluded that the two-stage approach has the highest utility. Although the two-stage approach is not without complications, it has been established as the current standard of care by resulting in the highest cure rate with lowest morbidity and mortality rates.

## Outcomes

Long-term outcomes after shunt infection have serious implications for the health and well-being of patients. After an initial infection, the risk for reinfection is higher, with 16 to 25% of patients admitted with reinfection within 12 months.[3,14] Although infections are usually insidious, nearly 20% of patients are admitted to neurosurgical intensive care units.[29] Infection can lead to the development of multiloculate hydrocephalus, with an increased need for repeat surgery and lifelong shunt dependence,[36] an increased risk for seizures and decreased intellectual performance and cognitive function, and a twofold higher increase in long-term mortality rate.[23,46,47]

## Prevention

Although preoperative antibiotics are widely employed,[18] many studies suggest that the common use of cephalosporins, such as cefazolin, may not decrease the risk for infection,[4,34] especially as first- and second-generation antibiotics do not have good BBB penetration. Intravenous vancomycin has been shown to be more effective (14% versus 4% infection rate) than cephalosporins, with lower mortality rates and shorter lengths of stay[18] in hospitals that have a high prevalence of methicillin-resistant *S. aureus* (MRSA). The intraoperative use of intraventricular antibiotics, specifically vancomycin and gentamicin, resulted in one study in a decrease in the infection rate from 6.5% to 0.412% with no adverse effects.[17] Meticulous operative technique and control of the operative theater are thought to be the best prevention,[1,48] with the inclusion of double gloving into standard surgical practice.[16] The introduction of antibiotic-impregnated ventricular catheters has provided some evidence for the prevention of infection[13]; however, results have been mixed.[49,50]

## ■ Spinal Instrumentation–Associated Infections

The multiple indications for spinal fusions include treatment of scoliosis, stenosis, spondylosis, spondylolisthesis, trauma, tumor, and instability. Because of the advancing age of the baby boomer generation, the percentage of the total population compris-

ing older adults in the United States will continue to increase, and it is estimated that there will be 87 million Americans past the age of 65 by the year 2050, representing more than 20% of the total population.[51] In turn, the growing number of older Americans with spinal pathology requiring operative intervention will lead to an increase in the number of fusion procedures performed. This trend in spinal surgery has already begun, and based on recent estimates, over 460,000 spinal fusions were performed in 2010, with a total cost of upward of $43 billion. In comparison, in 1997, roughly 130,000 spinal fusions were performed in the United States, with an estimated aggregate charge of slightly over $3 billion.[52]

## Definitions

The Centers for Disease Control and Prevention (CDC) classify surgical wound infections as either incisional site infections or organ/space infections, with further stratification of incisional surgical site infections (SSIs) based on the tissue compartment involved (**Table 16.2**).[53] A superficial incisional SSI involves the skin and/or subcutaneous tissues, whereas a deep incisional SSI involves the fascial and subfascial layers. In the lumbar spine (**Fig. 16.1**), deep infections occur subjacent to the lumbodorsal fascia with a posterior lumbar wound and below the anterior abdominal fascia with an anterior approach. The ligamentum nuchae and fascial layer serve as the anatomic landmarks to delineate the deep layers of the posterior cervical tissue, whereas deep wound infections after anterior cervical surgery are located deep to the platysma.[54] Of note, postoperative infections may also involve the intervertebral disks, the vertebral bodies, and/or the epidural space, resulting in diskitis, osteomyelitis, or epidural phlegmon/abscess.

## Epidemiology

The development of an infection is a known complication following surgery and is a common cause of patient morbid-

**Table 16.2** Criteria for defining a surgical site infection

**Superficial incisional SSI**

Infection occurs within 30 days after the operation and involves only skin or subcutaneous tissue of the incision and at least one of the following:

1. Purulent drainage, with or without laboratory confirmation, from the superficial incision.

2. Organisms isolated from an aseptically obtained culture of fluid or tissue from the superficial incision.

3. At least one of the following signs or symptoms of infection: pain or tenderness, localized swelling, redness, or heat, and superficial incision is deliberately opened by the surgeon, unless incision is culture-negative.

4. Diagnosis of superficial incisional SSI by the surgeon or attending physician.

**Deep incisional SSI**

Infection occurs within 30 days after the operation if no implant is left in place or within 1 year if implant is in place and the infection appears to be related to the operation and involves deep soft tissues (e.g., fascial and muscle layers) of the incision and at least one of the following:

1. Purulent drainage from the deep incision but not from the organ/space component of the surgical site.

2. A deep incision spontaneously dehisces or is deliberately opened by a surgeon when the patient has at least one of the following signs or symptoms: fever (> 38°C), localized pain, or tenderness, unless site is culture-negative.

3. An abscess or other evidence of infection involving the deep incision is found on direct examination, during reoperation, or by histopathologic or radiologic examination.

4. Diagnosis of a deep incisional SSI by a surgeon or attending physician.

*Abbreviation*: SSI, surgical site infection
*Source*: Adapted from Mangram AJ, Horan TC, Pearson ML, et al; Hospital Infection Control Practices Advisory Committee (HICPAC) and Centers for Disease Control and Prevention (CDC). Guidelines for prevention of surgical site infection. Infect Control Hosp Epidemiol 1999;24(4):247–278.

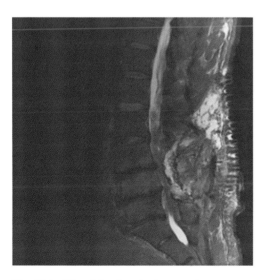

**Fig. 16.1** T2-weighted sagittal magnetic resonance image of a lumbar wound infection depicts hyperintensity within the soft tissues.

ity in the postoperative period. Wound infections, particularly deep wound infections of the spine, have significant consequences for patients and for the health care system at large. Postoperative spinal wound infections generally lead to longer in-hospital lengths of stay, higher costs, and the potential for reoperation. Moreover, these complications are known to increase patient morbidity and mortality.[55-59] Achieving a decrement in the rate of postoperative wound infections has been the premise behind many centers' adopting various guidelines for perioperative patient care; however, the prevention of wound infections involves consideration of pre-procedural, intra-procedural, and post-procedural sources of microbial colonization and thus requires a multifaceted approach to patient management.

Patient-specific risk factors, such as advanced age, a history of drug and alcohol abuse, smoking, diabetes, obesity, malnutrition, and immunologic compromise,[60] reduce the patient's ability to mount an adequate inflammatory response against pathogens.[61] Smoking and diabetes, specifically, are believed to lead to microvascular damage and tissue ischemia, which in turn increase the risk for SSI development.[62–66] In terms of preprocedural care, advocating for measures such as smoking cessation and improved preoperative diabetic control and nutritional status should be employed to optimize patient risk factors. In addition, surgeries performed for patients with traumatic spinal injuries or neoplastic processes are associated with an increased incidence of SSIs.[61]

As surgeries become more complex, with an increasingly wide variety of pathologies treated and instrumentation used, the likelihood of infectious complications increases.[67,68] Studies have estimated that the incidence of deep wound infections following instrumented lumbar fusion surgery ranges between 1 and 14%.[55–58,67,69–79] Repeat surgery, a greater number of levels fused, a posterior approach, longer operative times, blood transfusions, and increased intraoperative blood loss are all associated with postoperative SSI.[60,68,80–82] Another risk factor that has been identified is the presence of more people in the operating theater, a finding especially germane to spinal instrumentation surgeries, in which the surgeon, assistants, anesthesia team, circulators, and equipment representatives all share the operating room, increasing traffic and adding potential sources of infection.[83]

Minimally invasive approaches have been shown to compare favorably with traditional, open surgical approaches with respect to the incidence of wound infections.[84,85] Fewer postoperative deep wound infections are seen after instrumented cervical fusion surgery; however, as recent reports demonstrate, patients who undergo operative fixation and arthrodesis via an isolated posterior approach have a higher rate of wound infection than those treated anteriorly.[86,87] In patients who manifest with deep wound infections after undergoing anterior cervical diskectomy and fusion, the clinician must have a high index of suspicion for esophageal injury, which carries significant morbidity and mortality.[88]

Understanding surgery-specific risk factors, adhering meticulously to aseptic technique, and employing measures to decrease the potential for microbial colonization are crucial to minimizing the potential for developing subsequent deep wound infections, as highlighted by recommendations published by the CDC for SSI prevention.[53]

As previously noted, measures to reduce the risk for developing a postoperative wound infection are not relegated to the preoperative and immediate perioperative periods. As such, the postoperative management of patients is also important in preventing surgical site complications. Open and effective communication between the patient, nursing staff, and physicians is integral to optimizing patient outcomes. Protecting the surgical wound with a sterile dressing for 24 to 48 hours postoperatively, washing hands before and after dressing changes and when any contact with the surgical site is anticipated, and using sterile technique are recommended.[53] Administration of antibiotics is discouraged beyond 24 hours as there is scant evidence to support this practice. Additionally, prolonged administration of antibiotics has been shown to result in the selection of antibiotic-resistant bacterial species.[89] Although closed suction drainage has traditionally been employed because of its potential to promote wound healing and also prevent bacterial colonization and growth within the surgical bed, there is little evidence to support its use.[90] The results of recently published works illustrate that drains may not lead to any reduction in wound infections,[90,91] and with prolonged use, they are an independent risk factor for subsequent development of an SSI.[92]

## Microbiology

Most commonly, *S. aureus* is responsible for SSI development. Recent reviews have shown that the incidence of MRSA isolates in patients manifesting with SSI is upward of 34%.[83] *S. epidermidis*, *Enterococcus faecalis*, *Pseudomonas* species, *Enterobacter cloacae*, and *Proteus mirabilis* are other, less commonly isolated bacterial pathogens. Patients with traumatic injuries to the spine and those with urosepsis are particularly vulnerable to infection by gram-negative organisms.[61]

### Presentation and Diagnostic Work-Up

Patients with postoperative deep wound infections can present in a variety of ways. Increasing pain is often experienced and represents a subjective complaint that is important to take in context with the patient's general postoperative course. To avoid delays in diagnosis, one must consider how much time has passed since surgery and note whether the increased pain is disproportionate to the amount of discomfort that the patient has previously experienced during his or her recovery.[67] Patients typically present with signs and symptoms of infection between 2 and 4 weeks after surgery[63,92] and will frequently manifest with incisional drainage.[63,78] As noted by Beiner et al, systemic signs such as fever are often absent; however, local signs such as peri-incisional erythema and other manifestations of wound inflammation are frequently present.[67]

Laboratory studies of the white blood cell count, erythrocyte sedimentation rate (ESR), and C-reactive protein (CRP) level are performed as part of the diagnostic work-up of patients presenting with suspected postoperative SSI. All three acute phase reactants become elevated in states of systemic inflammation and are nonspecific markers of infection because their levels rise in association with other disease processes. Various publications have highlighted the utility of CRP level testing in cases of spinal SSIs.[93,94] Noting that the white blood cell count is an unreliable infectious biomarker,[95] Mok et al found that in their patient cohort, the CRP level was more reliable and applicable as a test for infection compared with ESR. The authors demonstrated that postoperative CRP levels followed a more predictable kinetic profile compared with the ESR, which demonstrated increased variability and typically peaked later in the postoperative period, and they showed that a second rise in CRP levels or their failure to decrease had good specificity and negative predictive value for postoperative deep wound infection.[93]

MR imaging with administration of intravenous gadolinium is the optimal imaging modality for evaluating patients for deep postsurgical infections. In cases of deep wound infections, T2-weighted sequences will demonstrate hyperintensity within the involved tissues. Diskitis and osteomyelitis manifest on MR imaging with decreased signal on T1-weighted sequences and increased signal on T2-weighted images within the disk space and vertebral bodies, respectively, with contrast enhancement after gadolinium administration. Epidural abscesses are isointense with the spinal cord on T1-weighted imaging and appear hyperintense on T2-weighted sequences. Contrast enhancement is also typically present[54] (**Fig. 16.2**). Given their ability to detail bony

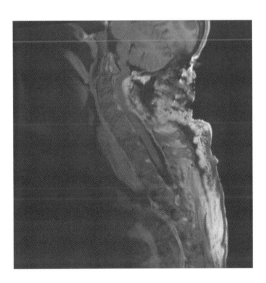

**Fig. 16.2** Sagittal T1-weighted magnetic resonance image of a cervical epidural abscess depicts avid contrast enhancement after administration of gadolinium.

anatomy, CT scans are useful in the work-up of patients with infections. In the setting of diskitis and osteomyelitis, CT scans often reveal narrowing of the disk spaces and erosion of the adjacent end plates. The presence of haloing around screws is indicative of hardware failure, which may be due to concomitant infection.

## Treatment

The treatment of deep SSIs requires identification of the particular tissue(s) or compartment(s) involved and the clinical state of the patient. Once these have been identified, quick and definitive treatment is compulsory to maximize the patient's chances of normal recovery and to minimize long-term sequelae of the infection. As mentioned previously, patients with deep wound infections have increased morbidity and mortality[55-59]; however, despite the development of this complication, such patients can still derive benefit from their initial surgery and experience a significant improvement over their preoperative health-related quality of life.[96,97]

The nonoperative management of postoperative deep SSI is rarely indicated because of the fact that such infections typically cannot be cleared with the administration of intravenous antibiotics alone.[61,67] At our center, unless the patient appears clinically ill with systemic signs of sepsis, administration of intravenous antibiotics is withheld until after intraoperative tissue cultures are obtained. Surgery involves opening the incision and obtaining wound cultures, followed by aggressive removal of the necrotic tissue and bone graft with wound debridement and thorough lavage of the wound with antibiotic irrigation. Because of a high diagnostic yield in the setting of infection, tissue specimens should be sent for microbiological analysis and culture.[98] In cases in which the wound can be closed, some authors recommend placing surgical drains before closure.[55,99]

No consensus exists in the literature regarding the utility of serial wound debridements and washouts and the necessity of wound closure in the setting of deep SSI in patients with spinal instrumentation. Given the added concern that arthrodesis will not have occurred, there is additional debate as to whether hardware removal is warranted in patients who present with deep SSI in the early postoperative period. Some authors state that hardware must be removed to clear the infection.[100] A study by Collins et al showed that among patients who presented with early postoperative deep SSIs, 40% of those who underwent repeat wound debridements and washouts with concomitant administration of intravenous antibiotics had active infection at the time of eventual hardware removal.[101] However, the efficacy of serial operations for wound debridement and washout without removal of instrumentation has been documented.[55,71,78]

The use of the vacuum-assisted closure of postoperative spinal wounds has gained popularity. This involves placing a sponge into the wound, covering it with an occlusive dressing, and then connecting the sponge to a suction device. By introducing negative pressure to the wound, the vacuum-assisted closure device (V.A.C. Dynamic Wound Therapy; KCI Medical, San Antonio, Texas) has been shown to promote the formation of granulation tissue while also optimizing tissue perfusion and decreasing interstitial edema, thus facilitating bacterial removal from the wound.[102] The specific manner in which the vacuum-assisted device has been used among patients with deep SSI following spinal hardware implantation varies in the literature; some authors have used a vacuum-assisted closure device after an initial irrigation and debridement procedure and allowed the wound to heal via secondary intention,[103] whereas others have utilized the device until granulation tissue forms over the retained hardware, at which time definitive wound closure is undertaken.[104,105] At our institution, the treatment paradigm requires that patients presenting with postoperative deep SSI undergo serial wound washout and debridement procedures; intraoperative wound cultures are taken with each procedure, and a vacuum-assisted closure dressing is left in place attached to continuous suction. Plastic surgeons, infectious disease specialists, and clinical nutritionists are consulted, and after sterile cultures have been obtained from the wound and the patient has been nutritionally optimized, primary closure is undertaken.

After the surgical treatment and inpatient management of patients with deep SSI, the multidisciplinary team approach must be continued on an outpatient basis. The CRP level has been demonstrated to be of utility in measuring the response to antibiotics of patients with wound infections after spinal surgery.[106] Patients are often kept on long-term oral suppressive antibiotic therapy at the recommendation of the infectious disease specialists. From the standpoint of the spine surgeon, close monitoring with serial imaging studies is also important to monitor for progression of instability or pseudoarthrosis.[107]

## Intrathecal Pump Infections

Implantable pumps are now commonly used to treat spasticity, dystonia, and intractable pain. These devices present a unique subset of challenges in terms of infection prevention and the treatment of infections when they do occur. The rate of infection after pump implantation has been estimated to be from 4.0 to more than 10%.[108–111] In addition to the issues associated with other implantable devices, these devices are often implanted in patients with numerous comorbidities, such as immunosuppression in patients with intractable cancer pain and pressure ulcers, gastrostomy tubes, and indwelling catheters in patients being treated for spasticity. These patients have often previously been exposed to multiple antibiotics; therefore, they are at increased risk for harboring resistant strains of bacteria and may have developed allergies to antibiotics commonly used in prophylaxis. Gastrostomy tubes, pediatric age, and incontinence have been associated with a higher risk for infection.[109]

Many techniques to prevent infection of intrathecal pumps have been described. Before surgery, the nutritional status of the patient should be assessed and optimized. Patients must be carefully assessed for the presence of active infections, and surgery should be delayed if they are found. The appropriate use and timing of presurgical antibiotic prophylaxis are necessary. Close attention to sterile operative technique is particularly important, and sterile preparation of the surgical site can be challenging because of the lateral positioning of the patient. At Children's Hospital of Pittsburgh of UPMC, pledgets soaked with Betadine are stapled to the wound edges immediately after incision to reduce the risk for contamination. The surgical site is also irrigated with a total of 1 L of saline and Betadine solution before closure. Meticulous attention to wound closure is also of key importance, as is the avoidance of tension on the wound, which may result from the bulk of the pump in what is often a malnourished patient. Subfascial placement of the pump may help reduce wound tension.

Infection of the intrathecal pump most often necessitates removal of the device. Systemic antibiotics may be used to suppress an infection while a drug delivered at high doses is withdrawn. Infection may occasionally be treated with antibiotics alone[112,113]; however, in the authors' experience, treatment with antibiotics alone does not typically eradicate an infection. Attempts to treat pump infections without an interruption in intrathecal drug delivery have included washout without removal of the device,[114] removal with replacement in the same setting, and intrathecal co-infusion of antibiotics.[115,116] In cancer patients with limited life expectancy who are receiving intrathecal opioids, palliative suppression of the infection without removal of the device should be considered.

## Deep Brain Stimulator Hardware Infections

Over the last quarter of a century, deep brain stimulation (DBS) has evolved from an experimental therapy to a well-accepted treatment for a wide variety of medical conditions. Most commonly, DBS is used to treat movement disorders, such as Parkinson disease,[117–122] essential tremor,[117,120–122] dystonia,[117,120–122] and Tourette syndrome[119,123]; psychological disorders, such as obsessive-compulsive disorder[124]; and other neurologic and pain disorders.[118,119,121,122,124,125]

A DBS system consists of a multicontact intracranial electrode, extension leads or wires with a connector, and an internal pulse generator. Surgical implantation of the electrode generally involves the use of a stereotactic frame[126] to target a predetermined region after appropriate imaging and physiologic mapping with the patient under minimal, if any, anesthesia.[122] Internal pulse generator implantation is most commonly subclavicular and may occur at the same time as electrode implantation (single procedure)[126] or in a second procedure following a period of temporary lead externalization and continuous test stimulation (staged procedure).[127]

DBS is a reversible procedure, with its effect based on electric modulation of the nervous system,[118] resulting in a functional rather than a structural lesion. In contrast to the ablative procedures (thalamotomy, pallidotomy) that may be used as alternative therapy for movement disorders, DBS offers the ability to adjust stimulation parameters noninvasively and tailor treatment to the patient's individual needs without creating an irreversible lesion,[119] but it precludes the use of potential neurorestorative therapies that may become available in the future.[127] Given these benefits and the low risk for permanent neurologic deficit associated with the procedure, the number of patients undergoing DBS has increased dramatically in recent years, and the number of those undergoing ablative therapy has proportionally decreased. However, treatment is lifelong, based on implantation of foreign material, and thus is subject to the inherent risk for complication.[128]

Complications associated with DBS can be classified as operation-, stimulation-, or hardware-related.[119,129,130] Overall complication rates reported in the literature vary widely, ranging from 3.8 to 37% of patients,[119,131–133] 4.3 to 19% of implants,[128,133,134] and 3.2 to 8.4% per electrode-year.[121,125,133] Serious operation-related complications, such as intracranial

hemorrhage, stroke, and even death, are rare, with reported rates ranging from 1 to 2%.[133,134] In contrast, hardware-related complications are extremely common, occurring in up to 25% of patients[124] and in 17% of procedures.[128] They are of particular importance because they usually require surgical correction or removal of the system with an associated loss of therapeutic benefit, need for hospitalization, and significant economic burden.[119] The most common hardware-related complications include electrode migration, lead fracture, infections, erosions, and internal pulse generator malfunction.[119,121,122,128,133] Although hardware failure may require costly replacement, infection remains one of the most significant potential complications, and the risk for infection persists long after the immediate perioperative period, making it the most common late complication of DBS therapy.[125,135]

## Epidemiology and Risk Factors

The reported incidence of DBS hardware-related infection varies with study design, definition of infection, and length of follow-up. Individual studies have described infection rates ranging from 0 to 15% of patients,[117,122,126,133,136–140] with most reporting rates of approximately 5 to 10% of patients and 3 to 7% of devices.[120,121,124,126,128,132,134,141–146] In a recent meta-analysis of more than 3,000 patients, Bhatia et al calculated an average infection rate of 4.7%[147]; similarly, in an earlier review, the authors reported rates of 3.3% of electrodes and 3.8% of patients, with a decline in the incidence after implantation.[141] Additionally, Baizabal Carvallo et al noted that the overall incidence has declined in recent years, with reported rates after 2010 ranging from 0.62 to 9.3%.[119]

Risk factors for infection following DBS are poorly understood. There are conflicting data about age as a predisposing factor,[120,125,127] with some authors identifying younger age as a risk factor,[138,144] but the majority of studies fail to associate age with an increased incidence of infection.[117,124] General patient characteristics and comorbidities traditionally identified as neurosurgical risk factors, particularly those that may impair wound healing (e.g., smoking, excessive alcohol consumption, systemic illness, diabetes mellitus, hypertension, and obesity) have not been demonstrated to increase risk in most studies of DBS outcomes.[119–121,124,125,127,139,144,146] Furthermore, operative factors, such as duration of surgery, unilateral versus bilateral lead placement, type of operating room (conventional versus MR imaging suite), number of personnel in the operating room, surgeon experience, and method of hair removal, have not been found to convey a significant increase in infection risk.[120,121,124,138,139,144,146] Importantly, DBS in which a staged implantation is used, with externalization and continuous stimulation of leads, has not been found to result in higher infection rates, even with longer time between surgeries; Piacentino et al reported that no infections occurred in wounds that were reopened and resutured during the second-stage procedure.[120,124,127,138] Specific devices, including brand or one dual-channel versus two small single-channel internal pulse generators, are not associated with infection risk.[117,124,138] One operative factor found to convey an increased risk for infection is the use of a straight incision directly over burr holes rather than a curvilinear incision; Constantoyannis et al reported an increase in incidence from 2 to 12.5% in patients with a straight incision ($p = 0.03$).[121] Perhaps the most commonly noted risk factor for infection, particularly in long-term follow-up and often reported undistinguished from frank infection, is skin erosion over hardware sites.[125] Although rates of infection decrease in the months to years postoperatively, of those who do experience complications, more than half have associated skin erosions,[121,126–128,134,138] and as noted by Oh et al, it may be difficult to distinguish the temporal relationship between erosion and infection because both complications present concomitantly.[125]

## Pathogenesis and Microbiology

Infection of DBS hardware can initially affect any part of the system and spread to adjacent tissue by following the track of the implanted device[119]; accordingly, bacterial inoculation may occur directly at the time of surgery, via hematogenous spread, or secondary to skin breakdown.[118] Distal inoculation at the connection site between electrodes and extension cables or at the internal pulse generator pocket is the most common route of hardware infection.[124,126,128,133,136,148] Most investigators report that a majority of infections present as suppurative cellulitis at the internal pulse generator pocket in association with skin erosion or less commonly trauma, with rapid spread to incisional sites in the retroauricular or scalp regions.[124,125,128,138] Although the vast majority of infections occur in the distal system components, infection at the burr hole incision is not uncommon and often secondary to, or coexistent with, distal hardware infection.[120,125] Intracranial infection of electrodes is rarely observed.[143] Reviews of the literature have identified just a handful of cases of intracranial infection,[133,139,143,149] with one particular case study describing an early diagnosis of *Enterobacter* abscess on postoperative day 10.[150]

Given the natural history of hardware infections associated with skin erosion,[127] the average time to diagnosis of infection tends to extend into the months following implantation. Reports of mean time to infection range from 1 to 4 months,[120,126,134,138,139] with varied identification of highest rate of infection in the first 3 months compared with the 3- to 6-month period after surgery.[121,124,140,141] Interestingly, in studies of pediatric patients, all infections were diagnosed at the internal pulse generator site and within 4 to 6 weeks after implantation, leading authors to postulate that pulse generators, originally designed for the larger subclavicular areas of adults, may cause undue tension at the chest wall and thus lead to an increased risk for infection.[137] Although diagnosis can rarely occur within the first week postoperatively, time to infection may also be months to years[121,125,126,128,134,139]; studies of long-term complications of DBS have noted that infections may occur at more than 1 year in 40%[126] and more than 2 years in 25% of patients following DBS,[128] thus underscoring the need for close long-term follow-up.

Constantoyannis et al classify DBS hardware infections and bacterial etiologies into two categories: external infections, which may begin as erythema or healing problems at the surgical site and are usually caused by skin flora, and internal infections, which are secondary to the hematogenous spread of bacteria and may result in meningismus or intracranial abscess.[122] Gram-positive cocci are the most common organisms responsible for infection, with *S. aureus* identified in 40 to 100% of culture-positive cases,[117,125,126,129,137,138,144] in addition to *S. epidermidis*,[126,136,143] other coagulase-negative staphylococci,[138,143,145] and less commonly other skin flora, such as *P. acnes* and *Micrococcus*.[126,137,138] Additional pathogens routinely identified, although with much lower frequency, include *Enterobacter*,[121,126,144] *Serratia*,[141] *Klebsiella*,[144] and *Pseudomonas*,[142,143] which may reflect the potential for patients to contract nosocomial infections. Polymicrobial infections have not been routinely described in the literature; fungal infections do account for a small percentage of pathogens, with *Candida*[117,141,144] most frequently isolated.

## Diagnosis

The definitions of *hardware-related infection* vary quite widely in the literature. Some definitions include patients with only superficial inflammatory changes at incisional sites and/or skin erosion, whereas other, stricter definitions are based on specimen cultures.[119] In contrast to what is observed with other types of implanted hardware, temporal proximity to surgery is of less importance because skin dehiscence may occur at any time and is highly correlated with infection risk.

Most authors use the presence of clinical or microbiological criteria to diagnose infection. Clinical evidence of infection may include superficial signs, such as induration, erythema, pain, warmth, and purulence at an incision over a hardware component,[117,142] or signs of deep infection, with purulence visualized through the subcutaneous level and in contact with portions of the hardware system.[124,126,138,144] Cultures obtained from exposed device components, wound drainage, or intraoperative specimens may be used to confirm the diagnosis of infection and identify pathogens to guide therapy[117,124,138]; however, a significant percentage of cultures may not provide positive results. In one case series, no organisms were identified by blood culture, but 10 of 12 surgical swabs provided positive cultures[127]; other series have described positive cultures in only half of clinically diagnosed infections.[121] Systemic signs and symptoms of infection are uncommon in DBS hardware–related infection; Fily et al reported mild fever in only one-quarter of patients and change in mental status in only one patient.[126] Although uncommon, intracranial infection may be apparent on CT or MR imaging of the head. In patients presenting with local infection near the external portion of the electrode and new neurologic symptoms, imaging may demonstrate abscess or edema around the electrodes, signified by signal change on T2-weighted MR images or hypodensity on CT scans.[126,143,150,151]

In addition to a thorough history and physical examination, one suggested algorithm for work-up includes CT of the head with contrast, complete blood count, ESR, CRP level, electrolyte levels, and urinalysis. Certain institutions may advocate the use of technetium-99m sulesomab immunoscintigraphy to evaluate for the presence and extent of infection and thus aid in surgical planning.[152] If the examination or imaging is concerning for intracranial infection, a neurosurgical consult should be obtained.[122] Because of the variability of culture results, particularly because cultures are often obtained after surgical treatment is undertaken, thereby somewhat negating their diagnostic value, and because of the subtlety or lack of systemic symptoms at presentation, a high level of clinical suspicion and a low threshold for the initiation of therapy are important for patients with potential hardware-related infections.

## Management

In patients presenting with likely DBS hardware infection, wide-spectrum empiric antibiotics may be started early.[117] Importantly, antibiotic therapy must target *S. aureus* and *P. acnes*,[123] but they can then be altered to address the subsequent final culture results and sensitivities. Reported success rates of management with antibiotics alone range from 4 to 75%.[122,144] Oral and topical antibiotics may be tried as primary therapy for patients with mild superficial skin infection without purulence or signs of inflammation along the hardware tract[119]; for those with more prominent local infections, successful therapy with 10 to 14 days of intravenous antibiotics followed by 7 to 14 days of oral antibiotics has also been described.[139] In one series, patients adequately treated with antibiotics alone presented earlier after the onset of symptoms compared with those requiring surgical therapy; on average, the eradication of infection was achieved following 3.5 weeks of antibiotics.[117]

The majority of hardware-related infections require surgical intervention, either as the initial management or following a failed trial of antibiotics with or without wound debridement.[125,126,141,142] Surgical management ranges from minimal removal of one component of a DBS system to complete removal of the internal pulse generator, lead extender, and intracranial electrodes. Rates of complete removal range from 11 to 73%.[124,141,142] If infection is located around the internal pulse generator or extension wires, however, removal of these distal parts of the system may be attempted with preservation of the intracranial electrodes. Salvage rates of 21 to 89% have been reported for partial hardware removal of just the internal pulse generator or the internal pulse generator and lead extenders,[126,141,142] although conversion to full removal may be necessary in up to one-third of cases.[138]

Continued controversy exists regarding initial management of DBS hardware infections; while some groups tend to utilize early surgical hardware removal, others opt for an initial attempt at conservative medical therapy.[119] A small percentage of patients may successfully be managed conservatively; in one series, 25% of patients with cranial wound infections initially treated with antibiotics and wound debridement avoided surgical intervention.[117] Similarly, in a pooled analysis of a large study sample, 20% of infections were successfully treated with antibiotics alone.[148] Factors associated with an increased risk for antibiotic failure include deep, purulent infections and the isolation of *S. aureus*.[141]

Partial removal of distal hardware components is frequently attempted in cases of infection localized to the internal pulse generator or extracranial lead extenders.[124,133,138,142] In cases of infection over the internal pulse generator secondary to skin erosion, surgical removal is nearly always necessary; however, some success has been reported with removal of the generator, sterilization, and immediate reimplantation in the contralateral subclavicular region.[118,133] Failure of partial removal, necessitating complete removal, can occur in patients managed in this manner[126] and has been associated with deep, purulent infections, positive *S. aureus* cultures, extensive cellulitis, and wound dehiscence.[133] Some investigators have noted that if infection of a cranial incision, which can easily spread to electrodes, or evidence of intracranial involvement is present, complete removal is likely necessary for effective therapy. This is compared with infection limited to the internal pulse generator site, in which case partial removal with prolonged antibiotic therapy is highly successful.[126]

Surgical removal of hardware is combined with extended courses of antibiotic therapy for complete eradication of device-related infection. The reported duration of antibiotic therapy following hardware removal varies, as does the mode of administration. Nearly all studies report using intravenous antibiotics in the immediate postoperative period, with the majority of courses ranging from 3 to 6 weeks[124,126,133,143,144]; subsequently, it is possible to switch to oral medication in patients without clinical or radiographic evidence of intracranial involvement.[126,144] After completion of antibiotics and an asymptomatic period, hardware replacement is generally possible, with reported time to reimplantation ranging from 3 to 11 months.[124,126,137]

Although consensus regarding the early management of DBS device-related infections has proved difficult, review of the literature supports an initial attempt at management with antibiotics in selected cases, followed by hardware removal if the infection persists.[121] Antibiotics alone may be sufficient to treat superficial, localized infections at the distal system components[121,143]; however, if deep infection with clear involvement of the internal pulse generator or external lead extenders is present, partial hardware removal with preservation of the intracranial leads is appropriate.[143] Additionally, in these cases, unaffected contralateral hardware may be left in place.[121,139] Patients who have diffuse infection of the system with extensive cellulitis or multiple purulent sites along the tract and those who have involvement of intracranial components will likely require early removal of the entire system for effective treatment.[121,138,143]

## Outcomes

Although most patients with infection requiring hardware removal eventually are able to undergo replacement, this management is not without serious repercussions. After removal, patients are left for an extended period of time (up to 11 months in some series) without treatment, and if they are unfortunate enough to develop an abscess, they may be unable ever to undergo replacement.[126] In addition to losing the benefits of stimulation, patients are subjected to further lengthy stereotactic procedures,[137] during which the risk for permanent neurologic deficit, although small, does exist; they are also subjected to additional hospitalizations, the long-term use of antibiotics, and additional cost.[125] Lastly, repeated infection

with associated sequelae may lead patients to refuse replacement of the hardware or choose to undergo ablative therapy, even though such methods have largely been abandoned.[135]

## Prevention

The prevention of DBS hardware-related infection largely centers on the careful modulation of perioperative factors. Clinicians routinely use a preoperative antibiotic, most commonly cefazolin or vancomycin (for those allergic to penicillin), to prevent postoperative infection.[117,119,124,125] Although some physicians prefer to prescribe a course of antibiotics after implantation, little evidence exists to suggest that postoperative antibiotics prevent infection,[117] nor does the use of intraoperatively pouch-installed antibiotics or the completion of implantation in one procedure rather than a staged procedure.[147] The use of a self-administered 70% ethyl alcohol wash above the waist on the evening and morning before surgery has been found to decrease the risk for infection significantly.[142] One series noted that shaving the head before surgery did not reduce the infection rate; therefore, the authors modified their clinical practice to eliminate head shaving.[140] Intraoperatively, the injection of a dilute povidone-iodine irrigation, which is superior to saline and is bactericidal against MRSA, has been successfully utilized.[153,154] Alternatively, irrigation with a solution of 40 mg of neomycin and 200,000 U of polymyxin B sulfate just after fascial closure but before skin closure has been shown to reduce the risk for infection in patients receiving neurosurgical hardware.[137] Additionally, the use of cement containing erythromycin and colistin for fixation of the intracerebral electrode has been advocated.[139] Depending on the type of hardware available, some surgeons may choose to drill troughs into the skull above the mastoid to lower the profile of the connector and reduce the risk for scalp erosion[135]; however, with the advent of low-profile connection cables, skin erosion and the risk for infection at this site have been greatly reduced.[128]

# References

1. Simpkins CJ. Ventriculoperitoneal shunt infections in patients with hydrocephalus. Pediatr Nurs 2005;31(6):457–462

2. Kestle JR. Pediatric hydrocephalus: current management. Neurol Clin 2003;21(4):883–895, vii

3. Kestle JRW, Garton HJL, Whitehead WE, et al. Management of shunt infections: a multicenter pilot study. J Neurosurg 2006;105(3, Suppl): 177–181

4. Korinek A-M, Fulla-Oller L, Boch A-L, Golmard J-L, Hadiji B, Puybasset L. Morbidity of ventricular cerebrospinal fluid shunt surgery in adults: an 8-year study. Neurosurgery 2011;68(4):985–994, discussion 994–995

5. Boaz JC. Central nervous system infectious diseases and therapy. In: Roos KL, ed. Neurological Disease and Therapy. New York, NY: Marcel Dekker; 1997:519–544

6. Nulsen FE, Spitz EB. Treatment of hydrocephalus by direct shunt from ventricle to jugular vain. Surg Forum 1951;399–403

7. Bondurant CP, Jimenez DF. Epidemiology of cerebrospinal fluid shunting. Pediatr Neurosurg 1995;23(5):254–258, discussion 259

8. Massimi L, Paternoster G, Fasano T, Di Rocco C. On the changing epidemiology of hydrocephalus. Childs Nerv Syst 2009;25(7):795–800

9. Cochrane DD, Kestle J. Ventricular shunting for hydrocephalus in children: patients, procedures, surgeons and institutions in English Canada, 1989-2001. Eur J Pediatr Surg 2002;12(Suppl 1): S6–S11

10. Fernell E, Hagberg G, Hagberg B. Infantile hydrocephalus—the impact of enhanced preterm survival. Acta Paediatr Scand 1990;79(11): 1080–1086

11. Drake JM, Kestle JR, Milner R, et al. Randomized trial of cerebrospinal fluid shunt valve design in pediatric hydrocephalus. Neurosurgery 1998;43(2):294–303, discussion 303–305

12. Kestle JRW, Drake JM, Cochrane DD, et al; Endoscopic Shunt Insertion Trial participants. Lack of benefit of endoscopic ventriculoperitoneal shunt insertion: a multicenter randomized trial. J Neurosurg 2003;98(2):284–290

13. Steinbok P, Milner R, Agrawal D, et al. A multicenter multinational registry for assessing ventriculoperitoneal shunt infections for hydrocephalus. Neurosurgery 2010;67(5): 1303–1310

14. Simon TD, Hall M, Dean JM, Kestle JRW, Riva-Cambrin J. Reinfection following initial cerebrospinal fluid shunt infection. J Neurosurg Pediatr 2010;6(3):277–285

15. Simon TD, Hall M, Riva-Cambrin J, et al; Hydrocephalus Clinical Research Network. Infection rates following initial cerebrospinal fluid shunt placement across pediatric hospitals in the United States. Clinical article. J Neurosurg Pediatr 2009;4(2):156–165

16. Tulipan N, Cleves MA. Effect of an intraoperative double-gloving strategy on the incidence of cerebrospinal fluid shunt infection. J Neurosurg 2006;104(1, Suppl):5–8

17. Ragel BT, Browd SR, Schmidt RH. Surgical shunt infection: significant reduction when using intraventricular and systemic antibiotic agents. J Neurosurg 2006;105(2):242–247

18. Tacconelli E, Cataldo MA, Albanese A, et al. Vancomycin versus cefazolin prophylaxis for cerebrospinal shunt placement in a hospital with a high prevalence of methicillin-resistant *Staphylococcus aureus*. J Hosp Infect 2008;69(4): 337–344

19. Cochrane DD, Kestle JRW. The influence of surgical operative experience on the duration of first ventriculoperitoneal shunt function and infection. Pediatr Neurosurg 2003;38(6):295–301

20. Wang K-W, Chang W-N, Shih T-Y, et al. Infection of cerebrospinal fluid shunts: causative pathogens, clinical features, and outcomes. Jpn J Infect Dis 2004;57(2):44–48

21. McGirt MJ, Zaas A, Fuchs HE, George TM, Kaye K, Sexton DJ. Risk factors for pediatric ventriculoperitoneal shunt infection and predictors of infectious pathogens. Clin Infect Dis 2003;36(7):858–862

22. McClinton D, Carraccio C, Englander R. Predictors of ventriculoperitoneal shunt pathology. Pediatr Infect Dis J 2001;20(6):593–597

23. Walters BC, Hoffman HJ, Hendrick EB, Humphreys RP. Cerebrospinal fluid shunt infection. Influences on initial management and subsequent outcome. J Neurosurg 1984;60(5): 1014–1021

24. Kulkarni AV, Drake JM, Lamberti-Pasculli M. Cerebrospinal fluid shunt infection: a prospective study of risk factors. J Neurosurg 2001;94(2): 195–201

25. Filka J, Huttova M, Tuharsky J, Sagat T, Kralinsky K, Krcmery V Jr. Nosocomial meningitis in children after ventriculoperitoneal shunt insertion. Acta Paediatr 1999;88(5):576–578

26. Stamos JK, Kaufman BA, Yogev R. Ventriculoperitoneal shunt infections with gram-negative bacteria. Neurosurgery 1993;33(5):858–862

27. Shapiro S, Boaz J, Kleiman M, Kalsbeck J, Mealey J. Origin of organisms infecting ventricular shunts. Neurosurgery 1988;22(5):868–872

28. Prusseit J, Simon M, von der Brelie C, et al. Epidemiology, prevention and management of ventriculoperitoneal shunt infections in children. Pediatr Neurosurg 2009;45(5):325–336

29. Conen A, Walti LN, Merlo A, Fluckiger U, Battegay M, Trampuz A. Characteristics and treatment outcome of cerebrospinal fluid shunt-associated infections in adults: a retrospective analysis over an 11-year period. Clin Infect Dis 2008;47(1):73–82

30. Lund-Johansen MSF, Svendsen F, Wester K. Shunt failures and complications in adults as related to shunt type, diagnosis, and the experience of the surgeon. Neurosurgery 1994;35(5):839–844, discussion 844

31. Kontny U, Höfling B, Gutjahr P, Voth D, Schwarz M, Schmitt HJ. CSF shunt infections in children. Infection 1993;21(2):89–92

32. Vanaclocha V, Sáiz-Sapena N, Leiva J. Shunt malfunction in relation to shunt infection. Acta Neurochir (Wien) 1996;138(7):829–834

33. Bayston RLJ, Lari J. A study of the sources of infection in colonised shunts. Dev Med Child Neurol 1974;16(6, Suppl 32):16–22

34. Bayston R, Ashraf W, Bhundia C. Mode of action of an antimicrobial biomaterial for use in hydrocephalus shunts. J Antimicrob Chemother 2004;53(5):778–782

35. McLaurin RL, Frame PT. Treatment of infections of cerebrospinal fluid shunts. Rev Infect Dis 1987;9(3):595–603

36. Duhaime AC. Evaluation and management of shunt infections in children with hydrocephalus. Clin Pediatr (Phila) 2006;45(8):705–713

37. Wong GKC, Wong SM, Poon WS. Ventriculoperitoneal shunt infection: intravenous antibiotics, shunt removal and more aggressive treatment? ANZ J Surg 2011;81(4):307

38. Brown EM, Edwards RJ, Pople IK. Conservative management of patients with cerebrospinal fluid shunt infections. Neurosurgery 2006;58(4):657–665

39. Anderson EJ, Yogev R. A rational approach to the management of ventricular shunt infections. Pediatr Infect Dis J 2005;24(6):557–558

40. Arnell K, Enblad P, Wester T, Sjölin J. Treatment of cerebrospinal fluid shunt infections in children using systemic and intraventricular antibiotic therapy in combination with externalization of the ventricular catheter: efficacy in 34 consecutively treated infections. J Neurosurg 2007;107(3, Suppl):213–219

41. Lutsar IMG, McCracken GH Jr, Friedland IR. Antibiotic pharmacodynamics in cerebrospinal fluid. Clin Infect Dis 1998;27(5):1117–1127, quiz 1128–1129

42. James HE, Bradley JS. Aggressive management of shunt infection: combined intravenous and intraventricular antibiotic therapy for twelve or less days. Pediatr Neurosurg 2008;44(2):104–111

43. James HE, Walsh JW, Wilson HD, Connor JD, Bean JR, Tibbs PA. Prospective randomized study of therapy in cerebrospinal fluid shunt infection. Neurosurgery 1980;7(5):459–463

44. Yogev R. Cerebrospinal fluid shunt infections: a personal view. Pediatr Infect Dis 1985;4(2):113–118

45. Schreffler RT, Schreffler AJ, Wittler RR. Treatment of cerebrospinal fluid shunt infections: a decision analysis. Pediatr Infect Dis J 2002;21(7):632–636

46. Hunt GMHA, Holmes AE. Factors relating to intelligence in treated cases of spina bifida cystica. Am J Dis Child 1976;130(8):823–827

47. Chadduck WAJ, Adametz J. Incidence of seizures in patients with myelomeningocele: a multifactorial analysis. Surg Neurol 1988;30(4):281–285

48. Bayston R, Ashraf W, Fisher L. Prevention of infection in neurosurgery: role of "antimicrobial" catheters. J Hosp Infect 2007;65(Suppl 2):39–42

49. Kan PKJ, Kestle J. Lack of efficacy of antibiotic-impregnated shunt systems in preventing shunt infections in children. Childs Nerv Syst 2007;23(7):773–777

50. Ritz RRF, Roser F, Morgalla M, Dietz K, Tatagiba M, Will BE. Do antibiotic-impregnated shunts in hydrocephalus therapy reduce the risk of infection? An observational study in 258 patients. BMC Infect Dis 2007;7(5):38

51. He W, Sengupta M, Velkoff VA, et al. 65+ in the United States: 2005. In: Current Population Reports. Washington, DC: US Government Printing Office; 2005:23–209. www.census.gov/prod/2006pubs/p23-209.pdf. Accessed December 22, 2012

52. Nationwide Inpatient Sample (NIS). Healthcare Cost and Utilization Project (HCUP). 2007–2009. Rockville, MD: Agency for Healthcare Research and Quality. www.hcup-us.ahrq.gov/nisoverview.jsp. Accessed December 22, 2012

53. Mangram AJ, Horan TC, Pearson ML, et al. Hospital Infection Control Practices Advisory Committee (HICPAC) and Centers for Disease Control and Prevention (CDC). Guidelines for prevention of surgical site infection. Infect Control Hosp Epidemiol 1999;24:247–278

54. Chaudhary SB, Vives MJ, Basra SK, Reiter MF. Postoperative spinal wound infections and postprocedural diskitis. J Spinal Cord Med 2007;30(5):441–451

55. Levi AD, Dickman CA, Sonntag VK. Management of postoperative infections after spinal instrumentation. J Neurosurg 1997;86(6):975–980

56. Rechtine GR, Bono PL, Cahill D, Bolesta MJ, Chrin AM. Postoperative wound infection after instrumentation of thoracic and lumbar fractures. J Orthop Trauma 2001;15(8):566–569

57. Rihn JA, Lee JY, Ward WT. Infection after the surgical treatment of adolescent idiopathic scoliosis: evaluation of the diagnosis, treatment, and impact on clinical outcomes. Spine (Phila Pa 1976) 2008;33(3):289–294

58. Veeravagu A, Patil CG, Lad SP, Boakye M. Risk factors for postoperative spinal wound infections after spinal decompression and fusion surgeries. Spine (Phila Pa 1976) 2009;34(17):1869–1872

59. Mok JM, Guillaume TJ, Talu U, et al. Clinical outcome of deep wound infection after instrumented posterior spinal fusion: a matched cohort analysis. Spine (Phila Pa 1976) 2009;34(6):578–583

60. Watanabe M, Sakai D, Matsuyama D, Yamamoto Y, Sato M, Mochida J. Risk factors for surgical site infection following spine surgery: efficacy of intraoperative saline irrigation. J Neurosurg Spine 2010;12(5):540–546

61. Meredith DS, Kepler CK, Huang RC, Brause BD, Boachie-Adjei O. Postoperative infections of the lumbar spine: presentation and management. Int Orthop 2012;36(2):439–444

62. Olsen MA, Mayfield J, Lauryssen C, et al. Risk factors for surgical site infection in spinal surgery. J Neurosurg 2003;98(2, Suppl):149–155

63. Pull ter Gunne AF, Cohen DB. Incidence, prevalence, and analysis of risk factors for surgical site infection following adult spinal surgery. Spine (Phila Pa 1976) 2009;34(13):1422–1428

64. Friedman ND, Sexton DJ, Connelly SM, Kaye KS. Risk factors for surgical site infection complicating laminectomy. Infect Control Hosp Epidemiol 2007;28(9):1060–1065

65. Capen DA, Calderone RR, Green A. Perioperative risk factors for wound infections after lower back fusions. Orthop Clin North Am 1996;27(1):83–86

66. Goodson WH III, Hung TK. Studies of wound healing in experimental diabetes mellitus. J Surg Res 1977;22(3):221–227

67. Beiner JM, Grauer J, Kwon BK, Vaccaro AR. Postoperative wound infections of the spine. Neurosurg Focus 2003;15(3):E14

68. Schimmel JJ, Horsting PP, de Kleuver M, Wonders G, van Limbeek J. Risk factors for deep surgical site infections after spinal fusion. Eur Spine J 2010;19(10):1711–1719

69. Cho KJ, Suk SI, Park SR, et al. Complications in posterior fusion and instrumentation for degenerative lumbar scoliosis. Spine (Phila Pa 1976) 2007;32(20):2232–2237

70. Fang A, Hu SS, Endres N, Bradford DS. Risk factors for infection after spinal surgery. Spine (Phila Pa 1976) 2005;30(12):1460–1465

71. Glassman SD, Dimar JR, Puno RM, Johnson JR. Salvage of instrumental lumbar fusions complicated by surgical wound infection. Spine (Phila Pa 1976) 1996;21(18):2163–2169

72. Kornberg M, Rechtine GR, Herndon WA, Reinert CM, Dupuy TE. Surgical stabilization of thoracic and lumbar spine fractures: a retrospective study in a military population. J Trauma 1984;24(2):140–146

73. Olsen MA, Nepple JJ, Riew KD, et al. Risk factors for surgical site infection following orthopaedic spinal operations. J Bone Joint Surg Am 2008;90(1):62–69

74. Sasso RC, Garrido BJ. Postoperative spinal wound infections. J Am Acad Orthop Surg 2008;16(6):330–337

75. Sierra-Hoffman M, Jinadatha C, Carpenter JL, Rahm M. Postoperative instrumented spine infections: a retrospective review. South Med J 2010;103(1):25–30

76. Smith JS, Shaffrey CI, Sansur CA, et al; Scoliosis Research Society Morbidity and Mortality Committee. Rates of infection after spine surgery based on 108,419 procedures: a report from the Scoliosis Research Society Morbidity and Mortality Committee. Spine (Phila Pa 1976) 2011;36(7):556–563

77. Sponseller PD, LaPorte DM, Hungerford MW, Eck K, Bridwell KH, Lenke LG. Deep wound infections after neuromuscular scoliosis surgery: a multicenter study of risk factors and treatment outcomes. Spine (Phila Pa 1976) 2000;25(19):2461–2466

78. Weinstein MA, McCabe JP, Cammisa FP Jr. Postoperative spinal wound infection: a review of 2,391 consecutive index procedures. J Spinal Disord 2000;13(5):422–426

79. Wimmer C, Gluch H, Franzreb M, Ogon M. Predisposing factors for infection in spine surgery: a survey of 850 spinal procedures. J Spinal Disord 1998;11(2):124–128

80. Thelander U, Larsson S. Quantitation of C-reactive protein levels and erythrocyte sedimentation rate after spinal surgery. Spine (Phila Pa 1976) 1992;17(4):400–404

81. Abdul-Jabbar A, Takemoto S, Weber MH, et al. Surgical site infection in spinal surgery: description of surgical and patient-based risk factors for postoperative infection using administrative claims data. Spine (Phila Pa 1976) 2012;37(15):1340–1345

82. Schwarzkopf R, Chung C, Park JJ, Walsh M, Spivak JM, Steiger D. Effects of perioperative blood product use on surgical site infection following thoracic and lumbar spinal surgery. Spine (Phila Pa 1976) 2010;35(3):340–346

83. Koutsoumbelis S, Hughes AP, Girardi FP, et al. Risk factors for postoperative infection following posterior lumbar instrumented arthrodesis. J Bone Joint Surg Am 2011;93(17):1627–1633

84. Parker SL, Adogwa O, Witham TF, Aaronson OS, Cheng J, McGirt MJ. Post-operative infection after minimally invasive versus open transforaminal lumbar interbody fusion (TLIF): literature review and cost analysis. Minim Invasive Neurosurg 2011;54(1):33–37

85. McGirt MJ, Parker SL, Lerner J, Engelhart L, Knight T, Wang MY. Comparative analysis of perioperative surgical site infection after minimally invasive versus open posterior/transforaminal lumbar interbody fusion: analysis of hospital billing and discharge data from 5170 patients. J Neurosurg Spine 2011;14(6):771–778

86. Campbell PG, Yadla S, Malone J, et al. Early complications related to approach in cervical spine surgery: single-center prospective study. World Neurosurg 2010;74(2-3):363–368

87. Fehlings MG, Smith JS, Kopjar B, et al. Perioperative and delayed complications associated with the surgical treatment of cervical spondylotic myelopathy based on 302 patients from the AOSpine North America Cervical Spondylotic Myelopathy Study. J Neurosurg Spine 2012;16(5):425–432

88. Fountas KN, Kapsalaki EZ, Nikolakakos LG, et al. Anterior cervical discectomy and fusion associated complications. Spine (Phila Pa 1976) 2007;32(21):2310–2317

89. Kanayama M, Hashimoto T, Shigenobu K, Oha F, Togawa D. Effective prevention of surgical site infection using a Centers for Disease Control and Prevention guideline-based antimicrobial prophylaxis in lumbar spine surgery. J Neurosurg Spine 2007;6(4):327–329

90. Scuderi GJ, Brusovanik GV, Fitzhenry LN, Vaccaro AR. Is wound drainage necessary after lumbar spinal fusion surgery? Med Sci Monit 2005;11(2):CR64–CR66

91. Diab M, Smucny M, Dormans JP, et al. Use and outcomes of wound drain in spinal fusion for

adolescent idiopathic scoliosis. Spine (Phila Pa 1976) 2012;37(11):966–973

92. Rao SB, Vasquez G, Harrop J, et al. Risk factors for surgical site infections following spinal fusion procedures: a case-control study. Clin Infect Dis 2011;53(7):686–692

93. Mok JM, Pekmezci M, Piper SL, et al. Use of C-reactive protein after spinal surgery: comparison with erythrocyte sedimentation rate as predictor of early postoperative infectious complications. Spine (Phila Pa 1976) 2008;33(4):415–421

94. Kang BU, Lee SH, Ahn Y, Choi WC, Choi YG. Surgical site infection in spinal surgery: detection and management based on serial C-reactive protein measurements. J Neurosurg Spine 2010;13(2):158–164

95. Takahashi J, Ebara S, Kamimura M, et al. Early-phase enhanced inflammatory reaction after spinal instrumentation surgery. Spine (Phila Pa 1976) 2001;26(15):1698–1704

96. Falavigna A, Righesso O, Traynelis VC, Teles AR, da Silva PG. Effect of deep wound infection following lumbar arthrodesis for degenerative disc disease on long-term outcome: a prospective study: clinical article. J Neurosurg Spine 2011;15(4):399–403

97. Petilon JM, Glassman SD, Dimar JR, Carreon LY. Clinical outcomes after lumbar fusion complicated by deep wound infection: a case-control study. Spine (Phila Pa 1976) 2012;37(16):1370–1374

98. El-Gindi S, Aref S, Salama M, Andrew J. Infection of intervertebral discs after operation. J Bone Joint Surg Br 1976;58(1):114–116

99. Bassewitz HL, Fishgrund JS, Herkowitz HN. Postoperative spine infections. Semin Spine Surg 2000;12:203–211

100. Richards BS. Delayed infections following posterior spinal instrumentation for the treatment of idiopathic scoliosis. J Bone Joint Surg Am 1995;77(4):524–529

101. Collins I, Wilson-MacDonald J, Chami G, et al. The diagnosis and management of infection following instrumented spinal fusion. Eur Spine J 2008;17(3):445–450

102. Venturi ML, Attinger CE, Mesbahi AN, Hess CL, Graw KS. Mechanisms and clinical applications of the vacuum-assisted closure (VAC) Device: a review. Am J Clin Dermatol 2005;6(3):185–194

103. van Rhee MA, de Klerk LW, Verhaar JA. Vacuum-assisted wound closure of deep infections after instrumented spinal fusion in six children with neuromuscular scoliosis. Spine J 2007;7(5):596–600

104. Vicario C, de Juan J, Esclarin A, Alcobendas M. Treatment of deep wound infections after spinal fusion with a vacuum-assisted device in patients with spinal cord injury. Acta Orthop Belg 2007;73(1):102–106

105. Mehbod AA, Ogilvie JW, Pinto MR, et al. Postoperative deep wound infections in adults after spinal fusion: management with vacuum-assisted wound closure. J Spinal Disord Tech 2005;18(1):14–17

106. Khan MH, Smith PN, Rao N, Donaldson WF. Serum C-reactive protein levels correlate with clinical response in patients treated with antibiotics for wound infections after spinal surgery. Spine J 2006;6(3):311–315

107. Weiss LE, Vaccaro AR, Scuderi G, McGuire M, Garfin SR. Pseudarthrosis after postoperative wound infection in the lumbar spine. J Spinal Disord 1997;10(6):482–487

108. Borowski A, Littleton AG, Borkhuu B, et al. Complications of intrathecal baclofen pump therapy in pediatric patients. J Pediatr Orthop 2010;30(1):76–81

109. Fjelstad AB, Hommelstad J, Sorteberg A. Infections related to intrathecal baclofen therapy in children and adults: frequency and risk factors. J Neurosurg Pediatr 2009;4(5):487–493

110. Motta F, Buonaguro V, Stignani C. The use of intrathecal baclofen pump implants in children and adolescents: safety and complications in 200 consecutive cases. J Neurosurg 2007;107(1, Suppl):32–35

111. Njee TB, Irthum B, Roussel P, Peragut JC. Intrathecal morphine infusion for chronic non-malignant pain: a multiple center retrospective survey. Neuromodulation 2004;7(4):249–259. doi: 10.1111/j.1094-7159.2004.04210.x

112. Kallweit U, Harzheim M, Marklein G, Welt T, Pöhlau D. Successful treatment of methicillin-resistant *Staphylococcus aureus* meningitis using linezolid without removal of intrathecal infusion pump. Case report. J Neurosurg 2007;107(3):651–653

113. Boviatsis EJ, Kouyialis AT, Boutsikakis I, Korfias S, Sakas DE. Infected CNS infusion pumps. Is there a chance for treatment without removal? Acta Neurochir (Wien) 2004;146(5):463–467

114. Hester SM, Fisher JF, Lee MR, Macomson S, Vender JR. Evaluation of salvage techniques for infected baclofen pumps in pediatric patients with cerebral palsy. J Neurosurg Pediatr 2012;10(6):548–554

115. Zed PJ, Stiver HG, Devonshire V, Jewesson PJ, Marra F. Continuous intrathecal pump infusion of baclofen with antibiotic drugs for treatment of pump-associated meningitis. Case report. J Neurosurg 2000;92(2):347–349

116. Galloway A, Falope FZ. *Pseudomonas aeruginosa* infection in an intrathecal baclofen pump: successful treatment with adjunct intra-reservoir gentamicin. Spinal Cord 2000;38(2):126–128

117. Fenoy AJ, Simpson RK Jr. Management of device-related wound complications in deep brain stimulation surgery. J Neurosurg 2012;116(6):1324–1332

118. Themistocleous MS, Boviatsis EJ, Stathis P, Stavrinou LC, Sakas DE. Infected internal pulse generator: treatment without removal. Surg Neurol Int 2011;2:33

119. Baizabal Carvallo JF, Simpson R, Jankovic J. Diagnosis and treatment of complications related to deep brain stimulation hardware. Mov Disord 2011;26(8):1398–1406

120. Voges J, Waerzeggers Y, Maarouf M, et al. Deep-brain stimulation: long-term analysis of complications caused by hardware and surgery—experiences from a single centre. J Neurol Neurosurg Psychiatry 2006;77(7):868–872

121. Constantoyannis C, Berk C, Honey CR, Mendez I, Brownstone RM. Reducing hardware-related complications of deep brain stimulation. Can J Neurol Sci 2005;32(2):194–200

122. Resnick AS, Foote KD, Rodriguez RL, et al. The number and nature of emergency department encounters in patients with deep brain stimulators. J Neurol 2010;257(1):122–131

123. Müller-Vahl KR, Cath DC, Cavanna AE, et al; ESSTS Guidelines Group. European clinical guidelines for Tourette syndrome and other tic disorders. Part IV: deep brain stimulation. Eur Child Adolesc Psychiatry 2011;20(4):209–217

124. Piacentino M, Pilleri M, Bartolomei L. Hardware-related infections after deep brain stimulation surgery: review of incidence, severity and management in 212 single-center procedures in the first year after implantation. Acta Neurochir (Wien) 2011;153(12):2337–2341

125. Oh MY, Abosch A, Kim SH, Lang AE, Lozano AM. Long-term hardware-related complications of deep brain stimulation. Neurosurgery 2002;50(6): 1268–1274, discussion 1274–1276

126. Fily F, Haegelen C, Tattevin P, et al. Deep brain stimulation hardware-related infections: a report of 12 cases and review of the literature. Clin Infect Dis 2011;52(8):1020–1023

127. Sixel-Döring F, Trenkwalder C, Kappus C, Hellwig D. Skin complications in deep brain stimulation for Parkinson's disease: frequency, time course, and risk factors. Acta Neurochir (Wien) 2010;152(2):195–200

128. Blomstedt P, Hariz MI. Hardware-related complications of deep brain stimulation: a ten year experience. Acta Neurochir (Wien) 2005;147(10): 1061–1064, discussion 1064

129. Chan DTM, Zhu XL, Yeung JHM, et al. Complications of deep brain stimulation: a collective review. Asian J Surg 2009;32(4):258–263

130. Benabid A, Koudsie A, Benazzouz A. Subthalamic nucleus deep brain stimulation. In: Lozano A, ed. Movement Disorders Surgery. Progress in Neurological Surgery. Basel, Switzerland: Karger; 2000:196–226

131. Seijo FJ, Alvarez-Vega MA, Gutierrez JC, Fdez-Glez F, Lozano B. Complications in subthalamic nucleus stimulation surgery for treatment of Parkinson's disease. Review of 272 procedures. Acta Neurochir (Wien) 2007;149(9):867–875, discussion 876

132. Paluzzi A, Belli A, Bain P, Liu X, Aziz TM. Operative and hardware complications of deep brain stimulation for movement disorders. Br J Neurosurg 2006;20(5):290–295

133. Boviatsis EJ, Stavrinou LC, Themistocleous M, Kouyialis AT, Sakas DE. Surgical and hardware complications of deep brain stimulation. A seven-year experience and review of the literature. Acta Neurochir (Wien) 2010;152(12): 2053–2062

134. Goodman RR, Kim B, McClelland S III, et al. Operative techniques and morbidity with subthalamic nucleus deep brain stimulation in 100 consecutive patients with advanced Parkinson's disease. J Neurol Neurosurg Psychiatry 2006;77(1):12–17

135. Bronstein JM, Tagliati M, Alterman RL, et al. Deep brain stimulation for Parkinson disease: an expert consensus and review of key issues. Arch Neurol 2011;68(2):165

136. Haridas A, Tagliati M, Osborn I, et al. Pallidal deep brain stimulation for primary dystonia in children. Neurosurgery 2011;68(3):738–743, discussion 743

137. Miller JP, Acar F, Burchiel KJ. Significant reduction in stereotactic and functional neurosurgical hardware infection after local neomycin/polymyxin application. J Neurosurg 2009;110(2): 247–250

138. Sillay KA, Larson PS, Starr PA. Deep brain stimulator hardware-related infections: incidence and management in a large series. Neurosurgery 2008;62(2):360–366, discussion 366–367

139. Temel Y, Ackermans L, Celik H, et al. Management of hardware infections following deep brain stimulation. Acta Neurochir (Wien) 2004;146(4):355–361, discussion 361

140. Umemura A, Jaggi JL, Hurtig HI, et al. Deep brain stimulation for movement disorders: morbidity and mortality in 109 patients. J Neurosurg 2003;98(4):779–784

141. Bhatia S, Zhang K, Oh M, Angle C, Whiting D. Infections and hardware salvage after deep brain stimulation surgery: a single-center study and review of the literature. Stereotact Funct Neurosurg 2010;88(3):147–155

142. Halpern CH, Mitchell GW, Paul A, et al. Self-administered preoperative antiseptic wash to prevent postoperative infection after deep brain stimulation. Am J Infect Control 2012; 40(5):431–433

143. Vergani F, Landi A, Pirillo D, Cilia R, Antonini A, Sganzerla EP. Surgical, medical, and hardware adverse events in a series of 141 patients undergoing subthalamic deep brain stimulation for Parkinson disease. World Neurosurg 2010;73(4):338–344

144. Gorgulho A, Juillard C, Uslan DZ, et al. Infection following deep brain stimulator implantation performed in the conventional versus magnetic resonance imaging-equipped operating room. J Neurosurg 2009;110(2):239–246

145. Kenney C, Simpson R, Hunter C, et al. Short-term and long-term safety of deep brain stimulation in the treatment of movement disorders. J Neurosurg 2007;106(4):621–625

146. Voges J, Hilker R, Bötzel K, et al. Thirty days complication rate following surgery performed for deep-brain-stimulation. Mov Disord 2007;22(10):1486–1489

147. Bhatia R, Dalton A, Richards M, Hopkins C, Aziz T, Nandi D. The incidence of deep brain stimulator hardware infection: the effect of change in antibiotic prophylaxis regimen and review of the literature. Br J Neurosurg 2011;25(5):625–631

148. Hamani C, Lozano AM. Hardware-related complications of deep brain stimulation: a review of the published literature. Stereotact Funct Neurosurg 2006;84(5-6):248–251

149. Merello M, Cammarota A, Leiguarda R, Pikielny R. Delayed intracerebral electrode infection after bilateral STN implantation for Parkinson's disease. Case report. Mov Disord 2001;16(1):168–170

150. Vanderhorst VG, Papavassiliou E, Tarsy D, Shih L. Early brain abscess: a rare complication of deep brain stimulation. Mov Disord 2009;24(9):1395–1397

151. Deligny C, Drapier S, Verin M, Lajat Y, Raoul S, Damier P. Bilateral subthalamotomy through DBS electrodes: a rescue option for device-related infection. Neurology 2009;73(15):1243–1244

152. Real R, Linhares P, Fernandes H, et al. Role of Tc-Sulesomab immunoscintigraphy in the management of infection following deep brain stimulation surgery. Neurology Research International 2011;2011:817-951. doi: 10.1155/2011/817951

153. Cheng MT, Chang MC, Wang ST, Yu WK, Liu CL, Chen TH. Efficacy of dilute betadine solution irrigation in the prevention of postoperative infection of spinal surgery. Spine (Phila Pa 1976) 2005;30(15):1689–1693

154. Chundamala J, Wright JG. The efficacy and risks of using povidone-iodine irrigation to prevent surgical site infection: an evidence-based review. Can J Surg 2007;50(6):473–481

# V

# Special Populations

# 17

# Pediatric Central Nervous System Infections

Ian Mutchnick and Thomas M. Moriarty

This chapter focuses on two of the most common pediatric infectious conditions requiring neurosurgical intervention: intracranial focal suppurative infections and cerebrospinal fluid (CSF) ventricular shunt infections. Limited space and the intended audience have directed content decisions. This chapter is targeted at the neurosurgeon, who will be managing the surgical issues within the context of a team of pediatric specialists representing infectious disease, neuroradiology, intensive care, and inpatient hospitalist services, who will provide depth in topics not covered in this chapter. Therefore, we have emphasized content more germane to the neurosurgeon—detailed clinical information required to bring clarity to the decision-making process and an explicit review of the literature on management.

## Focal Intracranial Infectious Lesions

An abscess of the brain was one of those cases which occurred but once in the course of a lifetime.
—Macewen, 1893

This section covers focal intracranial suppurative lesions: cranial epidural abscess, subdural empyema, and intraparenchymal abscess. Because specialists of the pediatric neurosurgical service usually see patients with these entities as consults, the sec-tion focuses on the diagnostic challenges that may influence the decision to operate and the treatment options available to the neurosurgeon, with an emphasis on the information required to choose the correct management pathway for the patient.

### Clinical Context

A recent review of large inpatient databases found that the rate of admission for all identifiable intracranial focal suppurative infections secondary to sinusitis or otitis (including epidural abscesses, subdural empyemas, and brain abscesses) was 2.74 to 4.38 per million children in the United States.[1] A busy neurosurgical service in the developed world with two pediatric neurosurgeons can therefore expect to see two to four of these patients in a given year.[1,2] Several key events have shaped our current approach to these lesions. The introduction of antibiotics to patient care reduced reported mortality from between 60 and 80% to between 20 and 40%.[3] This rate has been further reduced to between 0 and 10% in modern series both by the availability of computed tomography (CT) and magnetic resonance (MR) imaging and by improvements in antibiotic therapy.[1,2,4,5]

Extra-axial abscesses have a bimodal distribution based on patient age. This finding is consistent throughout the literature and was recently reiterated in a review of 70 patients treated for extra-axial abscesses at The Hospital for Sick Children in Toronto, Canada, between 1995 and 2009.[2] Fifty percent of these children were older than 11 years of age, and 21% were below 1 year of age. In children younger than 5 years of age, the extra-axial abscess was most often the consequence of meningitis or otitis media. All patients with post-meningitis extra-axial abscesses were younger than 1 year of age. All patients with post-sinusitis abscesses were older than 7 years of age because the frontal sinus is not pneumatized in younger children. Central nervous system (CNS) infection complicates 3 to 4% of hospital-admitted cases of sinusitis.[6] Valveless mucosal veins penetrate the inner lamina of this sinus and allow communication with both the diploë and the dura mater.[7] Unlike other etiologies, postoperative extra-axial abscesses were seen to span these age groups.

Infants who develop a post-meningitic abscess (often subdural) have signs and symptoms of meningitis that include a bulging fontanelle, and their condition often fails to improve despite adequate antibiotic therapy for their meningitis.[8] In the older child, Pott puffy tumor is a common finding in patients who have developed an intracranial extra-axial abscess; in the Toronto series, this was found in 16 of 38 (42.1%) patients with post-sinusitis abscesses.[2,9] In the absence of a Pott puffy tumor, the clinical presentation does not follow a consistent pattern; although headache, fever, emesis, and meningismus are often present, the specificity of these findings is far too low to be used for effective decision making.[8] However, the clinical presentation, in conjunction with a high degree of suspicion, often prompts imaging studies by the admitting and subsequently the consult-seeking service, whereupon intracranial mass lesions are revealed if present. Routine blood work is rarely useful in diagnosing these infectious lesions. Neither a leukocytosis nor a left shift is always present. The erythrocyte sedimentation rate (ESR) and C-reactive protein (CRP) level can be useful for monitoring response to therapy for established lesions but lack the positive or negative predictive value needed to be helpful in diagnosis.[8] Blood cultures are similarly of low yield, though, because of their ease of collection, they should be obtained on the slight chance of assisting in the microbial identification. CSF analysis for these lesions is neither sensitive nor specific, and results will often be normal.[8]

The identification of most extra-axial abscesses on CT and MR imaging is straightforward. On CT scans, the extra-axial abscess will show a hypodense collection of pus with enhancement along both the cortical and the dural border. T1-weighted MR imaging will show the pus collection to be iso- to hypointense, and on T2-weighted imaging it will be hyper- to isointense.[10] On post-contrast MR imaging, there is usually enhancement of the outer border on the medial, lateral, or both margins. Infants can pose a radiographic challenge in differentiating a post-meningitic subdural empyema from a sterile reactive subdural effusion. Although reactive subdural effusions can occur in 33% of infantile patients with meningitis and usually do not require intervention, subdural empyemas occur in only 1%.[11] On ultrasound, the reactive subdural effusion is usually anechoic, with the thickened hyperechoic inner membranes and echogenic cerebral sulci characteristic of meningitis. Chen et al were able to use ultrasound to correctly distinguish subdural empyema from reactive subdural effusion in 15 of 16 lesions. They found that subdural empyema tends to be anechoic with prominent traversing fibrinous strands in the early stages and hyperechoic in its entirety with frequent loculi as it matures.[12] CT scans of a subdural empyema can vary widely and lack high specificity or sensitivity, although some authors in the developing world have used CT as the sole radiographic modality because of its accessibility and low cost.[10,13,14] MR imaging is probably the best modality to differentiate these entities. Wong et al reported on 10 patients with a total of 12 lesions. Of the 12 lesions, 10 were subdural empyemas and 2 were reactive subdural effusions; MR images of 9 of the patients with subdural empyemas revealed restricted diffusion, while one image demonstrated mixed signal on diffusion-weighted imaging.

Both patients with reactive subdural effusions demonstrated low signal intensity on diffusion-weighted imaging.[15] In older children, imaging is more straightforward, with CT the nearly universal modality used to evaluate children with a suspected extra-axial suppurative process. MR imaging is often used to clarify anatomic detail or to characterize the abscess better in cases in which it will be followed with conservative treatment. In the previously cited Toronto series, MR imaging was used in only 12 of 38 patients with sinusitis-related extra-axial abscess; this may be related to the fact that the vast majority of these cases (64 of 70 patients) were managed operatively, necessitating only CT localization rather than the subtle definition of improvement with medical therapy.[2]

Abscesses of the brain parenchyma tend to have two main causes. Hematogenous spread occurs in children with congenital cyanotic heart disease and a left-to-right shunt, which bypasses the reticuloendothelium of the lung, or an infectious focus elsewhere in the body. Contiguous spread can occur, as with extra-axial abscesses, from sinus or middle ear disease. Cases arising from trauma or as a postsurgical complication are less common, while abscess in the context of immunosuppression is an increasingly frequent clinical situation.[8] Some 10 to 37% of intraparenchymal abscesses are idiopathic.[16] The clinical presentation of an intraparenchymal abscess lacks both sensitivity and positive predictive value for the disease. The classic triad of headache, fever, and neurologic deficit is present in only 17 to 30% of cases.[8,17] As with extra-axial abscesses, the clinical blood count (CBC), ESR, CRP level, and CSF evaluations are seldom helpful beyond tracking the effect of therapy in patients with a diagnosis. An exception to this rule is in the patient in whom the abscess has ruptured into the ventricle, who will usually have a positive CSF evaluation. Blood cultures return relevant results approximately 30% of the time and should be obtained if there is suspicion of this diagnosis.[18]

CT or MR imaging should be obtained with contrast and reveal either an edema-tous region with mass effect in the cerebritis stage or a ring-enhancing lesion with a hypodense interior in the later stages. Early abscesses can have a radiographic appearance similar to that of an ischemic stroke on CT without contrast; therefore, the index of clinical suspicion should guide the need for repeat CT with contrast or enhanced MR imaging.[19] Characteristics that distinguish mature abscess from tumor are gas within the center of the lesion, a rim of less than 5 mm (which tends to be thinner than that of a brain tumor), and ependymal enhancement that can be associated with ventriculitis or ventricular rupture. Diffusion-weighted images show restriction (hyperintensity) in the interior of the abscess, with a dark absolute diffusion coefficient (ADC).[18] If needed, further differentiation from a tumor can be made with perfusion MR imaging, which demonstrates hypovascularity in an abscess capsule and hypervascularity in a tumor capsule.[8] A radioactively labeled leukocyte scan can also be used to diagnose an infectious process in uncertain situations.[20] In infants with an open fontanelle, ultrasound can be used to diagnose and follow intraparenchymal abscesses.[21]

## Management Issues

### Medical Management

Although clear parameters for medical management of intracranial abscesses (epidural, subdural, and intraparenchymal) are still not defined, the method of treatment has been under investigation since 1970.[4] The widespread availability of both potent antibiotics and improved intracranial imaging has expanded the role of medical management. In most cases, intracranial abscesses that are less than 2.5 cm can be managed medically if they present in otherwise healthy patients without focal deficits, altered sensorium, or the imminent threat of either. In sick, high-risk patients or in patients with deep-seated abscesses, neurologic deficits may be unavoidable and can worsen with surgery.

Few specifics exist for the medical management of epidural abscesses. Nathoo et al first reported on this strategy in 1999, managing six patients without fever with antibiotic therapy and serial imaging. No information is available on lesion size or whether there was associated sinus disease that was treated by the otolaryngologic service.[22,23] Heran et al contributed to the literature on this topic in 2003, treating four patients who had isolated epidural abscesses with sinus drainage and antibiotics without intracranial intervention. There was no evidence of bony erosion, which would have allowed spontaneous drainage of the intracranial component into the extracranial space. None of these patients had focal neurologic deficits or an altered sensorium, and the average size of the abscesses was 2.9 × 2.6 × 1.4 cm, with a maximum size 3.5 × 3.5 × 1.2 cm in one that was infratentorial.[24] At our institution, we routinely treat epidural abscesses as a medical disease to great effect and rarely operate unless there is a decreased level of consciousness or focal neurologic deficits attributable to the lesion. Decisions regarding the treatment of primary sinus disease are left to the discretion of the otolaryngologists.

The medical management of subdural empyema was first explored in an article from 1979 by Rossaza et al, in which a child with an interhemispheric empyema and foot weakness was cured clinically and radiographically with antibiotics alone.[25] Steroids were used in this case to ameliorate the foot weakness. Leys et al provided more support for medical management in the 1980s, finding that individuals as young as 2 years of age with empyemas up to 44 mm thick in the supratentorial space, with an average Glasgow Coma Scale score of 11 (range, 7 to 13) and even with a severe neurologic deficit, could be medically treated with a good clinical outcome. Although the length of stay was shorter and the infectious organism was more often identified in both the aspiration and craniotomy groups of patients, medically treated patients had the same mortality rates and a lower probability of persistent neurologic deficits and seizures than those treated surgically.[26,27] Similar to Heran et al, Leys found that minor deterioration in neurologic status within 24 to 48 hours of the start of medical treatment often resolved without the need for surgical intervention. A few modern series have made reference to medically managed empyemas, but they do not include the details of these patients.[2,28] Salunke et al did describe one patient treated successfully with antibiotics alone who had a thin subtentorial empyema.[28] At our institution, we have even had success treating subdural empyemas of the posterior fossa with antibiotic therapy. Recently, we successfully treated an 8-day-old infant with Currarino triad; she had multiple infratentorial subdural empyemas that measured 1 and 0.6 cm, and at no time did she demonstrate a neurologic deficit. After 6 weeks of intravenous antibiotics, all empyemas had resolved, and she remained without neurologic deficit (**Fig. 17.1**).

Decisions regarding the medical management of intraparenchymal abscesses are similar to those for other intracranial abscesses and include abscess size, neurologic status of the patient, general medical condition of the patient, and the need for organism identification. In addition to these factors, the location of the intraparenchymal abscess must be considered because the indications for operating within eloquent brain must be justified. No specific criteria for the appropriate size of an intraparenchymal abscess have been established that will result in its successful medical treatment. A comprehensive review of the literature has provided a thoughtful, well-supported approach to patients with intraparenchymal abscess.[29] Patients with intraparenchymal abscesses smaller than 2.5 cm in maximum diameter are the best candidates for medical management, especially where their overall neurologic condition is good and microbiological speciation has been determined from another source. Although well supported in the literature, the size of 2.5 cm or less may be an unduly conservative requirement for medical management. In a review of reports of the medical treatment

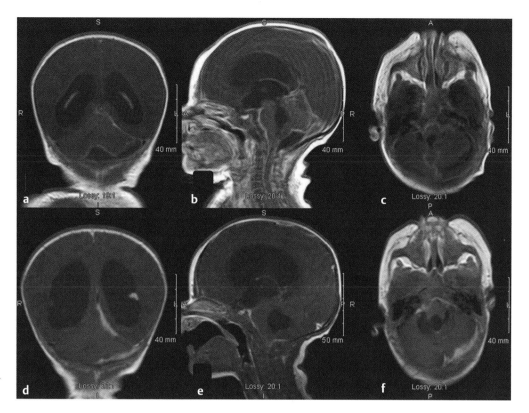

**Fig. 17.1a–f** **(a–c)** Post-contrast magnetic resonance (MR) imaging of the brain on day 18 of life of a girl who had Currarino triad with meningitis complicated by multiple subdural empyemas of the posterior fossa. At no point was there focal or global deficit. This patient was observed closely in the pediatric intensive care unit and received intravenous vancomycin and meropenem. **(d–f)** At day 48 of life, repeat MR imaging showed resolution of the empyemas with residual meningeal enhancement that resolved over the next month.

of intraparenchymal abscesses, Bamberger found that 100% of 113 brain abscesses less than 5 cm in maximum diameter and 74% of 30 intraparenchymal abscesses 5 cm or more in diameter were successfully treated medically.[30] At our institution, we routinely treat intraparenchymal abscesses more than 2.5 cm in maximum diameter medically, with only a rare conversion to operative management. Multiple abscesses can also be treated medically, with surgical excision of intraparenchymal abscesses larger than 2.5 cm or of smaller ones causing symptomatic mass effect. When a patient is being treated medically, surgery should be reconsidered if the patient's condition deteriorates clinically or if clinical or radiographic improvement is not observed within 1 to 2 weeks.

## Surgical Management

Although the indications for medical management of intracranial focal infections have expanded, the large majority of these lesions are handled operatively. In their large review of 70 patients with extra-axial abscesses, Gupta et al operated on all but six patients.[2] Similarly, most modern series reporting on extra-axial abscesses indicate that surgery is overwhelmingly the first choice of treatment.[14,28,31,32] The main cause for concern in approaching an extra-axial abscess operatively is the extent of exposure. Although it is clear that extra-axial abscesses can be treated with either burr hole drainage or limited craniotomy, the rate of recurrence—requiring reoperation to clear the infection—is potentially higher after burr hole drainage in larger extra-axial abscesses and in those with evidence of loculi.[5,16,22,31,33–37] Parafalcine or paratentorial empyemas may pose a higher risk for recurrence after burr hole drainage than after craniotomy.[28] In contrast, a series of post-meningitis empyemas demonstrated that these lesions might preferentially be treated safely with burr hole drainage rather than with craniotomy.[31] Certainly, in a decision to use a surgical approach to an infection, the clinical context must be considered. Those patients with significant focal or global neurologic deficits should be considered candidates for craniotomy, with craniectomy more appropriate for those at risk for postoperative hemispheric swelling. For the significant number of patients who have an associated sinusitis or mastoiditis, an otorhinologic consult should be obtained. If possible, definitive intracranial management should occur at the same time as otorhinologic treatment because several authors have reported lower rates of intracranial recurrence with concurrent management.[2,7,22]

Issues regarding management of the bone flap arise in these cases, with most authors advocating immediate replacement of the bone flap unless frank, extensive osteomyelitis is present. A report addressed the issue of devascularized bone flaps in the context of extra-axial abscesses without osteomyelitis.[38] In this series of 14 patients, all had successful immediate reimplantation of the bone flap following craniotomy for an extra-axial abscess. One of these patients had tetralogy of Fallot, and two had undergone chemotherapy and radiation therapy following resection of brain tumors. In each case, the surgeons removed all soft tissue from the bone flap, scrubbed the flap for 3 to 5 minutes in iodophor or bacitracin solution, then soaked the flap in an iodine or bacitracin solution until reimplantation. In addition, the surgical bed was scrubbed abrasively with surgical sponges, and the bone edges were débrided, with care taken not to injure the exposed brain. Two other reports used an implanted irrigation–drainage system to salvage devascularized bone flaps in the context of postsurgical infection but did not comment on the degree of osteomyelitis present in the flaps.[39,40] Unfortunately, there are no clear data on the possibility of immediate reimplantation of a bone flap affected with frank osteomyelitis, and the risks and benefits of aggressive débridement and immediate replacement of the osteomyelitis flap must be left to the surgeon. Of note, in the report by Gupta et al on 12 patients receiving a craniectomy for osteomyelitis, six did not require a cranioplasty because in situ bone growth with a good cosmetic result was present. No ages were provided for these patients.[2]

Although abundant literature is available on the management of intraparenchymal abscesses, it lacks patient stratification, clear management protocols, and consistent outcome measures, decreasing the usefulness of this body of information. In a review from Italy, the authors made several useful conclusions regarding intraparenchymal abscesses.[29] First, the choice of a surgical approach that includes either a burr hole or a craniotomy did not appear to impact outcome. Instead, the patient's initial neurologic condition and the rapidity with which therapeutic intervention is initiated are far more important prognostic factors. Those determinants of operation type are influenced by the preference and abilities of the surgeon and whether the patient will be able to tolerate the proposed procedure. It might be more reasonable to aspirate those intraparenchymal abscesses that are located deep within eloquent areas of the brain or that are small or multiple, even if they are recurrent. Those intraparenchymal abscesses that are superficial, are located in the posterior fossa, or result from posttraumatic or postoperative complications might better be treated by a craniotomy than by burr holes. It is not clear whether the size of the abscess and the neurologic status of the patient are independent determinants of what type of management is required. We recently encountered a 9-month-old girl with a 3-week history of progressive lethargy and decreased appetite. On her evaluation in the emergency department, she was fussy but consolable and had a bulging fontanelle. MR imaging revealed multiple abscesses occupying nearly the entire left hemisphere. Each abscess was aspirated through a separate burr hole with a ventricular catheter and a syringe that had a Luer connector. A catheter was left overnight in the largest abscess, and that abscess was reaspirated the next day. The patient was then treated with antibiotics and had a good clinical outcome (**Fig. 17.2**).

## Cerebrospinal Fluid Ventricular Shunt Infections

> Infections of the central nervous system in shunted hydrocephalic patients are the neurosurgeon's nightmare.
> —*Walters, Hoffman, Hendrick, and Humphreys, 1984*

Infection is the most serious complication of a ventricular CSF shunt, so that the treatment and prevention of shunt infections are of great importance to all neurosurgeons, especially those who specialize in pediatrics.[41] The risk for a shunt infection is estimated to be 10%, and the number of admissions to U.S. hospitals in 2003 for the treatment of shunt infections was approximately 2,300, or 6% of all hydrocephalus-related hospital admissions.[42,43] The impact on children struck by infection is considerable: treatment requires multiple-day hospital stays with limited mobility and long-term effects include lower IQ, seizures, and future shunt failure.[44] At an approximate cost of $49,000 per infection (making infection the most costly per-case complication of shunt systems), the estimated cost to the U.S. health care system in 2003 caused by infected shunts was $112,700,000.[44] It is therefore imperative for neurosurgeons to be well versed in the management of ventricular shunt infections.

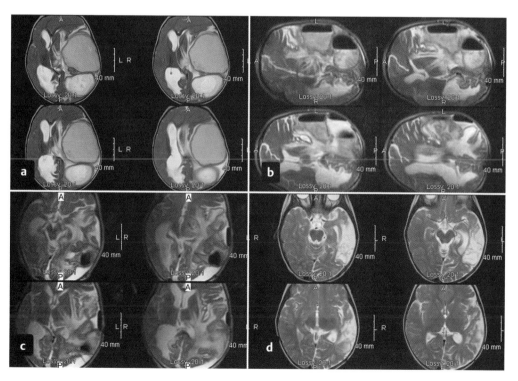

**Fig. 17.2a–d** **(a)** T2-weighted axial magnetic resonance (MR) imaging of the brain of a 9-month-old girl with lethargy and decreased oral intake showing large, multiple, left-sided brain abscesses taking up virtually the entire left hemisphere. **(b)** Intraoperative MR imaging–guided drainage of both abscesses on day 1. **(c)** Drainage on day 2. **(d)** Follow-up MR imaging 9 months after the MR imaging in **(a)**. After a lengthy intravenous antibiotic course, the patient has continued to do well.

## Clinical Context

The pediatric patient with a ventricular shunt infection does not have a stereotypic presentation because the possible infectious and neurologic signs and symptoms are numerous, highly variable, and nonspecific. For example, fever is common, but approximately 25% of patients with a confirmed case of ventricular shunt infection have no fever.[45] Equally challenging are the many shunt infections that present as mechanical malfunctions without overt infectious signs or symptoms. Walters et al noted that in their series of ventricular shunt infection, shunt malfunction was diagnosed as infection in only half of the cases, resulting in delayed treatment.[41,42] Because the number of shunt malfunctions without infection is much larger than the number of malfunctions with occult infection, it would be counterproductive to obtain cultures from all patients with a ventricular shunt malfunction. The overall clinical picture can be helpful in guiding the management of patients with ventricular shunt infection.

First, infections in the different components of the shunt system can present with localizable clinical findings. Patients with proximal catheter infections are more likely to present with neurologic findings that include nausea, mental status changes, seizures, and meningeal symptoms. Abdominal pain, gastrointestinal symptoms, and a possible pseudocyst may be present if a distal peritoneal catheter is involved. Patients with distal atrial catheter infections can present with bacteremia and evidence of systemic infections. Nearly all patients with infected ventriculoatrial shunts present with fevers because of the vascular position of the distal catheter.[41,46] In addition, these patients can develop shunt nephritis, presenting with hepatosplenomegaly, anemia, and cerebral manifestations.[47] This condition is relatively rare and arises from the deposition of immunoglobulin M and immunoglobulin G antigen–antibody complexes in the renal glomeruli secondary to persistent stimulation of the immune system due to chronic infection. Renal disease usually resolves with treatment of the shunt infection.

Second, the time from the last shunt manipulation to infection can be useful both in understanding the clinical picture and in predicting the possible infectious agent. Some 80% of all shunt infections occur within the first 3 months after placement, with the earliest infections occurring within 8 to 15 days.[45] Arnell et al found that of 25 patients presenting after revision or initial placement within 20 weeks, 21 were infected with coagulase-negative staphylococci (15 patients) or *Staphylococcus aureus* (6 patients).[48] All patients presenting with a visible wound infection had coagulase-negative staphylococci or *S. aureus* infection, with a mean time to infection of 3.5 weeks (range, 1.5 to 6 weeks after operation). Similarly, coagulase-negative staphylococci or *S. aureus* was the infectious agent in 8 of 9 initial shunt placements (mean time to infection, 3 weeks) and in 7 of 8 proximal revisions (mean time to infection, 1 week). A single patient with *Enterococcus* infection had an inguinal hernia repaired at the time of shunt placement, and a second patient grew *Propionibacterium acnes* after a proximal revision in which the valve was punctured. Although one easily presumes that contamination with skin flora at the time of surgery explains early infection, several studies have found that fewer than 50% of the microorganisms cultured from the wound or infected shunt could be traced directly to the patient.[49] A prospective study by Thompson et al carefully sampled the flora of the skin covering the operative site of a shunt placement, and the isolated bacteria matched a preoperative swab specimen in only 1 of the 7 patients who went on to develop ventricular shunt infection.[50] Although the timing of postoperative ventricular shunt infection strongly suggests a perioperative etiology, these consistent findings suggest that the method of contamination and subsequent infection may be more complex than simple intraoperative wound seeding. As the time from shunt surgery becomes longer than 20 weeks, infection with gram-negative rods and fungi becomes more likely as ventriculoperitoneal shunts are seeded hematogenously or via retrograde infection from the abdomen.[49] Fungal infections are rare in this population but should be more seriously considered with patients on antibiotic therapy, with immunocompromise, on steroids, or receiving hyperalimentation.[49]

In patients who present with the possibility of ventricular shunt infection, the evaluation can be as difficult as the presentation. As previously stated, the absence of fever does not rule out an infection, nor does a benign CBC or negative blood culture unless the patient has a ventriculoatrial shunt.[42,51] Even CSF protein, glucose, cell count, and Gram stain are imperfectly sensitive to the presence of infection.[52] Patients with coagulase-negative staphylococcal infections may not have CSF pleocytosis, and conversely, an increased CSF cell count may be seen in patients within approximately 14 days of intracranial procedures as well as in patients without any CNS infectious process.[45] Neuroimaging and shunt series are of limited use unless there is suspicion of shunt failure or there is evidence of meningitis or encephalitis. Several laboratory parameters have been described that have diagnostic power, but clarity is required to prevent their misuse. CSF eosinophilia comprising more than 5% of white blood cells has been shown to have a positive predictive value for infection in the 90th percentile range but may also arise as an allergic reaction to latex, shunt materials, or even the ethylene oxide used to sterilize shunts. The absence of CSF eosinophilia is of no diagnostic value.[45,53] Of greater diagnostic value is the combination of fever and CSF neutrophilia comprising more than 10% of white blood cells, as described by McClinton et al.[53] This combination had a 99% specificity, a 93% positive predictive value, a 95% negative predictive value, and a posttest probability of 92%. Recently, serum CRP levels have shown promise in helping to determine if patients have an infected shunt. Schuhmann et al found that patients with a serum CRP level above 7 mg/L had a posttest probability of ventricular shunt infection of 72.3% (an increase of 73% from a pretest probability of 41.7%), and the probability of missing ventricular shunt infection in an individual with a serum CRP level below 7 mg/L was only 2.7%.[52]

Perhaps the most important and controversial diagnostic maneuver for the patient with suspected ventricular shunt infection is a tap of the shunt for the purposes of obtaining CSF and evaluating shunt function. Although a lumbar puncture is also possible, CSF obtained this way is often sterile, even in patients who are later proven to have a ventricular shunt infection.[49] Only one paper exists regarding the complication rate of a shunt tap, published in 1984 by Noetzel et al.[54] In this study, a "neurosurgeon experienced in dealing with shunts" soak-scrubbed the area to be tapped, shaved the area for 2 inches in all directions, triple-washed the area with an alcohol and betadine solution, and then finally covered the area with a Steri-Drape so as to expose only the small area to be tapped. The authors had no mechanical or medical complications, and of the 53 patients whose shunts were tapped and whose cultures revealed no infection, two later became infected at 15 and 20 months after the tap, both with *Haemophilus influenzae*. The diagnostic yield was high; in 12 of 13 patients with infection proven in the end, infection was correctly diagnosed via shunt tap. It should be kept in mind that the administration of antibiotics before the tap decreases the positive culture rate from 96 to 53%.[51] Despite these findings, shunt taps remain a maneuver of debated importance, and many investigators, including those at our institution, feel that nearly all diagnostic challenges involving shunts can be safely addressed without performing a shunt tap.[55–57]

## Management Issues

The neurosurgical literature concerning ventricular shunt infection is divided into two main categories: procedural techniques to avoid ventricular shunt infection during shunt placement and strategies for managing ventricular shunt infection with minimal morbidity and mortality. Many preventive strategies for lowering ventricular shunt infection rates have been generated over the years and include, but are not limited to, perioperative antibiotic prophylaxis, limiting traffic through the operating room, not using a scrub nurse, no-touch operative technique, iodine solution irrigation, preoperative hair washes, and short operative times.[58-64] A multicenter study by Kestle et al has provided strong empiric evidence that procedural rigor can reduce the risk for ventricular shunt infection.[65] These authors found that the average rate of ventricular shunt infection in four separate institutions dropped from 8.5 to 5.7% ($p = 0.0028$) after a standard operative protocol for shunt insertion had been adopted. Brushless preoperative hand preparation by any member of the operative team was associated with a higher ventricular shunt infection rate than traditional brush scrub ($p = 0.025$). In addition, antibiotic-impregnated sutures for wound closure ($p = 0.026$), preoperative chlorhexadine hair wash ($p = 0.004$), and double gloving by all operating room personnel ($p = 0.043$) were all associated with lower ventricular shunt infection rates.

Double gloving is an easy measure to institute that has multiple sources of support in the literature. The Food and Drug Administration (FDA), which regulates the manufacture of sterile surgical gloves, has set the Acceptable Quality Level at 2.5 microperforations per sterile pair. Multiple studies have shown that the rate of tears in surgical gloves during surgery is anywhere from 10 to 60%.[66,67] Double gloving protects both the surgeon and the patient from manufacturing defects and frequent intraoperative glove damage. The literature suggests that gloves should be considered only temporarily sterile during a procedure, even if strict sterile protocol is maintained. In 2005, Al-Maiyah et al found that frequent glove changes reduce the risk for contamination during hip arthroplasty procedures.[68] Bukhari et al found not only that gloved fingertips become contaminated in 52% of operations but also that bacterial counts increase through the duration of surgery.[69] Sørensen found that all 10 pairs of the surgeon's gloves in a ventricular shunt implantation case grew *P. acnes* by the time it was appropriate to implant

the shunt, and 8 of the 10 grew coagulase-negative staphylococci.[70] Tulipan and Cleves made a more direct connection between wearing double gloves and ventricular shunt infection in 2006; they reported a decrease in the ventricular shunt infection rate from 15.2 to 6.7% when the operating room staff changed to a shunt insertion protocol that required double gloving.[71]

Evidence has also clarified the role of prophylactic antibiotics in the prevention of ventricular shunt infection. In a 2009 Cochrane review, Ratilal et al found in a meta-analysis of 17 trials with 2,134 participants that the use of systemic antibiotic prophylaxis perioperatively and for 24 hours postoperatively was associated with a decrease in the ventricular shunt infection rate (odds ratio [OR], 0.52; 95% confidence interval [CI], 0.36 to 0.74).[72] This same review also found a decrease in the ventricular shunt infection rate (OR, 0.21; 95% CI, 0.08 to 0.55) with the use of antibiotic-impregnated shunts. In a separate review from 2011, Parker et al[73] conducted a meta-analysis of 12 studies that included 5,613 shunt procedures (2,664 antibiotic-impregnated shunts versus 2,949 non–antibiotic-impregnated shunts). Antibiotic-impregnated shunts were associated with a reduction in the shunt infection rate from 7.2 to 3.3% ($p < 0.0001$). In a meta-analysis of 9 studies that included only pediatric patients and compared 854 procedures with antibiotic-impregnated shunts and 795 procedures without antibiotic-impregnated shunts, the ventricular shunt infection rates fell from 11.2 to 5.0% ($p < 0.0001$). Although it is clear that many procedural interventions can reduce the rate of ventricular shunt infection, further study must be done to determine the most cost-effective measures to institute.

Despite nearly 60 years of experience, the optimal treatment strategy for ventricular shunt infection is still a topic of great debate. In a large retrospective multicenter analysis from 2010, Simon et al reviewed collected data on 675 children who underwent an uncomplicated ventricular shunt placement, had 24 months of follow-up, and developed a ventricular shunt infection.[74] Of these children, 111 developed a second ventricular shunt infection within 12 months after treatment; however, no patient, hospital, or surgeon factors were identified that correlated significantly with a risk for reinfection. Of the 675 children, 483 had retrospectively identifiable treatment details that allowed an analysis of infection risk according to treatment strategy. All 675 children received antibiotics. The surgical strategies for these 483 patients were as follows: 286 (59.2%) had the shunt removed with placement of an external ventricular drain followed by placement of a new shunt once the CSF was cleared of infection; 59 (12.2%) had shunt externalization and placement of a new shunt once the CSF was cleared; 64 (13.3%) received nonsurgical management (antibiotic only); and 74 (15.3%) had the shunt removed without being replaced. Of these treatment strategies, nonoperative management had a significantly ($p = 0.03$) higher risk for reinfection, with 15 (23%) of the 64 patients becoming reinfected. As a measure of internal consistency, no patient who had a shunt removed permanently experienced reinfection. Although there was a trend ($p = 0.19$) toward a greater risk for infection in patients whose shunts were externalized, this was not a statistically significant finding; 12 of 59 patients with externalized shunts experienced reinfection, and 44 of 286 patients who had shunt removal with external ventricular drain replacement experienced reinfection. Even an extensive study such as this failed to determine the best treatment for ventricular shunt infection.

Two meta-analyses in the literature, one by Yogev and the other by Schreffler et al, have been influential in guiding operative treatment.[75,76] Schreffler et al constructed a decision tree based on the information from 17 published studies and concluded that the cure rates were 88% for a two-stage strategy (shunt removal with external ventricular drain placement followed by shunt replacement), 64% for one-stage treatment (shunt removal and immediate replacement), and 34% for nonoperative management. Yogev's assessment of 18 studies yielded similar results, with cure rates of 96%, 65%, and 36%, respectively, for the same three strategies. Although these results plus those of Simon et al strongly imply that any cure for ventricular shunt infection must include some form of surgical intervention, a few organisms have been identified for which only systemic antibiotics are required to achieve eradication successfully; these include *Streptococcus pneumoniae*, *Neisseria meningitidis*, and *H. influenzae*, the bacteria most commonly associated with community-acquired meningitis.[77–81]

The striking difference between the rates of reinfection following nonoperative treatment of ventricular shunt infection in the studies of Yogev and of Schreffler et al and the empiric reinfection rate of 23.4% in the study of Simon et al is somewhat puzzling but may be due to modifications in nonoperative management. An example of how this treatment modality has changed in recent years is provided by Brown et al, who in 2006 reported an 84% cure rate in 43 patients who were treated with systemic and intraventricular antibiotics. In 36 patients without *S. aureus* infection, the cure rate was 92%. Conservative management of *S. aureus* infection was discontinued when an early cure rate of only 50% was found. There was no increased risk for mechanical shunt failure in follow-up lasting 6 to 128 months when the infecting agents were coagulase-negative staphylococci (28/30 cured), *Enterococcus* species (3/3 cured), *P. acnes* (2/2 cured), *Streptococcus sanguis* (1/1 cured), and *Pseudomonas aeruginosa* (0/1 cured). There are a few important methodologic aspects of this study. First, rifampin was included in the treatment regimen because this agent has been shown to have good penetration into the biofilm created by coagulase-negative staphylococcal species. Second, intraventricular antibiotics were administered via a ventricular access device, which was already present in 33 of the patients but had to be implanted in 10. Although the requirement for a ventricular access device may limit the usefulness of this technique, this paper does establish the possibility of clearing ventricular shunt infection without the removal of shunt hardware. The strategy may be optimal for patients with a complex CSF diversion system or with retained hardware, in whom the risk of ventricular access device implantation to clear a ventricular shunt infection may be warranted.

Shunt externalization was also the subject of a study by Arnell et al in 2007, in which 34 consecutive ventricular shunt infections were treated with ventricular catheter externalization followed by systemic and intraventricular antibiotics. After a negative CSF culture had been obtained, the ventricular catheter was replaced, and a new subcutaneous route for the valve and distal catheter was used. Infecting organisms included coagulase-negative staphylococci, *S. aureus*, *P. acnes*, *Enterococcus* species, *Escherichia coli* and other gram-negative rods, and β-hemolytic streptococci; cure was obtained in all cases. Although technically a two-stage procedure, the single ventricular catheter replacement with use of the same burr hole may be of less risk to the CNS and can also reduce the number of operated sites in patients with shunts. Although individual investigators continue to pursue the optimal treatment of ventricular shunt infection, it may turn out that no one single treatment is best and that applying valid options to an individual patient's specific circumstances may yield the best results.

## References

1. Piatt JH Jr. Intracranial suppuration complicating sinusitis among children: an epidemiological and clinical study. J Neurosurg Pediatr 2011;7(6):567–574
2. Gupta S, Vachhrajani S, Kulkarni AV, et al. Neurosurgical management of extraaxial central nervous system infections in children. J Neurosurg Pediatr 2011;7(5):441–451
3. Morgan H, Wood MW, Murphey F. Experience with 88 consecutive cases of brain abscess. J Neurosurg 1973;38(6):698–704
4. Heineman HS, Braude AI, Osterholm JL. Intracranial suppurative disease. Early presumptive diagnosis and successful treatment without surgery. JAMA 1971;218(10):1542–1547
5. Madhugiri VS, Sastri BVS, Srikantha U, et al. Focal intradural brain infections in children: an analysis of management and outcome. Pediatr Neurosurg 2011;47(2):113–124
6. Glickstein JS, Chandra RK, Thompson JW. Intracranial complications of pediatric sinusitis. Otolaryngol Head Neck Surg 2006;134(5):733–736
7. Cochrane DD, Price AV, Dobson S. Intracranial epidural and subdural infections. In: Albright AL, Adelson PD, Pollack IF, eds. Principles and Practice of Pediatric Neurosurgery. 2nd ed. New York, NY: Thieme; 2007:1148–1155
8. Yogev R. Focal suppurative infections of the central nervous system. In: Long SS, Pickering LK, Prober CG, eds. Principles and Practice of Pediatric Infectious Diseases. 3rd ed. Philadelphia, PA: Saunders; 2009. http://www.mdconsult.com/books/page.do?eid=4-u1.0-B978-0-7020-3468-8.50054-7&isbn=978-0-7020-3468-8&type=bookPage&from=content&uniqId=290678879-2. Accessed December 23, 2012
9. Bambakidis NC, Cohen AR. Intracranial complications of frontal sinusitis in children: Pott's puffy tumor revisited. Pediatr Neurosurg 2001;35(2):82–89
10. Kirmi O, Sheerin F, Patel N. Imaging of the meninges and the extra-axial spaces. Semin Ultrasound CT MR 2009;30(6):565–593
11. Yikilmaz A, Taylor GA. Sonographic findings in bacterial meningitis in neonates and young infants. Pediatr Radiol 2008;38(2):129–137
12. Chen CY, Huang CC, Chang YC, Chow NH, Chio CC, Zimmerman RA. Subdural empyema in 10 infants: US characteristics and clinical correlates. Radiology 1998;207(3):609–617
13. Banerjee AD, Pandey P, Devi BI, Sampath S, Chandramouli BA. Pediatric supratentorial subdural empyemas: a retrospective analysis of 65 cases. Pediatr Neurosurg 2009;45(1):11–18
14. Venkatesh MS, Pandey P, Devi BI, et al. Pediatric infratentorial subdural empyema: analysis of 14 cases. J Neurosurg 2006;105(5, Suppl):370–377
15. Wong AM, Zimmerman RA, Simon EM, Pollock AN, Bilaniuk LT. Diffusion-weighted MR imaging of subdural empyemas in children. AJNR Am J Neuroradiol 2004;25(6):1016–1021
16. Hall WA, Truwit CL. The surgical management of infections involving the cerebrum. Neurosurgery 2008;62(Suppl 2):519–530, discussion 530–531
17. Tseng J-H, Tseng M-Y. Brain abscess in 142 patients: factors influencing outcome and mortality. Surg Neurol 2006;65(6):557–562, discussion 562
18. Bernardini GL. Diagnosis and management of brain abscess and subdural empyema. Curr Neurol Neurosci Rep 2004;4(6):448–456
19. Fitzpatrick MO, Gan P. Lesson of the week: contrast enhanced computed tomography in the early diagnosis of cerebral abscess. BMJ 1999;319(7204):239–240
20. Frazier JL, Ahn ES, Jallo GI. Management of brain abscesses in children. Neurosurg Focus 2008;24(6):E8
21. Moorthy RK, Rajshekhar V. Management of brain abscess: an overview. Neurosurg Focus 2008;24(6):E3
22. Nathoo N, Nadvi SS, van Dellen JR, Gouws E. Intracranial subdural empyemas in the era of computed tomography: a review of 699 cases.

Neurosurgery 1999;44(3):529–535, discussion 535–536

23. Nathoo N, van Dellen JR, Nadvi SS. Conservative neurological management of intracranial epidural abscesses in children. Neurosurgery 2004;55(1):263–264, author reply 264

24. Heran NS, Steinbok P, Cochrane DD. Conservative neurosurgical management of intracranial epidural abscesses in children. Neurosurgery 2003;53(4):893–897, discussion 897–898

25. Rosazza A, de Tribolet N, Deonna T. Nonsurgical treatment of interhemispheric subdural empyemas. Helv Paediatr Acta 1979;34(6):577–581

26. Leys D, Christiaens JL, Derambure P, et al. Management of focal intracranial infections: is medical treatment better than surgery? J Neurol Neurosurg Psychiatry 1990;53(6):472–475

27. Leys D, Destee A, Petit H, Warot P. Management of subdural intracranial empyemas should not always require surgery. J Neurol Neurosurg Psychiatry 1986;49(6):635–639

28. Salunke PS, Malik V, Kovai P, Mukherjee KK. Falcotentorial subdural empyema: analysis of 10 cases. Acta Neurochir (Wien) 2011;153(1):164–169, discussion 170

29. Arlotti M, Grossi P, Pea F, et al; GISIG (Gruppo Italiano di Studio sulle Infezioni Gravi) Working Group on Brain Abscesses. Consensus document on controversial issues for the treatment of infections of the central nervous system: bacterial brain abscesses. Int J Infect Dis 2010;14(Suppl 4):S79–S92

30. Bamberger DM. Outcome of medical treatment of bacterial abscesses without therapeutic drainage: review of cases reported in the literature. Clin Infect Dis 1996;23(3):592–603

31. Liu Z-H, Chen N-Y, Tu P-H, Lee S-T, Wu C-T. The treatment and outcome of postmeningitic subdural empyema in infants. J Neurosurg Pediatr 2010;6(1):38–42

32. Yilmaz N, Kiymaz N, Yilmaz C, et al. Surgical treatment outcome of subdural empyema: a clinical study. Pediatr Neurosurg 2006;42(5):293–298

33. Ak HE, Ozkan U, Devecioglu C, Kemaloglu MS; AK HE. Treatment of subdural empyema by burr hole. Isr J Med Sci 1996;32(7):542–544

34. Bok AP, Peter JC. Subdural empyema: burr holes or craniotomy? A retrospective computerized tomography-era analysis of treatment in 90 cases. J Neurosurg 1993;78(4):574–578

35. Druhan SM, Shiels WE II, Kang DR, Elton SW, Koranyi K. Successful sonographically guided drainage of epidural abscess. AJR Am J Roentgenol 2006;187(5):W512–W514

36. Eviatar E, Lavi R, Fridental I, Gavriel H. Endonasal endoscopic drainage of frontal lobe epidural abscess. Isr Med Assoc J 2008;10(3):239–240

37. Tummala R, Chu R, Hall W. Subdural empyema in children. Neurosurg Q 2004;14(4):257–265

38. Widdel L, Winston KR. Pus and free bone flaps. J Neurosurg Pediatr 2009;4(4):378–382

39. Auguste KI, McDermott MW. Salvage of infected craniotomy bone flaps with the wash-in, washout indwelling antibiotic irrigation system. Technical note and case series of 12 patients. J Neurosurg 2006;105(4):640–644

40. Delgado-López PD, Martín-Velasco V, Castilla-Díez JM, Galacho-Harriero AM, Rodríguez-Salazar A. Preservation of bone flap after craniotomy infection. Neurocirugia (Astur) 2009;20(2):124–131

41. Walters BC, Hoffman HJ, Hendrick EB, Humphreys RP. Cerebrospinal fluid shunt infection. Influences on initial management and subsequent outcome. J Neurosurg 1984;60(5):1014–1021

42. Campbell J. Shunt infections. In: Albright AL, Adelson PD, Pollack IF, eds. Principles and Practice of Pediatric Neurosurgery. 2nd ed. New York, NY: Thieme; 2007:1141–1147

43. Simon TD, Hall M, Riva-Cambrin J, et al; Hydrocephalus Clinical Research Network. Infection rates following initial cerebrospinal fluid shunt placement across pediatric hospitals in the United States. Clinical article. J Neurosurg Pediatr 2009;4(2):156–165

44. Attenello FJ, Garces-Ambrossi GL, Zaidi HA, Sciubba DM, Jallo GI. Hospital costs associated with shunt infections in patients receiving antibiotic-impregnated shunt catheters versus standard shunt catheters. Neurosurgery 2010;66(2):284–289, discussion 289

45. Prusseit J, Simon M, von der Brelie C, et al. Epidemiology, prevention and management of ventriculoperitoneal shunt infections in children. Pediatr Neurosurg 2009;45(5):325–336

46. Kontny U, Höfling B, Gutjahr P, Voth D, Schwarz M, Schmitt HJ. CSF shunt infections in children. Infection 1993;21(2):89–92

47. Haffner D, Schindera F, Aschoff A, Matthias S, Waldherr R, Schärer K. The clinical spectrum of shunt nephritis. Nephrol Dial Transplant 1997;12(6):1143–1148

48. Arnell K, Cesarini K, Lagerqvist-Widh A, Wester T, Sjölin J. Cerebrospinal fluid shunt infections in children over a 13-year period: anaerobic cultures and comparison of clinical signs of infection with Propionibacterium acnes and with other bacteria. J Neurosurg Pediatr 2008;1(5):366–372

49. Tunkel AR, Drake JM. Cerebrospinal fluid shunt infections. In: Mandell GL, Bennett JE, Dolin R, eds. Mandell, Douglas, and Bennett's Principles and Practice of Infectious Diseases. 7th ed. Philadelphia, PA: Churchill Livingstone/Elsevier; 2010:1231–1236

50. Thompson DNP, Hartley JC, Hayward RD. Shunt infection: is there a near-miss scenario? J Neurosurg 2007;106(1, Suppl):15–19

51. Anderson EJ, Yogev R. A rational approach to the management of ventricular shunt infections. Pediatr Infect Dis J 2005;24(6):557–558

52. Schuhmann MU, Ostrowski KR, Draper EJ, et al. The value of C-reactive protein in the management of shunt infections. J Neurosurg 2005;103(3, Suppl):223–230

53. McClinton D, Carraccio C, Englander R. Predictors of ventriculoperitoneal shunt pathology. Pediatr Infect Dis J 2001;20(6):593–597

54. Noetzel MJ, Baker RP. Shunt fluid examination: risks and benefits in the evaluation of shunt malfunction and infection. J Neurosurg 1984;61(2):328–332

55. Miller JP, Fulop SC, Dashti SR, Robinson S, Cohen AR. Rethinking the indications for the ventriculoperitoneal shunt tap. J Neurosurg Pediatr 2008;1(6):435–438

56. Oakes WJ. Ventriculoperitoneal shunt tap. J Neurosurg Pediatr 2008;1(6):433, 433–434

57. Rocque BG, Lapsiwala S, Iskandar BJ. Ventricular shunt tap as a predictor of proximal shunt malfunction in children: a prospective study. J Neurosurg Pediatr 2008;1(6):439–443

58. Choi S, McComb JG, Levy ML, Gonzalez-Gomez I, Bayston R. Use of elemental iodine for shunt infection prophylaxis. Neurosurgery 2003;52(4):908–912, discussion 912–913

59. Choux M, Genitori L, Lang D, Lena G. Shunt implantation: reducing the incidence of shunt infection. J Neurosurg 1992;77(6):875–880

60. Haines SJ, Walters BC. Antibiotic prophylaxis for cerebrospinal fluid shunts: a meta-analysis. Neurosurgery 1994;34(1):87–92

61. Kanev PM, Sheehan JM. Reflections on shunt infection. Pediatr Neurosurg 2003;39(6):285–290

62. Langley JM, LeBlanc JC, Drake J, Milner R. Efficacy of antimicrobial prophylaxis in placement of cerebrospinal fluid shunts: meta-analysis. Clin Infect Dis 1993;17(1):98–103

63. Rotim K, Miklic P, Paladino J, Melada A, Marcikic M, Scap M. Reducing the incidence of infection in pediatric cerebrospinal fluid shunt operations. Childs Nerv Syst 1997;13(11-12):584–587

64. Moriarty T, Angelini M, Carpenter J, et al. Rigid standardization of technique to affect outcome: ventricular shunt infection rate. J Neurosurg Pediatr. 2008;1(4):A356

65. Kestle JRW, Riva-Cambrin J, Wellons JC III, et al; Hydrocephalus Clinical Research Network. A standardized protocol to reduce cerebrospinal fluid shunt infection: the Hydrocephalus Clinical Research Network Quality Improvement Initiative. J Neurosurg Pediatr 2011;8(1):22–29

66. Palmer JD, Rickett JW. The mechanisms and risks of surgical glove perforation. J Hosp Infect 1992;22(4):279–286

67. Laine T, Aarnio P. How often does glove perforation occur in surgery? Comparison between single gloves and a double-gloving system. Am J Surg 2001;181(6):564–566

68. Al-Maiyah M, Bajwa A, Mackenney P, et al. Glove perforation and contamination in primary total hip arthroplasty. J Bone Joint Surg Br 2005;87(4):556–559

69. Bukhari SS, Harrison RA, Sanderson PJ. Contamination of surgeons' glove fingertips during surgical operations. J Hosp Infect 1993;24(2):117–121

70. Sørensen P, Ejlertsen T, Aaen D, Poulsen K. Bacterial contamination of surgeons' gloves during shunt insertion: a pilot study. Br J Neurosurg 2008;22(5):675–677

71. Tulipan N, Cleves MA. Effect of an intraoperative double-gloving strategy on the incidence of cerebrospinal fluid shunt infection. J Neurosurg 2006;104(1, Suppl):5–8

72. Ratilal BO, Costa J, Sampaio C. Antibiotic prophylaxis for surgical introduction of intracranial ventricular shunts. Cochrane Database Syst Rev 2006;19(3):CD005365. http://onlinelibrary.wiley.com/doi/10.1002/14651858.CD005365.pub2/abstract. Accessed December 23, 2012

73. Parker SL, Anderson WN, Lilienfield S, et al. Cerebrospinal shunt infection in patients receiving antibiotic-impregnated versus standard shunts. J Neurosurg Pediatr 2011;8(3):859–865

74. Simon TD, Hall M, Dean JM, Kestle JRW, Riva-Cambrin J. Reinfection following initial cerebrospinal fluid shunt infection. J Neurosurg Pediatr 2010;6(3):277–285

75. Schreffler RT, Schreffler AJ, Wittler RR. Treatment of cerebrospinal fluid shunt infections: a decision analysis. Pediatr Infect Dis J 2002;21(7):632–636

76. Yogev R. Cerebrospinal fluid shunt infections: a personal view. Pediatr Infect Dis 1985;4(2):113–118

77. Drake J, Sainte-Rose C. Cerebrospinal fluid shunt complications. In: Drake J, Sainte-Rose C, eds. The Shunt Book. Cambridge, MA: Blackwell Science; 1995:69–121

78. Klein D, Scott R. Shunt infections. In: Hydrocephalus: Concepts in Neurosurgery. Baltimore, MD: Williams & Wilkins; 1990:88

79. Leggiadro RJ, Atluru VL, Katz SP. Meningococcal meningitis associated with cerebrospinal fluid shunts. Pediatr Infect Dis 1984;3(5):489–490

80. Lerman SJ. *Haemophilus influenzae* infections of cerebrospinal fluid shunts. Report of two cases. J Neurosurg 1981;54(2):261–263

81. Patriarca PA, Lauer BA. Ventriculoperitoneal shunt-associated infection due to *Haemophilus influenzae*. Pediatrics 1980;65(5):1007–1009

# 18

# Central Nervous System Infections in Immunocompromised Hosts

Ouzi Nissim, Gahl Greenberg, Zvi R. Cohen, and Roberto Spiegelmann

The pool of patients with underlying conditions associated with immune compromise is continuously expanding. Improved medical management of malignancies and chronic illnesses and the extensive use of immunosuppressive medications has led to a dramatic increase in the need to treat this patient population.

Immune dysfunction is characterized by the emergence of infections with opportunistic microorganisms that under normal conditions are less virulent and that exploit this breach in immunocompetence.

The unique characteristics of dysfunction in a specific arm of this multi-component immune system generates a unique pattern of susceptibility to a specific class of pathogens. Patients with defects in antibody or complement function more often have infections with pyogenic encapsulated bacteria, whereas those with deficient cell–mediated immune deficiency are more susceptible to fungal, viral, mycobacterial, and protozoal infections. This principle is clearly illustrated in primary immunodeficiency states that stem from genetic abnormalities selectively affecting specific arms of the immune system. For example, in chronic granulomatous disease and in Chédiak-Higashi syndrome, there is a selective abnormality of phagocytosis. The infectious agents affecting these patients differ from those seen in patients with another genetic disorder, severe combined immunodeficiency (SCID), in which T-lymphocyte abnormalities damage both the humoral and cell-mediated arms of the immune system.

In secondary immunodeficiency states, a primary illness or the treatment of an illness results in immunosuppression. This category includes human immunodeficiency virus (HIV) infection, cancer, and the use of corticosteroids or immunosuppressive medications to treat patients with conditions like collagen vascular diseases and the recipients of organ transplants. Again, the mechanism of immunosuppressive action of these drugs will affect the type of infections that can arise.[1] In the growing group of patients with malignancies, there is usually interplay between several factors: the effects of the primary disease, myelosuppression from chemotherapy, and at times corticosteroid-induced immune dysfunction, each of them contributing to the overall immune dysfunction.

Central nervous system (CNS) infections in immunocompromised patients cause considerable morbidity and mortality. The CNS resides in a unique environment that affects the pathogenesis of infections. The brain is protected from infection by the calvaria and meninges, which serve as a mechanical barrier, and also by the chemical and mechanical filtering capabilities of the blood–brain barrier. However, the composition of the CSF makes it an excellent culture medium. In addition, the brain and subarachnoid space are considered immunologically sequestered because of the absence of lymphatics.[2]

The clinical manifestations of CNS infections in the immunocompromised host can reflect cerebral parenchymal and/or leptomeningeal involvement. With localized involvement in the form of solid mass lesions (abscesses, granulomas, or cysts) or more localized encephalitis, a clinical picture of focal neurologic deficits is expected to predominate. Brain abscesses in immunocompromised patients (as opposed to those in the general population) are caused more frequently by nonpyogenic microorganisms, such as fungi, protozoa, and mycobacteria. Meningeal or ependymal involvement will induce more generalized neurologic dysfunction, manifested by headache, photophobia, seizures, reduced level of consciousness, or other signs of elevated intracranial pressure (papilledema, sixth cranial nerve palsy).[3] In addition to the characteristic infectious profile that emerges, immunosuppression can alter the host response to the offending agents, thus obscuring diagnostic clues. Investigation for the presence of infection should therefore be diligently pursued in the appropriate setting of progressive neurologic dysfunction.[4]

## ■ Principles of Treatment

As patterns of infection are relatively defined in many subgroups of the immunocompromised population, prophylactic measures play a major role in disease prevention. The treatment of invasive infections in immunocompromised hosts is primarily pharmacologic. Definitive culture is ideal, but this can be time- and resource-consuming. Considering the high morbidity and mortality rates in immunocompromised patients with infectious diseases and the dire consequences of delaying therapy, empiric treatment is frequently considered the standard of care.

With CNS involvement, the management of discrete CNS space-occupying lesions is directed by several principles:

1. The need to obtain tissue samples for prompt and definite diagnosis
2. Reduction of the size of the lesion to enhance treatment efficacy
3. When needed, alleviation of mass effect

Stereotactic or image-guided needle biopsy is a minimally invasive method of establishing a definite diagnosis and allows the institution of appropriate treatment. This surgical technique is especially well suited for deep-seated lesions, such as those in the brainstem or hypothalamus. An open surgical excision is an appropriate option for large, accessible lesions with multiple loculi that cause brain herniation and also for those that do not respond to aspiration.

This chapter focuses on CNS infections in immunocompromised patients from a neurosurgical perspective. First, the causative fungal, protozoal, bacterial, and viral microorganisms causing intraparenchymal masses or cerebritis are reviewed. A patient-oriented perspective follows, in which issues relevant to specific underlying causes of immunodeficiency (HIV infection and organ transplant) are addressed.

## ■ Fungal Infections

Fungi are ubiquitous in the environment and exist as yeast, molds, and dimorphic forms. Fungal exposure occurs mostly through inhalation, ingestion, or direct contact. Although invasive fungal infections do occur in immunocompetent patients (primary mycoses, mostly in endemic regions and by trauma-induced inoculations), they are far more prevalent and considerably more life-threatening in immunocompromised patients, and they occur predominantly when the underlying cause of immunodeficiency is cell-mediated immune dysfunction. Fungi can reach the CNS by hematogenous dissemination from the primary site of inoculation or by direct spread from a contiguous site of infection (nasal sinusitis, osteomyelitis, after surgical procedures, and following the introduction of foreign bodies like indwelling catheters). Clinical syndromes associated with CNS fungal infections depend on the pathologic reaction elicited by the fungus. The three cardinal manifestations of fungal infection are meningitis, the formation of mass lesions (abscesses or granulomas) in the brain, and brain infarction. Meningitis has been reported in almost two-thirds of subjects with CNS fungal infections and is caused mostly by small yeastlike forms (*Candida* and *Cryptococcus*). These organisms reach the arterioles and capillaries to produce subpial ischemic lesions. From there, spread to the subarachnoid space occurs, causing meningitis. In this setting, in addition to the signs of meningeal irritation, increased intracranial pressure can develop. Space-occupying lesions are predominantly caused by molds (filamentous fungi). When brain abscesses are formed, signs and symptoms of focal neurologic dysfunction will predominate. Rarely, fungal infections can lead to granuloma formation.[5] Large hyphal forms, such as *Aspergillus* and Zygomycetes, can invade and obstruct large and intermediate-size arteries to cause brain infarction and strokelike symptoms.[6,7] The incidence of CNS fungal infections seems to be underestimated because of their nonspecific clinical presentations and the insufficient diagnostic work-up that these patients sometimes undergo.[8]

## Treatment

The treatment of invasive fungal infections is primarily pharmacologic. The extensive use of antifungal medications, either for treatment or for prophylaxis, has resulted in the emergence of new, previously less encountered causative agents. The resistance of these pathogens to conventional treatment poses new challenges. Thus, diagnosis by culture with identification of susceptibility patterns should be accomplished whenever possible.[9] The approach to any space-occupying lesion is directed by the aforementioned principles of care.

## ■ Aspergillosis

*Aspergillus*, a mold with septate hyphae, is clinically the most important fungal pathogen. Of the more than 100 *Aspergillus* species that are known, the most virulent pathogen is *A. fumigatus*, although infections occur also with *A. niger*, *A. flavus*, and *A. terreus*.

Aerosolized spores usually gain entry to the CNS through the sinopulmonary system. Invasive aspergillosis develops mostly in hosts with neutrophil- or T-cell–mediated dysfunction, including bone marrow, stem cell, or solid organ transplant recipients; those treated with high-dose corticosteroids; and those with hematologic malignancies, liver disease, or sarcoid.[9] Patients with HIV-associated aspergillosis typically have CD4+ cell counts below 100/μL and a history of other acquired immunodeficiency syndrome (AIDS)–defining opportunistic infections, and they typically are not receiving highly active antiretroviral therapy (HAART).

*Aspergillus* is an angioinvasive mold, and CNS seeding typically occurs after hematogenous dissemination from a pulmonary site. Additionally, direct spread from the primary site of infection may occur: from the nasal sinuses to the adjacent frontal and temporal lobes, by extension of an ear infection, or by invasion of the thoracic vertebrae and eventually the spinal epidural space. CNS involvement is diagnosed in 10 to 20% of patients with systemic dissemination; however, it is discovered at autopsy in as many as 44 to 94% of cases.[10]

Cerebral aspergillosis frequently causes single or multiple brain abscesses and rarely granulomas. *Aspergillus* granulomas are characterized by abundant fibrosis, an ill-defined epithelioid granuloma, and many foreign body and Langhans-type giant cells. Uncommonly, basal meningitis, dural abscesses, mycotic aneurysms, and multifocal cerebritis can occur. Carotid artery invasion can cause cerebral ischemia or hemorrhagic infarction. Pulmonary infections extending to thoracic vertebrae and the epidural space are capable of causing spinal cord compression and myelitis.

The clinical presentation of *Aspergillus* infection is nonspecific. This type of infection should be suspected with the development of facial pain, fever, headache, altered mental status, seizures, or focal neurologic deficits, but severely immunocompromised patients are less likely to develop symptoms. Orbital infiltration is suspected with periorbital pain, proptosis, blurred vision, or diplopia. Strokelike syndromes can develop, especially if the internal carotid artery is involved.[6] With case-fatality rates in CNS aspergillosis reported to be as high as 88%, the prompt diagnosis of invasive aspergillosis is crucial, but difficult.[11]

The radiologic appearance of cerebral aspergillosis is variable, showing regions of edema, hemorrhage, infarction (which can be poorly defined with minimal mass effect), or focal reticular or ring-enhancing mass lesions.[12] Standard CSF analysis is generally nondiagnostic and cultures are almost always negative, but recently developed serologic methods hold promise for early diagnosis. These tests rely on the detection of cell wall components, galactomannan, and 1,3-β-D-glucan in serum or CSF. Galactomannan has an overall reported sensitivity of 71% and specificity of 89% for *Aspergillus* infections. Additionally, the usefulness of a variety of molecular polymerase chain reaction (PCR) tests is being investigated.[13]

### Pharmacologic Treatment

The recommended treatment for invasive aspergillosis in patients without HIV infection is voriconazole. Amphotericin B deoxycholate and lipid-formulation amphotericin B are alternatives.[9] Unfortunately, with the increasing use of voriconazole for prophylaxis, the empiric, preemptive, and targeted treatment of invasive aspergillosis has resulted in an increase in the incidence of voriconazole-resistant zygomycosis. More recently, a combination of therapeutic approaches has been explored.[14,15]

### ◼ Zygomycosis

Zygomycetes are filamentous fungi with nonseptate branching hyphae. These microorganisms are ubiquitous saprophytes found in soil, plants, and decaying food. The three orders in this category are Mucorales (including the genera *Mucor*, *Rhizopus*, and *Rhizomucor*), Cunninghamella, and Absidia.[6]

### Epidemiology and Clinical Manifestations

Mucormycosis is the second most common mycosis caused by molds and is especially known to infect patients with poorly controlled diabetes mellitus, although another population at high risk comprises patients with hematologic malignancies.[16,17] Additionally, recipients of bone marrow transplants, patients with prolonged neutropenia or renal disease, and those receiving corticosteroid therapy are susceptible to infection. High glucose levels in patients with poorly controlled diabetes reduce the binding of iron to transferrin. The increased levels of free iron promote an accelerated growth of the fungus.

The major mode of infection is by inhalation. *Mucor* organisms then lodge in the lungs or sinuses to establish the primary site of infection. Among intravenous drug users, hematogenous transmission can occur. The clinical spectrum of CNS involvement can be part of a fulminant, disseminated disease or occur as an isolated cerebral or rhinocerebral mucormycosis. Rhinocerebral mucormycosis most often develops by direct spread from the paranasal sinuses to adjacent structures, which include the palate, face, and orbit. Cerebral infection often occurs after direct extension from the ethmoid sinus through the meninges or via a perineural route. Mucormycosis, like aspergillosis, has a tendency to invade blood vessels and cause tissue necrosis or serve as a vehicle for further propagation of the infection.[18]

Patients with rhinocerebral mucormycosis present with headache or facial pain that is often localized to the frontal or retro-orbital regions. A dark sinus discharge occurs, and necrotic tissue can be seen as a black eschar. Intracranial involvement can lead to cranial nerve palsies, acute motor or sensory deficits from infarction caused by major arterial thrombosis, lethargy and seizures.[19] Orbital cellulitis, together with proptosis, ophthalmoplegia, and visual impairment, signifies intraorbital or cavernous sinus involvement and represents a medical emergency.[6]

## Diagnosis

CSF analysis results are usually nonspecific. The growth of Zygomycetes organisms in blood cultures or tissue exudate is rare. Core tissue samples are preferable but nondiagnostic in 40% of the cases. Computed tomography (CT) and especially magnetic resonance (MR) imaging of the brain are quite sensitive for the diagnosis of mucormycosis. The MR signal intensity of *Mucor* species lesions tends to be isointense or hypointense on all sequences. After the administration of gadolinium, the lesions have variable enhancement patterns ranging from homogeneous to heterogeneous or have no enhancement. MR imaging can also clearly demonstrate cavernous sinus and dural involvement.[20,21]

MR spectroscopy shows markedly elevated lactate, depleted *N*-acetyl aspartate, and metabolite resonance attributable to succinate and acetate, which is essentially the same as that of pyogenic bacterial abscess without the commonly seen elevations of amino acids valine, leucine, and isoleucine.[22]

## Treatment

Disseminated mucormycosis with CNS involvement has a 98% mortality rate. For localized cerebral or rhinocerebral disease, the mortality can reach 62%. Appropriate drug therapy together with aggressive surgical débridement of tissue and treatment of underlying risk factors provides the best chance for a good outcome.[16,17]

## ■ Primary (Endemic) Mycoses

These fungi are endemic in certain geographic locations and affect primarily immunocompetent individuals. In individuals with immunosuppression, the disease has a very high probability of becoming disseminated from the primary site, which is usually the respiratory system, to reach the CNS and cause severe debilitation. Additionally, under these conditions, clinically evident disease can reflect reactivation of a dormant past infection. Aside from meningitis, which is the most common presentation, brain abscesses and granulomas can appear, causing mass effect and localized signs.[6,9]

## ■ Coccidioidomycosis

There are two species of the dimorphic fungus *Coccidioides*. *C. immitis* is endemic in California, and *C. posadasii* is endemic in northern Mexico, the southwestern United States (California and Arizona), Central America, and South America. The two species cause clinically indistinguishable disease. They are abundant in soil, and primary pulmonary infection results primarily after outdoor exposure. In immunocompetent hosts, the infection can be clinically silent. When it is evident, signs and symptoms suggest mild respiratory involvement. On the other hand, in immunocompromised patients with deficient cellular immunity, the rate of disseminated disease is as high as 22%.

Disseminated disease mostly involves the skin, joints, bones, and spleen, but approximately 50% of patients will have meningeal involvement. In some cases, subclinical, chronic meningitis will develop, only to become manifest clinically after a delayed period of weeks to months.

With meningitis, headache, fever, nausea and vomiting, nuchal rigidity, seizures, and papilledema can be present. Hydrocephalus will develop in approximately 50% of patients. CNS infection can progress infrequently to the development of a compressive space-occupying lesion, such as brain abscess or granuloma.

### Diagnosis and Treatment

Although CSF analysis will show nonspecific biochemical changes compatible with meningitis and lymphocytic pleocytosis, the presence of eosinophilia is highly suggestive of *Coccidioides* infection. Cultures will be positive in approximately 50% of cases. The diagnosis can be made by examining skin biopsies or by serologic tests. In the past, intrathecal amphotericin B was used. Amphotericin B has been replaced by fluconazole as the drug of choice. Those responding to therapy remain on lifelong treatment because of the high relapse rate.[9]

## Histoplasmosis

*Histoplasma capsulatum*, a dimorphic fungus, is the only species of the genus *Histoplasma*. *H. capsulatum* var. *capsulatum* is associated with North American histoplasmosis. The organism is found in bird droppings and bat guano, and in the United States it is endemic in the states bordering the Ohio and lower Mississippi River valleys. Primary infection involves the respiratory system. Although disseminated histoplasmosis is rare, it develops after infection in as many as 80% of immunocompromised patients. Most reports are from patients with HIV infection and lymphoma. CNS involvement occurs in 5 to 20% of those with disseminated disease but can occur in isolation. The clinical spectrum of disease is chronic meningitis with the development of hydrocephalus, or less commonly focal parenchymal mass lesions or strokes due to emboli.

### Diagnosis and Treatment

With the exception of patients with HIV infection, serologic antibody tests in immunocompromised patients are of little value. The diagnosis can be made by detecting the antigen in serum, urine, or CSF samples. Additionally, the fungus can be cultured from sputum or blood. The treatment of choice for CNS histoplasmosis is amphotericin B.[9]

## Blastomycosis

The dimorphic fungus *Blastomyces* is endemic in the southeastern and central southern United States, the Great Lakes region of Canada and the bordering Midwestern states, and an area along the Saint Lawrence River in New York and Canada. The lungs are the primary site from which disseminated disease can evolve. In 6 to 35% of those with disseminated disease, there is CNS involvement. In immunocompromised patients, the risk for CNS spread is considerably higher. CNS seeding can result in either meningitis or brain mass lesions (including abscesses). Additionally, spinal epidural abscesses can develop by direct extension from infected vertebrae.

### Diagnosis and Treatment

Serology is usually noninformative, but the fungus can be isolated directly from infected tissue specimens or from CSF samples if a lesion is based in the dura. Amphotericin B is the drug of choice for treatment.[9] Effective surgical resection has been reported in small series.

## Candidiasis

*Candida* species (primarily *C. albicans*) are opportunistic yeasts. They are a major cause of bloodstream infections, especially in surgical and critical care hospital settings. Immunodeficiency, especially phagocyte dysfunction, predisposes patients to both systemic candidiasis and CNS involvement.[16] *Candida* CNS infections are reported in 18 to 25% of those with disseminated disease and are likely underdiagnosed. Infection can develop in patients with diabetes or cancer, organ transplant recipients, those receiving cytotoxic or prolonged corticosteroid therapies, and patients who have undergone invasive procedures. From an immunologic perspective, patients with HIV infection are not at higher risk for infection because their defective cellular immunity is due to T-lymphocyte dysfunction.

CNS involvement usually manifests as multiple microabscesses measuring less than 1 mm in diameter. These occur primarily within the supratentorial cortex and less often in the basal ganglia and white matter.[23] Less commonly, meningitis (> 20%) and rarely macroabscesses can develop.[24] Vascular complications (infarction, mycotic aneurysms, and subarachnoid hemorrhage) have also been documented.

Microabscess formation usually presents as a diffuse, vague encephalopathy. These lesions are below CT resolution but can be visualized on MR imaging.[25] Meningitis usually presents with a subacute onset of headache and fever, confusion, and altered sensorium but can be fulminant and result in hydrocephalus. Macroabscesses will present with localizing signs and seizures.

### Diagnosis

Because CSF serology and cultures are unreliable, the diagnosis is often made indirectly, by funduscopic examination, blood cultures, and infrequently by samples from other tissues. CSF 1,3-β-D-glucan has better sensitivity than serum assays, ranging from 70 to 90%. PCR tests are being introduced but are of limited use because of a lack of availability and clinical validation and their high cost.[15]

## ■ Nocardiosis

*Nocardia*, an aerobic actinomyces, is a gram-positive branching rod found in soil, decaying vegetables, and aquatic media. *N. asteroides,* which causes human disease, has been redefined to include a complex of four members: *N. asteroides* sensu stricto, *N. farcinica*, *N. nova*, and *N. transvalensis.* Of those, *N. nova* and *N. farcinica* are the most virulent. *Nocardia* does not normally colonize human tissue and is considered an opportunistic microorganism, particularly in patients with cell-mediated immune dysfunction. *Nocardia* has the capacity to evade clearance by the immune system by several mechanisms that disrupt phagocytic activity, and about one-third of infected individuals have an intact immune system.[26] Organ transplant recipients constitute around 20% of patients with *Nocardia* infection, with an incidence of 0.1 to 3.5%. Steroid-sparing regimens have reduced the risk in this population.[27] The prevalence of nocardiosis in HIV-positive patients is low (0.2 to 2.0%), and nocardiosis appears mostly in severely immunocompromised (CD4+ cell count < 35/μL) patients. However, in cases of invasive nocardiosis, patients with HIV infection comprise a major risk group.

HIV patients can benefit from the administration of trimethoprim-sulfamethoxazole prophylaxis against *Pneumocystis jiroveci* pneumonia, which is also effective against *Nocardia* infections.[28,29] Because of the enlarging pool of susceptible patients, the incidence of nocardiosis is increasing, so that nocardiosis is now viewed as an emerging infectious disease.[30]

The most common site of primary infection is pulmonary (approximately 40% of patients), but nocardiosis can be transmitted transcutaneously via penetrating trauma, animal scratches, or bites and can also be spread iatrogenically. *Nocardia* frequently erodes into blood vessels and thus has the potential for hematogenous spread. Although any organ can be involved, the incidence of CNS nocardiosis is disproportionately high during dissemination (44%) or as an isolated primary site of infection (38%). The hallmark of CNS involvement is brain abscess formation without a predilection for any specific cerebral region (**Fig. 18.1**). Although constitutional symptoms can be found, the presentation can be solely that of a space-occupying lesion causing mass effect. A clinical presentation of subacute or chronic meningitis is infrequent.

### Diagnosis

CNS nocardiosis should be suspected in any immunocompromised patient whose clinical and radiologic presentation is compatible with a brain mass and concurrent pulmonary involvement. Additionally, a proven cutaneous or pulmonary nocardiosis infection in an immunocompromised patient, even without the suspicion of CNS involvement, warrants brain MR imaging to rule out occult CNS disease. The definitive diagnosis of nocardiosis requires identification of the pathogen in a collected specimen. Delay in diagnosis is common because of the nonspecific clinical presentation and difficulties in obtaining adequate specimens. Growing the bacteria is difficult, and blood cultures are rarely diagnostic. PCR provides rapid results and is highly sensitive and specific, but its availability is limited and its cost is high.

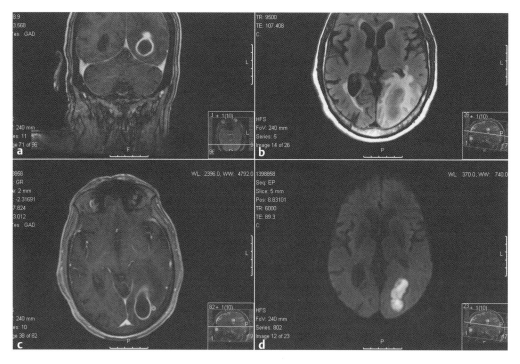

**Fig. 18.1** Magnetic resonance (MR) imaging. *Nocardia* abscess in a 74-year-old man on corticosteroid treatment for chronic obstructive pulmonary disease. T2-weighted MR image demonstrates a hypointense lesion in the occipital region with surrounding edema **(b)**. Coronal and axial T1-weighted MR images with gadolinium show a ring-enhancing lesion **(a,c)**. The lesion shows restriction on diffusion-weighted sequence **(d)**.

## Treatment

Because the sensitivity of isolated strains to antibiotics is highly variable, defining patterns of susceptibility is mandatory in each case. While these results are awaited, combination therapy is frequently used for the empiric treatment of nocardiosis. Trimethoprim-sulfamethoxazole and ceftriaxone are used primarily,[27] often with great success. The treatment of brain abscesses generally follows the guidelines set before for the treatment of infectious space-occupying lesions.[31]

## ■ Parasitic Infections

Many parasitic infections, including malaria, schistosomiasis, microsporidiosis, leishmaniasis, and trypanosomiasis, can involve the CNS in both immunocompetent and im-munocompromised patients.[32] In addition, some parasites, such as *Strongyloides stercoralis*, can rarely cause CNS infection in immunocompromised hosts. We discuss the more common opportunistic pathogens that selectively affect immunocompromised patients.

## Toxoplasmosis

*Toxoplasma gondii* is an obligatory intracellular protozoan. This parasite is able to develop in a variety of vertebrate hosts, but its definitive host is the house cat and other members of the family Felidae. Infection in humans occurs after the ingestion of cysts contained in uncooked meat or after exposure to oocytes shed in cat feces. Serologic markers reveal a variable geographic prevalence of toxoplasmosis. In Europe, 50 to 90% of the healthy adult population is seropositive, whereas the rate is estimated to be 15 to 35% in the United States.[33]

In immunocompetent adults and children past the neonatal period, the infection is usually asymptomatic. In a small percentage of patients, the clinical picture resembles that of infectious mononucleosis. Hematogenous spread from the intestine can seed any nucleated cell but most commonly affects the lungs, lymphoid system, heart, and CNS. Multiplication of the parasite within invaded cells leads to cellular disruption and death. Focal areas of necrosis and cyst formation result.[32]

Most cases of clinically apparent toxoplasmosis in immunocompromised patients are the result of reactivation of a previously acquired latent infection. The vast majority of cases of cerebral toxoplasmosis have been documented in AIDS patients, in whom it is the most frequent opportunistic brain infection, occurring in approximately 20 to 30% of individuals.[34] Toxoplasmosis is the leading cause of a mass lesion in AIDS patients. However, patients with malignancies may also develop cerebral toxoplasmosis, in particular those who undergo an allogeneic stem cell transplant (SCT) or a T-cell–depleting treatment regimen containing alemtuzumab or fludarabine. In addition to fungal infection, cerebral toxoplasmosis has become one of the leading causes of cerebral abscesses in patients after allogeneic SCT.[35,36] In solid organ transplant recipients, a primary infection can develop if a donor organ containing encysted *T. gondii* is transplanted into a seronegative recipient. Seronegative patients receiving cardiac or renal allografts from seropositive donors are at the highest risk for toxoplasmosis.[37,38]

In the CNS, toxoplasmosis produces multiple necrotic brain abscesses that develop at the corticomedullary junction and in the basal ganglia. These lesions manifest clinically as seizures and localized signs of a mass lesion, such as focal neurologic deficits and cranial nerve palsies. Lesions are solitary in approximately 30% of patients. Systemic manifestations include hepatosplenomegaly, pneumonitis, myositis, myocarditis, and skin rash.

## Diagnosis

The diagnosis is based on the demonstration of the pathogen (tachyzoites or cysts) in tissue sections or by CSF staining. MR imaging typically shows multiple ring-enhancing or smaller nodular lesions surrounded by cerebral edema. Less commonly, MR imaging demonstrates signs of meningoencephalitis. Although these MR imaging findings are nonspecific, the extent of CNS involvement is well demonstrated. A small eccentric nodule (eccentric target sign) in the enhancing ring is suggestive of toxoplasmosis, although the sensitivity of this finding is less than 30%. Rarely, the lesions can be hemorrhagic (**Fig. 18.2**). In immunosuppressed patients without HIV infection, the degree of perilesional enhancement has been found to be inversely related to the extent of immunosuppression. The radiologic differential diagnosis for toxoplasmosis in the CNS includes CNS lymphoma (typically subependymal lesions that lack the eccentric target sign), metastatic disease, and other nonpyogenic infections.[3]

The definitive diagnosis of toxoplasmosis can be established by identifying tachyzoites in tissue samples. Serologic investigations of the CSF may be useful, particularly for immunoglobulin G by enzyme-linked immunosorbent assay (ELISA). Immunoglobulin M antibody detection has a negligible value in the diagnosis of neurotoxoplasmosis because most cases are not newly acquired. The detection of specific DNA by PCR in the CSF, claimed to have high sensitivity and specificity, has produced inconsistent results and thus cannot be relied on for making the diagnosis. The presence of multiple ring-enhancing lesions in the basal ganglia or cerebrum on neuroimaging, in the presence of anti-*Toxoplasma* immunoglobulin G antibodies, is suggestive of CNS toxoplasmosis and is sufficient to start empiric pharmacologic treatment.[32]

## Treatment

See later section on HIV coinfections.

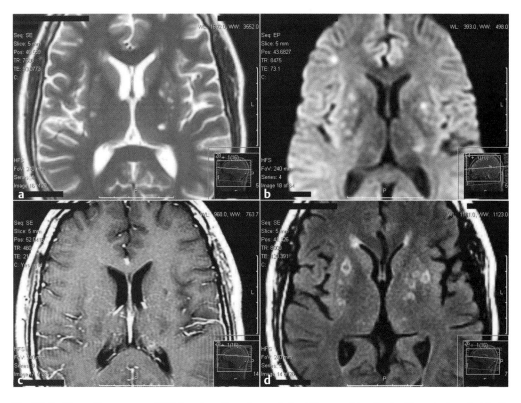

**Fig. 18.2** Magnetic resonance (MR) imaging. Toxoplasmosis in a 29-year-old patient with acute lymphoblastic leukemia. Diffusion-weighted **(b)**, T2-weighted **(a)**, and fluid-attenuated inversion recovery (FLAIR) **(d)** sequences demonstrate multiple scattered bilateral lesions in the globus pallidus, left thalamus, and right subcortical white matter. Lesions are nonenhancing on T1-weighted MR imaging with gadolinium **(c)**.

## Neurocysticercosis

Neurocysticercosis is caused by the larvae of *Taenia solium*. This is the most common helminthic infection of the CNS and the primary cause of acquired epilepsy in the world. Cysticercosis is endemic in most areas of the developing world where pigs are raised, including Latin America, most of Asia, sub-Saharan Africa, and parts of Oceania, but its frequency has increased in developed countries owing to emigration from these areas. Humans are infected by the accidental ingestion of *Taenia* eggs during fecal–oral contamination.[32] Considering the high prevalence of neurocysticercosis, reports of this disease in immunocompromised patients are surprisingly scarce, and it occurs generally as a coinfection in patients infected with HIV. Only a few cases

of neurocysticercosis in transplant recipients have been published.

Patients who have HIV infection present most frequently with a clinical picture resulting from multiple parenchymal lesions that represent enhancing or nonenhancing cysts. Uncommonly, solitary lesions, giant cysts, and mixed forms (parenchymal, subarachnoidal, and ventricular) of intracranial involvement are seen. An intracystic scolex can sometimes be visualized. Patients may exhibit findings compatible with those of other, concomitant CNS infections.

A clinical manifestation of neurocysticercosis has been recognized in the context of an immune reconstitution syndrome that develops in HIV patients under HAART. A paradoxical clinical deterioration, initiated by an intense inflammatory response to various subclinical or previously recognized infectious agents, can develop in these patients.[39] The current consensus is that HIV does not increase the tendency to develop neurocysticercosis, and that because of its high prevalence, neurocysticercosis is merely a coincidental finding. Still, neurocysticercosis is a condition that should be included in the differential diagnosis of CNS involvement and cystic lesions in an immunocompromised patient.

## Strongyloidiasis

*Strongyloides stercoralis* is a human intestinal nematode with an estimated prevalence of tens of millions worldwide. Although most individuals are asymptomatic, *Strongyloides* is capable of causing fulminant disease under conditions associated with compromised host immunity.

Strongyloidiasis is often considered a disease of tropical and subtropical regions in Asia and Africa, but foci of endemicity are also seen in temperate regions of South America and the southeastern United States. Additionally, infection with human T-lymphotropic virus type 1 (HTLV-1) is associated with an increased prevalence of *S. stercoralis* infection. The common mode of transmission is by transcutaneous penetration. The infective filariform larvae then migrate to the small intestine, enter the bloodstream, reach the lungs, and ascend the tracheobronchial tree to enter the gastrointestinal tract. Thus, a subclinical cycle can be established that allows the disease to persist in the host indefinitely. CNS involvement can appear when chronic strongyloidiasis transforms to a state of hyperinfection, with an increased larval load and possible dissemination attributed to accelerated autoinfection. Immunocompromised patients, especially those treated with corticosteroids for their underlying illness, are more prone to develop this syndrome.[40] The predominant manifestation of CNS involvement is meningitis. Rarely, the occurrence of discrete mass lesions has been reported in HIV patients, in those requiring autologous STCs, and in the recipients of kidney transplants before the cyclosporine era. In the past, *S.*

*stercoralis* hyperinfection was considered an opportunistic AIDS-defining illness, but the rarity of its occurrence despite the vast numbers of people who are likely coinfected suggests that HIV patients are not exceptionally predisposed.[41-43]

## American Trypanosomiasis

American trypanosomiasis, or Chagas disease, is a zoonotic disease caused by *Trypanosoma cruzi*, a hemoflagellate protozoan. *T. cruzi* develops successfully in several insects, but the domesticated reduviid bugs, also known as cone nose bugs or triatomids, are the only vectors of importance. Dogs and cats are important reservoirs in Brazil. In regions where the disease is endemic, from the southern United States to the south of Argentina and Chile, its impact has been staggering. With urbanization, population migration, and frequent traveling, the population at risk is growing, and nonzoonotic forms of transmission are emerging. In Latin America, the disease affects approximately 25% of the population, with 8 to 11 million people infected. Beyond the acute stage and after a variable latency period that can last 20 years, a chronic form of the disease appears in approximately 30% of those primarily affected.[32] In distinction to the cardiac and intestinal manifestations in immunocompetent individuals, the primary expression of disease in patients with immunodeficiency is CNS involvement. Most reports focus on HIV patients, in whom the disease is considered to represent reactivation.[44] The neurologic presentation in these cases is that of a space-occupying lesion (usually evident in the subcortical or central white matter), encephalitis, or meningoencephalitis. Toxoplasmosis can coexist with Chagas disease in HIV-positive individuals. Although the two lesions have similar radiologic features, toxoplasmosis on MR imaging is more likely to demonstrate lesions of the cortex or basal ganglia. Two epidemiologic criteria are useful for suspecting chagasic encephalitis at the time of initial presentation in patients with HIV infection and space-occupying lesions: a history of travel from an area where Chagas disease is endemic and a history of blood transfusions or intravenous drug abuse.[45]

## Leishmaniasis

Leishmaniasis is an obligate intracellular protozoan infection introduced by the bite of a female sand fly. Besides this natural vector, infection can be transmitted by syringe sharing in drug users. Leishmaniasis is endemic in 88 countries, and nearly 2 million people become infected each year. Most infections are due to species of the *Leishmania donovani* group, specifically *Leishmania infantum*. In regions where leishmaniasis is endemic, such as India, Nepal, Bangladesh, and Sudan, disseminated infection is more common in immunosuppressed hosts. In HIV-infected people, symptomatic leishmaniasis may represent reactivation of latent infection rather than primary infection. The most common neurologic manifestation of leishmaniasis is a peripheral neuropathy. CNS leishmaniasis is uncommon regardless of host immune status and usually occurs via the extension of contiguous infection, most often in the paranasal sinuses.[46] Leishmaniasis has been reported in immunosuppressed patients, usually in conjunction with disseminated infection. Dysfunctions of the optic and other cranial nerves and meningitis have been reported.[47,48]

## Schistosomiasis (Bilharziasis)

*Schistosoma* is a blood fluke. Infection follows contact with freshwater in which infected snails have liberated cercariae that penetrate the skin. Schistosomiasis is, after malaria, the second most prevalent tropical disease. Immunosuppression appears to have little effect on the natural history of schistosomiasis, but transmission by organ transplant has been described.[49] Neurologic complications are the most severe clinical consequence of *Schistosoma* infection. Three *Schistosoma* species are capable of causing CNS infection: *S. mansoni*, *S. haematobium* (African form), and *S. japonicum*. Although only a minority of patients (< 5%) will develop CNS involvement, schistoso-

miasis is potentially a public health risk to those traveling to areas within Africa and Asia where it is endemic.[46,50]

Because of a smaller egg size, the Asian schistosome *S. japonicum* causes 60% of all schistosomal brain infections. *S. haematobium* can infect either the brain or the spinal cord, whereas the larger egg size of *S. mansoni* usually limits infection to the spinal cord. CNS infection is thought to occur either through egg embolization or in situ egg deposition following the aberrant migration of adult worms to the brain or spinal cord. The encephalopathy that ensues typically presents with focal or generalized tonic-clonic epilepsy. The presence of numerous eggs can induce granuloma formation in the cortex, subcortex, basal ganglia, or internal capsule. These granulomas eventually become exudative and necrotic, create mass effect, and present with focal neurologic deficits and cranial nerve abnormalities.[51]

## ■ Human Immunodeficiency Virus Coinfections

Despite the availability of HAART and the application of prophylactic antimicrobial regimens, opportunistic infections continue to be a leading cause of morbidity in HIV patients. At least 10% of patients with AIDS present with neurologic involvement, and more than one-third will develop neurologic complications during the course of the disease.[52] Apart from the adverse clinical impact of these secondary infections, treating them effectively is important because opportunistic infections can enhance HIV activity, as evidenced by an increased viral load.

The selective loss of CD4+ cells during HIV infection results in clinical manifestations that often differ from those seen in other immunocompromised hosts. The majority of opportunistic CNS infections are due to *T. gondii*, Epstein-Barr virus (which also may cause primary CNS lymphoma), JC virus (progressive multifocal leukoencephalopathy [PML]), and *Cryptococcus neoformans*. Parasitic infections aside from toxoplasmosis and tuberculosis (TB) are most commonly found in HIV-infected people from developing countries, but they are becoming increasingly common in developed nations as the result of international travel and immigration.[34]

The risk for CNS infection usually varies with the CD4+ cell count. With the exception of TB and JC viral infections, CNS infection increases substantially with CD4+ cell counts of less than 200/mm[3]. In addition to infectious causes, the differential diagnosis of focal neurologic disease in patients with AIDS should include central CNS lymphoma.[53] Because of the attenuated cellular immune response in severely immunocompromised HIV patients, findings on neuroimaging usually differ from those seen in other immunocompromised hosts or in HIV hosts whose immune system has been reconstituted under HAART.

## Toxoplasmosis

Patients with primary HIV infection and toxoplasmosis are almost uniformly seropositive for anti-*Toxoplasma* immunoglobulin G antibodies. Clinical disease is rare among patients with CD4+ cell counts above 200/mL. The greatest risk for infection occurs among patients with a CD4+ cell count below 50/mL.[34,54] Prophylactic therapy has been effective in reducing the incidence of the disease. The majority of clinicians rely initially on an empiric diagnosis, which can be established as an objective response on the basis of clinical and radiographic responses to specific anti–*T. gondii* therapy in the absence of a likely alternative diagnosis. Brain biopsy is reserved for patients who fail to respond to specific therapy. The initial therapy of choice for toxoplasmosis is pharmacologic and consists of the combination of pyrimethamine, sulfadiazine, and leucovorin.[34,55] A brain biopsy, if not previously performed, should be strongly considered for patients who fail to respond to initial therapy for toxoplasmosis, as defined by clinical or radiologic deterioration during the first week despite adequate therapy, or lack of clinical improvement within 2 weeks.

## Cryptococcosis

*C. neoformans* (serotypes A, D, and the hybrid AD) is a yeastlike fungus ubiquitous in soil and bird excreta that is responsible for most infections worldwide. In Australia, *Cryptococcus gattii* is found in the vicinity of eucalyptus trees and is also a source of infection, mostly in immunocompetent individuals. *Cryptococcus* is transmitted by inhalation into the respiratory system.[6]

Usually, cryptococcal pulmonary involvement develops unnoticed, and the first clinical expression of infection is isolated meningitis. Other organs at risk for infection are the skin, prostate, and eyes. Cryptococcal meningitis is the most common fungal infection in patients with reduced cellular immunity. In HIV patients with CD4+ cell counts below 100 to 200/mL, it is the most frequent fungal infection (prevalence of 1 to 8%) and ranks third (after HIV encephalitis and toxoplasmosis) as a cause of CNS disease.[32] Cryptococcosis of the CNS occurs in 2.6 to 8% of organ transplant recipients. Infections involving the CNS are associated with higher mortality rates, which reach 40%.[9,56] In addition to meningitis, CNS involvement includes discrete parenchymal or intraventricular lesions (abscesses or granulomas), pseudocysts of the basal ganglia and thalami, and infarction. The latter are a complication of basal meningitis and arteritis of penetrating vessels. Cryptococcal meningitis reportedly causes hydrocephalus in up to two-thirds of patients.[57] Cryptococcomas are mass lesions that contain mucinous material, inflammatory cells, and the microorganism. They develop with blood–brain barrier disruption and extension of the fungus from the perivascular spaces into the parenchyma.[5,58]

## Diagnosis

In the setting of AIDS, CSF biochemical or cellular markers of inflammation are mildly elevated (suppressed), but CSF cryptococcal antigen is detected in more than 90%. With India ink staining of the CSF, the fungus can be seen surrounded by a halo created by its inert capsule. The rate of a positive India ink test ranges from very low (immunocompetent patients) to 91%. A definitive diagnosis can be reached by CSF cultures. However, it is suggested that PCR has a higher sensitivity, of more than 90%. Radiologic features include meningeal enhancement, hydrocephalus, and the demonstration of discrete lesions (cryptococcomas or abscesses), all of which are nonspecific.

The MR imaging features of cryptococcal mass lesions are variable. They are usually hypointense on T1-weighted imaging and hyperintense on T2-weighted imaging sequences, with peripheral edema and nodular or ring-shaped enhancement after gadolinium injection. Enhancement is seen more frequently in patients with an intact immune response. More suggestive of the diagnosis are pseudocysts of the basal ganglia and thalami, which appear as punctate hyperintensities on T2 sequences. At times, these lesions can enhance with gadolinium. Intraventricular cystic lesions can develop, although uncommonly. The differential diagnosis includes tumors and bacterial and protozoan mass lesions. From a neurosurgical perspective, these patients come to attention when a ventricular catheter or a permanent shunt is installed to treat hydrocephalus, or when surgical resection is needed for a lesion causing mass effect.[6]

## Tuberculosis

TB is acquired predominantly by the inhalation of mycobacteria-containing droplets. In immunocompetent individuals, this primary infection is of short duration, although latent infection remains. HIV patients are predisposed to the development of TB; new infection is responsible for approximately one-third of TB cases in HIV patients, whereas the transformation of latent disease accounts for the remainder. The rate of reactivation of latent TB is 3 to 12 times higher in HIV patients than in individuals without HIV infection; the rate is estimated to be 35 to 160 cases per 1,000 patient-years. Solid organ transplant recipients are also at much higher risk (0.2 to 0.5%).[34,59,60] In these settings, the rate of dissemination and the development of CNS disease is also higher than in the general population. About 20 to 36% of HIV patients develop neurotuberculosis, mostly meningitis, usually in the context of a disseminated disease.

Contrary to what is observed in other coinfections, the incidence of active TB does not depend on the CD4+ cell count, but the severity of the disease does, with a higher probability of extrapulmonary involvement occurring with lower CD4+ cell counts. Without profound immunodeficiency (CD4+ cell count > 350 /mL), HIV-related TB clinically resembles the TB seen among non-HIV patients, and the majority of patients have disease limited to the lungs. In the setting of severe immunodeficiency, extrapulmonary TB, including lymphadenitis, pleuritis, pericarditis, and meningitis, may develop with or without pulmonary involvement. Extrapulmonary involvement is detected in the majority of TB patients with CD4+ cell counts below 200/mL. Such patients may have severe systemic disease, rapid progression, and sepsis, but they also may be only mildly affected or asymptomatic. After the initiation of HAART, immunologic recovery can unveil subclinical TB, resulting in pronounced inflammatory reactions at the sites of infection. In solid organ transplant recipients, infection generally occurs within the first year. Especially susceptible to TB infection are kidney and lung transplant patients. CNS involvement manifests primarily as meningitis. Space-occupying lesions, tuberculomas (more common) or abscesses, develop in 10 to 25% of patients. In intravenous drug users, cerebral TB mass lesions are much more frequent (the second most common cause of cerebral lesions after cerebral toxoplasmosis).[61] The type of lesion that develops depends on the degree of immunodeficiency. Patients with relatively intact immune function typically have granulomatous inflammation. With progressive immunodeficiency, granulomas become poorly formed or can be completely absent. Tuberculous brain abscesses contain encapsulated pus with viable bacilli. The more common tuberculomas (granulomas) are usually small and contain caseous debris.

Mycobacterial infections can emerge in approximately 40% of HIV patients who develop an immune reconstitution inflammatory syndrome (IRIS) after the initiation of HAART. A vigorous granulomatous reaction can occur, with caseation or with suppuration and necrotizing inflammation. This syndrome can manifest as early as 2 weeks after the start of HAART, with neurologic manifestations occurring in more than 12% of TB cases with IRIS.[62,63] Tuberculous brain abscesses are usually supratentorial. Multiple lesions are found in one-third of cases. The radiologic features of TB brain abscesses are indistinguishable from those of other bacterial pyogenic abscesses. Tuberculomas have a variable appearance on T2-weighted sequences, depending on their composition. When central (caseating) necrosis is present, tuberculomas are hypointense to brain parenchyma on T2-weighted images with post-contrast ring enhancement.

A helpful clue leading to the diagnosis of TB is the presence of associated lesions, such as basal meningitis, multiple granulomas, and deep cerebral infarcts.[64] The evaluation of suspected cases of CNS TB should include MR imaging of the spine. MR spectroscopy can aid in the correct diagnosis by showing the absence of the 0.9-ppm amino acid peak present in pyogenic abscesses not caused by mycobacteria.[65]

## Treatment

Experience with the treatment of TB brain abscesses is limited. Complete recovery with pharmacologic treatment has been described, but in most reported cases, early surgical drainage and chemotherapy are considered appropriate.[66,67] Stereotactic or image-guided needle aspiration can be therapeutic as well as diagnostic. Early triple chemotherapy must be considered in all cases of suspected TB abscess, even before surgery, to reduce the risk for postoperative meningitis.

## JC Virus Infection and Progressive Multifocal Leukoencephalopathy

Classically, PML is a highly fatal and rapidly progressive demyelinating disease. It was described first in hematologic malignancies, and the later association of PML with the JC polyoma virus was made 44 years ago. The incidence of PML rose exponentially with the HIV epidemic. Although the introduction of HAART has lowered its occurrence and improved the prognosis, PML still manifests clinically in 1 to 5% of the HIV-positive population (in approximately 10% in pathologic studies), and HIV infection accounts for approximately 80 to 90% of all PML cases.[32,68] Other groups at risk for PML are patients with hematologic malignances, transplant recipients, those receiving chemotherapy (notably fludarabine), and a recently growing new group of patients treated with immunomodulatory antibodies for various autoimmune disorders, such as multiple sclerosis, rheumatoid arthritis, systemic lupus erythematosus, Crohn disease, and psoriasis.[69,70] JC virus is ubiquitous. Among young adults in developed countries, 50 to 91% of the urban population is seropositive. No distinct clinical syndrome or mode of transmission has been defined for the initial infection. The pathogenesis of PML in immunocompromised hosts results predominantly from activation of this previously acquired infectious state. Virulence is postulated to require the rearrangement of the viral genome from the old "archetypical" form to produce a neurotropic strain. Several factors have been proposed to explain the exceptional rate at which HIV patients develop PML. These include[1] facilitated entry of infected B lymphocytes into the brain by HIV-induced disruption of the blood–brain barrier or by the creation of vascular endothelium adhesion molecules,[2] and transactivation of JC virus by HIV proteins or by chemokines elaborated by microglia in response to HIV.[71] Unlike some of the other CNS opportunistic infections, which are almost wholly prevented when CD4+ cell counts are maintained above 100 to 200/mL, PML can still appear in such patients and in those on HAART. Moreover, PML can develop in the setting of initiating HAART and immune reconstitution.[72,73]

### Clinical Manifestations

PML manifests as focal neurologic deficits, usually with a slow onset but accelerating progression that lasts weeks or months. Any region of the CNS can be involved, but the subcortical occipital lobes (resulting in hemianopsia), the frontal and parietal lobes (hemiparesis and hemisensory deficits), and the cerebellar peduncles and deep white matter (dysmetria and ataxia) are affected most often. Spinal cord involvement is rare. Although the lesions are multifocal, often one lesion predominates clinically. Rarely, pyramidal cell disease with encephalopathy and dementia or a cerebellar syndrome (secondary to granular cell involvement) can develop. Even though PML is a white matter disease, seizures can appear in 20% of cases.[74]

### Diagnosis

The progression of disease over several weeks often provides a clue to the diagnosis, as the other major opportunistic focal brain disorders (cerebral toxoplasmosis and primary CNS lymphoma) characteristically progress more rapidly, over hours or a few days. A definitive diagnosis can be made by demonstrating the presence of JC virus in a specimen collected by brain biopsy. New CSF PCR methods have become reliable, less invasive means, with 90 to 100% specificity. Sensitivity, though, is up to 80%, and a PCR test can be negative at the first stages of the disease, necessitating additional samples. PCR results coupled with characteristic MR imaging findings in the appropriate clinical setting are diagnostic. T2-weighted MR imaging and fluid-attenuated inversion recovery (FLAIR) sequences reveal bilateral, asymmetric focal areas of high signal intensity, which become larger and confluent over time and lack any significant associated cerebral edema or mass effect. The disorder tends to involve the peripheral white matter, giving the lesions a scalloped outer margin (**Fig. 18.3**). Contrast enhancement or edema is the exception (6 to 10% of patients), although the presence of faint enhancement at the periphery of the lesion is not uncommon. In the context of IRIS, enhancement, edema, and even mass effect can develop.[74] The introduction of HAART has significantly decreased the incidence and improved the prognosis of this disease. Whereas PML was once an almost uniformly fatal disease, with death occurring within 6 months after diagnosis, patients now have a median survival of more than 2 years. Outcome correlates with the ability to reduce the JC viral load and improve immune function (CD4+ cell counts). Patients with contrast-enhancing lesions on MR imaging may also have a relatively favorable outcome, probably because abnormal enhancement reflects an improved immune response ("inflammatory PML").[75]

## ■ Infections in Transplant Recipients

Although clinically evident CNS infections occur in 1.3 to 6% of transplant recipients, the autopsy-proven prevalence of CNS involvement can reach 15%. The timing of the appearance and the nature of the offending pathogens affecting hematopoietic and solid organ transplant recipients have some distinguishing features. The risk for acquiring infections after either a solid organ transplant or a hematopoietic stem cell transplant (HSCT) and the specific microorganisms involved follow a relatively predictable pattern. The type of infection that develops is determined mainly by the organ transplanted, patient factors (age, comorbid state, previous infections), exposure to environmental hazards, and additional medical interventions. The introduction of new immunosuppressive protocols, organ screening, the use of prophylactic medications, and longer recipient survival are changing the patterns of infection.[76] Still, as a diagnostic framework, a time line can be plotted to reflect a patient's chrono-

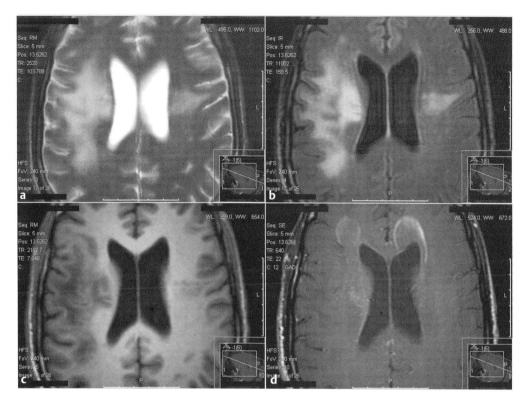

**Fig. 18.3** Magnetic resonance (MR) imaging. Progressive multifocal leukoencephalopathy in a 39-year-old patient with human immunodeficiency virus (HIV) infection presenting with left hemiparesis. Diffuse white matter involvement is seen on T2-weighted MR **(a)** and fluid-attenuated inversion recovery (FLAIR) **(b,c)** sequences. On T1-weighted MR image with gadolinium **(d)**, faint enhancement is seen in a small right periventricular region.

logic "net immunosuppression" status and susceptibility to specific infections. Conventionally, the emergence of infections is divided into three periods: the early or perioperative period, up to 1 month after transplant; the intermediate period, lasting 1 to 6 months after transplant; and the late period, starting at 6 months after transplant. Because immunosuppression has not fully taken effect, opportunistic infections are usually not observed during the first month after transplant. From month 1 to month 6, immunosuppression is most pronounced. CNS infection during this period is most often due to herpesviruses, especially cytomegalovirus (CMV) and Epstein-Barr virus (EBV), fungi, and atypical bacteria or parasites. Herpesvirus (es-

pecially CMV) infections can increase the patient's vulnerability to other infections, either by their adverse immunomodulatory effect or by precipitating graft rejection, which necessitates more intense pharmacologic immunosuppression. After this period, as the level of immunosuppression is usually reduced, the risk becomes lower unless aggressive immunosuppression is reinstituted to treat graft-versus-host disease. Fungi, *Toxoplasma*, *Nocardia*, rarely TB mycobacteria, and other bacteria cause nearly all space-occupying lesions.[77,78] In the differential diagnosis of focal CNS lesions in transplant recipients, one should include EBV-induced CNS lymphoma (posttransplant lymphoproliferative disorder). The incidence of B-cell lymphoma in patients with an HSCT is 2.0 to 7.7%, and 1 to 6% of these will exhibit CNS involvement. Additionally, as a result of exposure to high-dose radiation, HSCT patients can develop other, secondary malignant tumors that include gliomas and meningiomas. Space-occupying tumefacient demyelinating lesions can also develop in the chronic phase after HSCT. Finally, immunosuppressive drug–induced lesions (tacrolimus) can appear.[79]

## Hematopoietic Stem Cell Transplant

HSCT is employed to treat various hematologic malignancies and hematopoietic and autoimmune disorders. HSCT protocols vary according to the source of stem cells and the intensity of pretransplant myeloablation. In turn, these factors affect the pattern and susceptibility of HSCT recipients to infections. Before HSCT, the recipient receives chemotherapy or radiotherapy to eliminate defective bone marrow or residual cancer cells (conditioning). Then, blood- or bone marrow–derived hematopoietic progenitor cells taken either from a human leukocyte antigen (HLA)–matched donor (allogeneic) or from the patient (autologous) are implanted. The duration and degree of posttransplant myeloaplasia depend on the conditioning regimen. Immune reconstitution takes at least 4 months, and complete recovery is expected to happen after 1 year. Graft-versus-host disease can appear acutely (early) or several months after transplant (chronic graft-versus-host disease). Additional immunosuppressive therapy for acute or subacute graft-versus-host disease can cause severe, life-threatening immunosuppression. After allogeneic HSCT, there is the need for chronic immunosuppression to prevent graft-versus-host disease, which puts these patients at risk for opportunistic infections. Cerebral infections occur in approximately 0.3 to 4.5% of HSCT recipients.[80] The most notable infections in HSCT patients are due to viral, fungal, and protozoal agents. In the initial posttransplant period,

the patients are neutropenic, and the major risk is for the acquisition of fungal (*Candida*, *Aspergillus*) or bacterial infections (mostly iatrogenic) and the reactivation of latent viral infections.

At a later stage (beyond 1 month), defective cellular immunity exposes the patients mostly to viral, fungal, and protozoal infections. Infections with invasive molds (mostly *Aspergillus* species) have a high rate of CNS involvement (40 to 50%), and these are the most frequent agents, with an overall incidence of 3 to 4.5%.[81] *Toxoplasma* CNS infections occur in 0.3 to 3% of HSCT patients, depending on seroprevalence; however, the incidence has decreased because of the prophylactic use of trimethoprim-sulfamethoxazole. *T. gondii* infections, when they do occur in HSCT patients, can cause life-threatening complications, with an estimated mortality rate of 60 to 90%.[82,83]

Although aspergillosis can develop at any stage, most HSCT patients exhibit a bimodal susceptibility to *Aspergillus* infection—first in the early posttransplant neutropenic phase and later during the post-engraftment period, when high levels of immunosuppression are maintained to prevent graft-versus-host disease. Although they were initially thought to have lower rates of invasive fungal infection, recipients of nonmyeloablative allogeneic transplants are also reported to be at high risk.

## Solid Organ Transplant

Solid organ transplants are increasing in numbers. Patterns of infection under immunosuppression are essentially similar to those in HSCT recipients. During the initial month after transplant, CNS infection is infrequent. Infection is most often caused by common bacterial pathogens or opportunistic pathogens present in the environment or host (e.g., *Candida* and *Aspergillus* species or *Mycobacterium tuberculosis*). An additional risk associated with solid organ transplant is that a latent, unrecognized infectious agent can be inadvertently introduced through the implanted organ and reactivated in the recipient. This set of events has been observed in regions where *Trypanosoma cruzi* is endemic but has also been described for viral pathogens. The majority of infections in solid organ transplant recipients occur more than 90 days after transplant and are mostly of viral, fungal, or parasitic origin. Mass lesions are most often formed by invasive fungi. The highest incidence of invasive fungal infections is reported in recipients of small-bowel transplants (11.6%); this is followed by 8.6% (especially aspergillosis) in lung and heart–lung recipients, 4.7% in liver recipients, 4.0% in pancreas and kidney–pancreas recipients, and 3.4% in heart transplant recipients. Kidney transplant recipients have the lowest overall risk for infection of 1.3%. Most of these infections are caused by invasive *Candida* and *Aspergillus* species.

Importantly, a substantial number of fungal infections (up to 25%), especially cryptococcosis, mold infections other than aspergillosis, and endemic fungal infections can appear more than 3 years after transplant.[56] *Nocardia* infections have been reported in 0.1 to 3.5% of solid organ transplant recipients, more often in lung transplants and less often in kidney and liver transplants. Although the rate of infection has declined thanks to the prophylactic use of trimethoprim-sulfamethoxazole, at increased risk for infection are patients on high-dose steroids, those with recent CMV infection, and those with high calcineurin inhibitor levels. The risk for infection is highest during the first year after transplant—higher in lung (3.5%) and heart (2.5%) transplants and lower in kidney and liver transplants (1 to 2%).[27] Solid organ transplant patients are also at greater risk for developing TB (0.2 to 0.5%). Infection generally occurs within the first year. Especially susceptible are kidney and lung transplant patients.[34,59,60]

In this late posttransplant period, PML caused by infections with JC virus also rarely appear.

## References

1. Hayden RT, Carroll KC, Tang Y, Wolk DM, eds. Diagnostic Microbiology of the Immunocompromised Host. Washington, DC: ASM Press; 2009
2. Engelhardt B, Sorokin L. The blood-brain and the blood-cerebrospinal fluid barriers: function and dysfunction. Semin Immunopathol 2009;31(4):497–511
3. Karampekios S, Hesselink J. Cerebral infections. Eur Radiol 2005;15(3):485–493
4. Cunha BA. Central nervous system infections in the compromised host: a diagnostic approach. Infect Dis Clin North Am 2001;15(2):567–590
5. Dubey A, Patwardhan RV, Sampth S, Santosh V, Kolluri S, Nanda A. Intracranial fungal granuloma: analysis of 40 patients and review of the literature. Surg Neurol 2005;63(3):254–260, discussion 260
6. Rauchway AC, Husain S, Selhorst JB. Neurologic presentations of fungal infections. Neurol Clin 2010;28(1):293–309
7. Scully EP, Baden LR, Katz JT. Fungal brain infections. Curr Opin Neurol 2008;21(3):347–352
8. Bodey G, Bueltmann B, Duguid W, et al. Fungal infections in cancer patients: an international autopsy survey. Eur J Clin Microbiol Infect Dis 1992;11(2):99–109
9. Black KE, Baden LR. Fungal infections of the CNS: treatment strategies for the immunocompromised patient. CNS Drugs 2007;21(4):293–318
10. Kleinschmidt-DeMasters BK. Central nervous system aspergillosis: a 20-year retrospective series. Hum Pathol 2002;33(1):116–124
11. Lin SJ, Schranz J, Teutsch SM. Aspergillosis case-fatality rate: systematic review of the literature. Clin Infect Dis 2001;32(3):358–366
12. Jain KK, Mittal SK, Kumar S, Gupta RK. Imaging features of central nervous system fungal infections. Neurol India 2007;55(3):241–250
13. Posteraro B, Torelli R, De Carolis E, Posteraro P, Sanguinetti M. Update on the laboratory diagnosis of invasive fungal infections. Mediterr J Hematol Infect Dis 2011;3(1):e2011002
14. Low CY, Rotstein C. Emerging fungal infections in immunocompromised patients. F1000 Med Rep 2011;3:14–21
15. Singh N, Pursell KJ. Combination therapeutic approaches for the management of invasive aspergillosis in organ transplant recipients. Mycoses 2008;51(2):99–108
16. Mattiuzzi G, Giles FJ. Management of intracranial fungal infections in patients with haematological malignancies. Br J Haematol 2005;131(3):287–300
17. Roden MM, Zaoutis TE, Buchanan WL, et al. Epidemiology and outcome of zygomycosis: a review of 929 reported cases. Clin Infect Dis 2005;41(5):634–653
18. Thajeb P, Thajeb T, Dai D. Fatal strokes in patients with rhino-orbito-cerebral mucormycosis and associated vasculopathy. Scand J Infect Dis 2004;36(9):643–648
19. Pagano L, Offidani M, Fianchi L, et al; GIMEMA (Gruppo Italiano Malattie EMatologiche

dell'Adulto) Infection Program. Mucormycosis in hematologic patients. Haematologica 2004; 89(2):207–214

20. Horger M, Hebart H, Schimmel H, et al. Disseminated mucormycosis in haematological patients: CT and MRI findings with pathological correlation. Br J Radiol 2006;79(945):e88–e95

21. Herrera DA, Dublin AB, Ormsby EL, Aminpour S, Howell LP. Imaging findings of rhinocerebral mucormycosis. Skull Base 2009;19(2):117–125

22. Luthra G, Parihar A, Nath K, et al. Comparative evaluation of fungal, tubercular, and pyogenic brain abscesses with conventional and diffusion MR imaging and proton MR spectroscopy. AJNR Am J Neuroradiol 2007;28(7):1332–1338

23. Nakayama H, Shibuya K, Kimura M, Ueda M, Iwabuchi S. Histopathological study of candidal infection in the central nervous system. Nippon Ishinkin Gakkai Zasshi 2010;51(1):31–45

24. Mendes V, Castro S, Linhares P, Ribeiro-Silva ML. Tumoriform presentation of cerebral candidiasis in an HIV-infected patient. J Clin Neurosci 2009;16(4):587–588

25. Jain KK, Mittal SK, Kumar S, Gupta RK. Imaging features of central nervous system fungal infections. Neurol India 2007;55(3):241–250

26. Beaman BL, Beaman L. *Nocardia* species: host-parasite relationships. Clin Microbiol Rev 1994; 7(2):213–264

27. Peleg AY, Husain S, Qureshi ZA, et al. Risk factors, clinical characteristics, and outcome of *Nocardia* infection in organ transplant recipients: a matched case-control study. Clin Infect Dis 2007;44(10):1307–1314

28. Pintado V, Gómez-Mampaso E, Cobo J, et al. Nocardial infection in patients infected with the human immunodeficiency virus. Clin Microbiol Infect 2003;9(7):716–720

29. Minero MV, Marín M, Cercenado E, Rabadán PM, Bouza E, Muñoz P. Nocardiosis at the turn of the century. Medicine (Baltimore) 2009;88(4): 250–261

30. Ambrosioni J, Lew D, Garbino J. Nocardiosis: updated clinical review and experience at a tertiary center. Infection 2010;38(2):89–97

31. Valarezo J, Cohen JE, Valarezo L, et al. Nocardial cerebral abscess: report of three cases and review of the current neurosurgical management. Neurol Res 2003;25(1):27–30

32. Walker M, Zunt JR. Parasitic central nervous system infections in immunocompromised hosts. Clin Infect Dis 2005;40(7):1005–1015

33. Jones JL, Dargelas V, Roberts J, Press C, Remington JS, Montoya JG. Risk factors for *Toxoplasma gondii* infection in the United States. Clin Infect Dis 2009;49(6):878–884

34. Kaplan JE, Benson C, Holmes KH, Brooks JT, Pau A, Masur H; Centers for Disease Control and Prevention (CDC); National Institutes of Health; HIV Medicine Association of the Infectious Diseases Society of America. Guidelines for prevention and treatment of opportunistic infections in HIV-infected adults and adolescents: recommendations from CDC, the National Institutes of Health, and the HIV Medicine Association of the Infectious

Diseases Society of America. MMWR Recomm Rep 2009;58(RR-4):1–207, quiz CE1–CE4

35. Denier C, Bourhis JH, Lacroix C, et al. Spectrum and prognosis of neurologic complications after hematopoietic transplantation. Neurology 2006;67(11):1990–1997

36. Schmidt-Hieber M, Zweigner J, Uharek L, Blau IW, Thiel E. Central nervous system infections in immunocompromised patients: update on diagnostics and therapy. Leuk Lymphoma 2009; 50(1):24–36

37. Gourishankar S, Doucette K, Fenton J, Purych D, Kowalewska-Grochowska K, Preiksaitis J. The use of donor and recipient screening for toxoplasma in the era of universal trimethoprim sulfamethoxazole prophylaxis. Transplantation 2008;85(7): 980–985

38. Martina MN, Cervera C, Esforzado N, et al. *Toxoplasma gondii* primary infection in renal transplant recipients. Two case reports and literature review. Transpl Int 2011;24(1):e6–e12

39. Serpa JA, Moran A, Goodman JC, Giordano TP, White AC Jr. Neurocysticercosis in the HIV era: a case report and review of the literature. Am J Trop Med Hyg 2007;77(1):113–117

40. Keiser PB, Nutman TB. *Strongyloides stercoralis* in the immunocompromised population. Clin Microbiol Rev 2004;17(1):208–217

41. Orlent H, Crawley C, Cwynarski K, Dina R, Apperley J. Strongyloidiasis pre and post autologous peripheral blood stem cell transplantation. Bone Marrow Transplant 2003;32(1):115–117

42. Morgello S, Soifer FM, Lin CS, Wolfe DE. Central nervous system *Strongyloides stercoralis* in acquired immunodeficiency syndrome: a report of two cases and review of the literature. Acta Neuropathol 1993;86(3):285–288

43. Gompels MM, Todd J, Peters BS, Main J, Pinching AJ. Disseminated strongyloidiasis in AIDS: uncommon but important. AIDS 1991;5(3): 329–332

44. Cordova E, Boschi A, Ambrosioni J, Cudos C, Corti M. Reactivation of Chagas disease with central nervous system involvement in HIV-infected patients in Argentina, 1992-2007. Int J Infect Dis 2008;12(6):587–592

45. Diazgranados CA, Saavedra-Trujillo CH, Mantilla M, Valderrama SL, Alquichire C, Franco-Paredes C. Chagasic encephalitis in HIV patients: common presentation of an evolving epidemiological and clinical association. Lancet Infect Dis 2009; 9(5):324–330

46. Walker M, Kublin JG, Zunt JR. Parasitic central nervous system infections in immunocompromised hosts: malaria, microsporidiosis, leishmaniasis, and African trypanosomiasis. Clin Infect Dis 2006;42(1):115–125

47. Albrecht H, Sobottka I, Emminger C, et al. Visceral leishmaniasis emerging as an important opportunistic infection in HIV-infected persons living in areas nonendemic for *Leishmania donovani*. Arch Pathol Lab Med 1996;120(2):189–198

48. Karak B, Garg RK, Misra S, Sharma AM. Neurological manifestations in a patient with visceral

leishmaniasis. Postgrad Med J 1998;74(873): 423–425

49. Kayler LK, Rudich SM, Merion RM. Orthotopic liver transplantation from a donor with a history of schistosomiasis. Transplant Proc 2003; 35(8):2974–2976

50. Li Y, Ross AG, Hou X, Lou Z, McManus DP. Oriental schistosomiasis with neurological complications: case report. Ann Clin Microbiol Antimicrob 2011;10:5

51. Carod-Artal FJ. Neurological complications of *Schistosoma* infection. Trans R Soc Trop Med Hyg 2008;102(2):107–116

52. Gray F, Chrétien F, Vallat-Decouvelaere AV, Scaravilli F. The changing pattern of HIV neuropathology in the HAART era. J Neuropathol Exp Neurol 2003;62(5):429–440

53. Bayraktar S, Bayraktar UD, Ramos JC, Stefanovic A, Lossos IS. Primary CNS lymphoma in HIV positive and negative patients: comparison of clinical characteristics, outcome and prognostic factors. J Neurooncol 2011;101(2):257–265

54. Abgrall S, Rabaud C, Costagliola D; Clinical Epidemiology Group of the French Hospital Database on HIV. Incidence and risk factors for toxoplasmic encephalitis in human immunodeficiency virus-infected patients before and during the highly active antiretroviral therapy era. Clin Infect Dis 2001;33(10):1747–1755

55. Dedicoat M, Livesley N. Management of toxoplasmic encephalitis in HIV-infected adults (with an emphasis on resource-poor settings). Cochrane Database Syst Rev 2006;3(3):CD005420

56. Pappas PG, Alexander BD, Andes DR, et al. Invasive fungal infections among organ transplant recipients: results of the Transplant-Associated Infection Surveillance Network (TRANSNET). Clin Infect Dis 2010;50(8):1101–1111

57. Singh N, Lortholary O, Dromer F, et al; Cryptococcal Collaborative Transplant Study Group. Central nervous system cryptococcosis in solid organ transplant recipients: clinical relevance of abnormal neuroimaging findings. Transplantation 2008; 86(5):647–651

58. Li Q, You C, Liu Q, Liu Y. Central nervous system cryptococcoma in immunocompetent patients: a short review illustrated by a new case. Acta Neurochir (Wien) 2010;152(1):129–136

59. Nelson CA, Zunt JR. Tuberculosis of the central nervous system in immunocompromised patients: HIV infection and solid organ transplant recipients. Clin Infect Dis 2011;53(9):915–926

60. Torre-Cisneros J, Doblas A, Aguado JM, et al; Spanish Network for Research in Infectious Diseases. Tuberculosis after solid-organ transplant: incidence, risk factors, and clinical characteristics in the RESITRA (Spanish Network of Infection in Transplantation) cohort. Clin Infect Dis 2009;48(12):1657–1665

61. Bishburg E, Eng RHK, Slim J, Perez G, Johnson E. Brain lesions in patients with acquired immunodeficiency syndrome. Arch Intern Med 1989;149(4):941–943

62. Pepper DJ, Marais S, Maartens G, et al. Neurologic manifestations of paradoxical tuberculosis-associated immune reconstitution inflammatory syndrome: a case series. Clin Infect Dis 2009;48(11): e96–e107

63. Marais S, Scholtz P, Pepper DJ, Meintjes G, Wilkinson RJ, Candy S. Neuroradiological features of the tuberculosis-associated immune reconstitution inflammatory syndrome. Int J Tuberc Lung Dis 2010;14(2):188–196

64. Bernaerts A, Vanhoenacker FM, Parizel PM, et al. Tuberculosis of the central nervous system: overview of neuroradiological findings. Eur Radiol 2003;13(8):1876–1890

65. Luthra G, Parihar A, Nath K, et al. Comparative evaluation of fungal, tubercular, and pyogenic brain abscesses with conventional and diffusion MR imaging and proton MR spectroscopy. AJNR Am J Neuroradiol 2007;28(7):1332–1338

66. Bottieau E, Noë A, Florence E, Colebunders R. Multiple tuberculous brain abscesses in an HIV-infected patient successfully treated with HAART and antituberculous treatment. Infection 2003;31(2):118–120

67. Cárdenas G, Soto-Hernández JL, Orozco RV, Silva EG, Revuelta R, Amador JL. Tuberculous brain abscesses in immunocompetent patients: management and outcome. Neurosurgery 2010;67(4):1081–1087, discussion 1087

68. d'Arminio Monforte A, Cinque P, Mocroft A, et al; EuroSIDA Study Group. Changing incidence of central nervous system diseases in the EuroSIDA cohort. Ann Neurol 2004;55(3):320–328

69. Amend KL, Turnbull B, Foskett N, Napalkov P, Kurth T, Seeger J. Incidence of progressive multifocal leukoencephalopathy in patients without HIV. Neurology 2010;75(15):1326–1332

70. Carson KR, Focosi D, Major EO, et al. Monoclonal antibody-associated progressive multifocal leucoencephalopathy in patients treated with rituximab, natalizumab, and efalizumab: a Review from the Research on Adverse Drug Events and Reports (RADAR) Project. Lancet Oncol 2009;10(8):816–824

71. Kedar S, Berger JR. The changing landscape of progressive multifocal leukoencephalopathy. Curr Infect Dis Rep 2011;13(4):380–386

72. Tan K, Roda R, Ostrow L, McArthur J, Nath A. PML-IRIS in patients with HIV infection: clinical manifestations and treatment with steroids. Neurology 2009;72(17):1458–1464

73. Sidhu N, McCutchan JA. Unmasking of PML by HAART: unusual clinical features and the role of IRIS. J Neuroimmunol 2010;219(1-2):100–104

74. Tan CS, Koralnik IJ. Progressive multifocal leukoencephalopathy and other disorders caused by JC virus: clinical features and pathogenesis. Lancet Neurol 2010;9(4):425–437

75. Hernández B, Dronda F, Moreno S. Treatment options for AIDS patients with progressive multifocal leukoencephalopathy. Expert Opin Pharmacother 2009;10(3):403–416

76. Low CY, Rotstein C. Emerging fungal infections in immunocompromised patients. F1000 Med Rep 2011;3:14–21

77. Fishman JA. Infection in solid-organ transplant recipients. N Engl J Med 2007;357(25): 2601–2614

78. Czartoski T. Central nervous system infections in transplantation. Curr Treat Options Neurol 2006;8(3):193–201

79. Nishiguchi T, Mochizuki K, Shakudo M, Takeshita T, Hino M, Inoue Y. CNS complications of hematopoietic stem cell transplantation. AJR Am J Roentgenol 2009;192(4):1003–1011

80. Bleggi-Torres LF, de Medeiros BC, Werner B, et al. Neuropathological findings after bone marrow transplantation: an autopsy study of 180 cases. Bone Marrow Transplant 2000;25(3):301–307

81. Jantunen E, Volin L, Salonen O, et al. Central nervous system aspergillosis in allogeneic stem cell transplant recipients. Bone Marrow Transplant 2003;31(3):191–196

82. Martino R, Bretagne S, Rovira M, et al. Toxoplasmosis after hematopoietic stem cell transplantation. Report of a 5-year survey from the Infectious Diseases Working Party of the European Group for Blood and Marrow Transplantation. Bone Marrow Transplant 2000;25(10):1111–1114

83. Fricker-Hidalgo H, Bulabois CE, Brenier-Pinchart MP, et al. Diagnosis of toxoplasmosis after allogeneic stem cell transplantation: results of DNA detection and serological techniques. Clin Infect Dis 2009;48(2):e9–e15

# 19

# Systemic Infections in the Neurologic Intensive Care Unit

Michael F. Regner, Christopher D. Baggott, Barry C. Fox, and Joshua E. Medow

Evidence-based management guidelines have been reported in recent years, with the hope of inspiring effective and cost-efficient algorithms for the work-up and treatment of infectious diseases in the critical care unit.[1-7] Thoughtful application of these guidelines in the neurologic intensive care unit (ICU) is appropriate and important, given the impact of infection and fever on patient outcomes. We intend to present concise, guideline-based management principles for the critical care unit, while addressing idiosyncrasies in the care of neurologically injured patients.

## ■ General Principles of Fever Management

### Body Temperature and Neurologic Outcome

Hyperthermia and hypothermia are both important clinical indicators that an infectious process may be present in a critically ill patient. In units caring for neurologically injured patients, body temperature has a clear association with neurologic outcome.[8] Hyperthermia within the first 24 hours has a negative impact on neurologic outcome in stroke, probably because of increased metabolic demand in the ischemic pneumbra.[9] Conversely, hypothermia is associated with increased morbidity, particularly in the context of infection, hypotension, and arrhythmias.[10] Ultimately,

neurologic patients probably benefit from induced normothermia, which prevents the hypermetabolic state of hyperthermia while avoiding the complications associated with hypothermia. Avoiding hypothermia requires the close monitoring of patient temperature and the establishment of appropriate triggers to prompt an infectious work-up, appropriate systems-based identification of infectious and noninfectious sources, and measures to prevent hypothermia or hyperthermia.

### Monitoring

In order of preference, temperature monitoring should be achieved by intravascular, esophageal, or bladder thermometry. If these methods are not available, measurements can be collected at rectal, oral, or tympanic membrane sites. Axillary measurements, temporal artery estimates, and chemical dot thermometers should not be used.[3]

### Triggers Prompting Infectious Work-up

Although temperature is an important indicator of possible infectious status, automatic laboratory or radiologic investigations based on temperature alone should be avoided. The new onset of a temperature of 38.3°C or higher or of 36.0°C or lower in the absence of a known cause of pyrexia or hypothermia is an appropriate trigger for clinical assessment.[3] Careful clinical assessment drives decision making. Routine "panculturing" should not be performed without a clinical assessment, and microbiological specimens should be obtained at various time points for culture. The likelihood of infectious versus noninfectious processes arises from the clinical circumstance, and the site of infection may become apparent from the history and physical examination. Antibiotics should not be considered the antipyretics of choice[3] (**Table 19.1**).

## Suspected Bloodstream Infection

Bloodstream infections are a serious problem, and any suspicion of this type of infection should be investigated thoroughly and adequately addressed. It is very important that the clinician and laboratory personnel communicate effectively and regularly regarding infection evaluation protocols to improve their diagnostic value and to reduce technical errors as technology rapidly

**Table 19.1** Overview of clinical work-up for infection[3,11]

| Organ System | Symptoms | Signs |
|---|---|---|
| Central nervous system | Headaches, vision changes, motor disturbance, sensory disturbance, neck pain/stiffness, convulsions, changes in mood/perception, psychiatric symptoms | Decreased arousal, cranial nerve deficits, abnormal funduscopic examination, focal neurologic signs, meningismus |
| Cardiovascular | Precordial pain; dyspnea (exertional, positional, nocturnal); palpitations; syncope; edema; cyanosis | Murmurs, ectopic heart sounds, rubs, hypertension, increased jugular venous pressure, Janeway lesions, splinter hemorrhages |
| Pulmonary | Chest pain, shortness of breath, hemoptysis, wheezing, stridor, cough, night sweats | Decreased/adventitial sounds on auscultation (crackles, wheezes, rhonchi, stridor, pleural rub); secretions |
| Gastrointestinal | Diarrhea, constipation, abnormal stools, appetite changes, nausea, vomiting, hematemesis, abdominal pain | Diarrhea, constipation, hematochezia/melena, emesis, hematemesis, distention, rebound tenderness |
| Genitourinary | Urgency, increased frequency, dysuria, hematuria, polyuria/oliguria, flank tenderness, genital discharge | Erythema, genital discharge, foul odor, epithelial changes, cutaneous lesions |
| Skin/soft tissue | Rash, itching, redness, pigmentation changes, texture changes | Erythema, induration, swelling, discharge, purulence |
| Bones/joints | Pain, swelling, redness, decreased range of motion, stiffness | Erythema, swelling, discharge, purulence, sinus tracts, sensory deficits |
| Other/constitutional | Weight loss, reduced sense of well-being, leg swelling, withdrawal symptoms, facial pain/sinus headache, recent transfusion, recent travel history, recent surgery | Weight loss, Homan sign, cutaneous stigmata, diaphoresis, palpitations, pupillary size, Janeway lesions, heart murmurs, splinter hemorrhages, purulent nasal discharge, psychiatric disturbance, many others |

*Abbreviations*: ARDS, acute respiratory distress syndrome; BOOP, bronchiolitis obliterans–organizing pneumonia; CVA, cerebrovascular accident; IBS, irritable bowel syndrome; SLE, systemic lupus erythematosus; UTI, urinary tract infection evolves.[12] Some important clinical triggers for obtaining a blood culture are listed in **Table 19.2**. Standing orders should not be written for obtaining blood cultures; they should be indicated either after clinical assessment or in the presence of a known bloodstream infection. Such test-of-cure cultures, when indicated, may be discontinued after three consecutive days of negative cultures.[6]

Blood cultures are most useful if they are drawn during a febrile episode, espe-cially before the fever dissipates. However, in the case of suspected endocarditis or the more common intravascular device–related sepsis, blood cultures should be drawn as soon as possible. When attempts have been made to achieve normothermia in a patient, blood cultures should be considered for an elevation in the patient's white blood cell count. These blood cultures ideally are drawn from two separate sites by percutaneous venipuncture. Samples both by ve-

**Table 19.1** (*Continued*)   Overview of clinical work-up for infection[3,11]

| Infectious Diseases | Noninfectious Diseases |
|---|---|
| Meningitis; encephalitis (bacterial, viral, fungal, opportunistic); ventriculitis; cerebritis/abscess | Posterior fossa syndrome, central fever, seizures, cerebral infarction, intracranial hemorrhage, CVA |
| Central line infection, infected pacemaker, endocarditis, sternal osteomyelitis, viral pericarditis, myocardial/perivalvular abscess | Myocardial infarction, Dressler syndrome, vasculitis, balloon pump syndrome |
| Pneumonia, mediastinitis, tracheobronchitis, empyema | Pulmonary emboli, ARDS (fibroproliferative phase), atelectasis, BOOP, bronchogenic carcinoma, pneumonitis (SLE or others) |
| *C. difficile* colitis; intra-abdominal abscess; gastroenteritis (viral, bacterial); cholangitis; cholecystitis; peritonitis | Pancreatitis, acalculous cholecystitis, bowel ischemia, bleeding, cirrhosis, ischemic colitis, IBS |
| UTI, catheter-associated bacteriuria, pyelonephritis, cystitis, sexually transmitted infections | |
| Decubitus ulcers, cellulitis, wound infection | Drug rash/fever, autoimmune processes (low-grade) |
| Osteomyelitis, septic arthritis | Acute gout, heterotopic ossification |
| Bacteremia, sinusitis | Adrenal insufficiency, phlebitis/thrombophlebitis, neoplastic fever, alcohol/drug withdrawal, delirium tremens, drug fever, fat emboli, deep venous thrombosis, postoperative fever (48 hours), blood product transfusion, cytokine storm, immune reconstitution inflammatory syndrome, Jarisch-Herxheimer reaction, thyroid storm, transplant rejection, tumor lysis syndrome |

**Table 19.2** Triggers for blood culture

| Fever and any one of the following: |
| --- |
| • Rigors |
| • Mental status change |
| • Leukocytosis/unexplained leukopenia |
| • Oliguria |
| • Hypoxia |
| • Tachypnea |
| • Metabolic acidosis |
| • Hypotension |
| • Significant change in white blood cell count |
| Test of cure: |
| • Endocarditis |
| • *Staphylococcus aureus* sepsis |
| • Fungal sepsis |
| • Continued signs/symptoms of sepsis |

nipuncture and from an existing vascular catheter are preferred only when vascular access has exceeded 4 days. Inflammation at the catheter exit site is not a reliable predictor of intravascular catheter–related infection because the contamination of catheter lumens is often involved in the pathogenesis of intravascular infections.[13] If venous access is not an option, samples should be drawn from two separate vascular catheters and carefully labeled.[6]

Blood cultures for bacteria and yeast should consist of two samples in aerobic and anaerobic bottles from each site. Current blood culture media allow the detection of yeast without the need for special fungal blood cultures. Quantitative blood cultures in which special isolator blood culture tubes are used may be indicated for the diagnosis of bacteremia associated with cuffed Hickman or Broviac catheters or subcutaneous central venous ports.[6] The more common method of diagnosis of catheter-related infection is the differential time to positivity of blood cultures taken from catheter and peripheral blood sites. When the differential time exceeds 2 hours between the catheter culture and the peripheral culture, the inside of the catheter is usually considered the source of bacteremia, and the catheter should be removed if possible.[3]

**Table 19.3** summarizes some important guidelines to be considered when blood cultures are obtained. Additional recommendations are to avoid collecting from more than two sites at a time, collecting more than three cultures per day, and collecting more than four cultures per febrile episode.

**Table 19.3** Blood culture "do's" and "don'ts"

| Do: | Don't: |
| --- | --- |
| • Sample from two sites | • Send < 5 mL to the laboratory |
| • Draw from venipuncture if possible | • Send an anaerobic bottle without an aerobic bottle |
| • Draw during a febrile episode unless suspected endocarditis or intravascular-related sepsis | • Send adult specimens in pediatric bottles, or vice versa |
| | **Avoid:** |
| | • Line-drawn specimens (± venipuncture) without a simultaneous peripheral culture |
| | • > 2 sites collected at a time |
| | • > 3 cultures collected per day |
| | • > 4 cultures per febrile episode |

Diagnosing and treating the cause of a fever in a patient with catheters can be complicated, but a standardized management algorithm has been proposed in **Fig. 19.1**.

Treat resulting cultures per the Infectious Diseases Society of America guidelines reported by Mermel et al for the catheters and pathogenic species involved.[6] Although the tips of long intravascular catheters, such as percutaneously inserted central venous catheters, are often sent for culture, the preferred segment of the catheter to send to the laboratory is the "intracutaneous" segment. This is the catheter segment just inside the blood vessel that is not contaminated by the skin. The pathophysiology of external (rather than intraluminal) colonization and infection has a bacterial gradient highest at the intracutaneous site and lowest at the catheter tip. Hence, more false-negative results are likely to be obtained by sending the long line catheter tip than by sending the intracutaneous segment.

## Suspected Noninfectious Fever

Noninfectious fevers can often be difficult to diagnose, necessitating a careful and thorough history and physical examination. All recent medication changes and blood products received should be considered in the febrile patient. Establishing a temporal relationship between the initiation or change of a suspected drug and the fever can be helpful in establishing a causal relationship. If a particular medication is suspected as the causative agent, it should be stopped, or a comparable substitution should be made. Drug-induced fevers may require several days to resolve, depending on the drug pharmacokinetics and patient profile. Phenytoin is notorious for causing

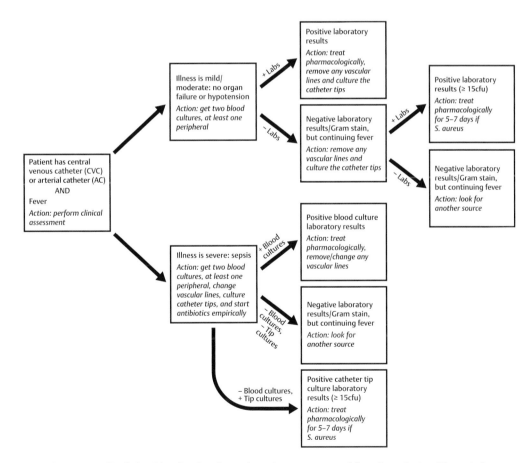

**Fig. 19.1** Generalized algorithm for the diagnosis and management of fever in patients with central venous catheters or arterial catheters.

drug fever and hepatitis in neurosurgical patients. Some nonpharmacologic, noninfectious causes of fevers are listed in the last column of **Table 19.1**.

### Suspected Postoperative Fever

A chest radiograph, urinalysis, and urine culture are usually not necessary for fever during the first 72 postoperative hours if the fever is observed as an isolated event.[3] Patients with an indwelling bladder catheter and fever for longer than 72 hours postoperatively should have a urinalysis, and a blood culture should be drawn.[3] The careful daily examination of surgical wounds is important in the setting of fever, and cultures should be obtained if signs of symptoms of infection exist. In any case of postoperative fever, clinicians should be suspicious of deep vein thrombosis, superficial thrombophlebitis, and pulmonary embolism.[3] Suspicion for a thrombotic fever should be greater in sedentary patients, those with malignancies, those on oral contraceptives, or those with limb immobility.[3]

Fever assessment in the neurologic ICU must include a daily examination of the surgical site for signs of infection, such as erythema, purulence, swelling, and tenderness. Clinicians should maintain a moderate threshold for opening and culturing an incision suspected of being infected and for aspirating any deep fluid collections. Any expressed purulence from within a deep incision consistent with a deep organ space or surgical space infection should be sent for Gram stain and culture. Tissue biopsy and aspiration are recommended methods to obtain infected material.[3] In contrast, superficial surgical site infections may be adequately treated with incision, drainage, and local antiseptic care without systemic antibiotic therapy. Superficial incision site swabs are not recommended.[3]

### Suspected Central Nervous System Infection

#### Assessment

Some of the characteristics that should trigger a clinical assessment for central nervous system (CNS) infection are listed in **Table 19.4**.

Assessment of a suspected CNS infection must be rapid. The new onset of fever, unexplained altered consciousness, or focal neurologic signs should trigger a diagnostic lumbar puncture unless there are contraindications.[7] If the symptoms and signs suggest a focal neurologic process proximal to the spinal cord, imaging studies are indicated before a lumbar puncture is performed to prevent cerebral herniation. If a mass is found, a neurology or neurosurgery consultation should be considered to determine the optimal diagnostic approach. Febrile patients with an intracranial device should have a cerebrospinal fluid (CSF) analysis conducted urgently. Patients with a ventriculostomy who develop the signs or symptoms listed in **Table 19.4** and a CSF pleocytosis suggestive of possible microbiological infection should usually have their intracranial catheter removed and the catheter tip cultured.

CSF analysis should involve a cytocentrifuged Gram stain and culture. The intracellular organisms on Gram stain should exclude for the clinician the likelihood of a contaminant. Urgent glucose quantification, protein quantification, and cell count with differential can be used as secondary measures to help determine the presence of infection. However, patients with recent

Table 19.4 Triggers of assessment for central nervous system infection

| Fever and at least one of the following: |
| --- |
| • Altered consciousness |
| • Papilledema |
| • Focal neurologic deficit |
| • Headache |
| • Nuchal rigidity |
| • New onset of seizure |
| • Imaging findings (meningeal enhancement) |
| • Recent neurosurgical procedure |
| • Basilar skull fracture |
| • Cerebrospinal fluid leak |

trauma, stroke (hemorrhagic or nonhemorrhagic), neoplasm, or surgery may have derangements of the cell count and protein levels that are not related to infection, and therefore trends or spot checks with these parameters alone may not be helpful. A CSF lactate determination may better assess for infection because an elevated lactate level may provide more specific and sensitive information on infection in the absence of the results of Gram stain and culture.[14] Additional tests for infectious pathogens and neoplastic cells should be conducted as indicated by the clinical situation.

## Infectious Meningitis

If infectious meningitis is suspected, empiric therapy should be initiated before confirmatory cultures are obtained. Such therapy consists of dexamethasone and empiric antimicrobial pharmacotherapy, such as ceftriaxone and vancomycin. Potential nosocomial bacterial meningitis should be treated with different antibiotic components, usually an agent active against methicillin-resistant *Staphylococcus aureus* (MRSA) and *Pseudomonas aeruginosa*. Clinicians should have a low threshold to initiate acyclovir therapy to treat herpes simplex virus infection empirically if the diagnosis is uncertain.

Postoperative CNS infections most commonly include meningitis, subdural empyema, and brain abscess. The incidence of such sequelae after neurologic procedures has been reported in the literature to be anywhere from 0.8 to 7%.[15-18] Surgical prophylaxis is most important for *S. aureus*, *Staphylococcus epidermidis*, and *Propionibacterium acnes*, usually with a cephalosporin antibiotic. Patients known to be colonized with MRSA generally should receive prophylaxis with vancomycin. Patients who have been hospitalized and who have received extended β-lactam antibiotics are at risk for infection with *Staphylococcus* species that are β-lactam–resistant and should be considered candidates for vancomycin prophylaxis. Prophylactic antimicrobial pharmacotherapy before craniotomy has been reported to decrease the incidence of postoperative meningitis by as much as 50%.[19]

## Aseptic Meningitis

Aseptic meningitis is common after neurosurgical procedures, particularly those involving the posterior fossa. There are no clear clinical findings or laboratory analyses that distinguish between bacterial meningitis and aseptic meningitis.[20] There is preliminary evidence that CSF lactate may be a sensitive and specific indicator of bacterial meningitis, but this requires further investigation.[21] Empiric antimicrobial pharmacotherapy should be initiated in all patients with postoperative meningitis; however, if the CSF culture results are negative, it is usually appropriate to withdraw treatment after 48 to 72 hours while monitoring closely for clinical signs and symptoms of infection.

## Ventriculitis

The standardized management of intraventricular catheters has been shown to reduce the incidence of intraventricular catheter–related ventriculitis.[22] The utility of routine CSF surveillance cultures has yet to be determined. Interestingly, patients who have catheters impregnated with antimicrobial agents have outcomes similar to those of patients who have nonimpregnated catheters and receive systemic antimicrobial treatment.[23] It remains to be seen whether antibiotic-impregnated catheters have any advantage over nonimpregnated catheters. Evidence from randomized controlled trials suggests that changing the ventricular catheter does not reduce the risk for CSF infection, and there are no prospective randomized controlled trials to demonstrate that prophylactic catheter exchange is efficacious.[24–26] Despite evidence suggesting that the duration of ventricular or lumbar CSF drainage is an independent risk factor for infection,[27] there is no evidence to support the practice of prophylactic ventricular catheter exchange.[26,28] The subcutaneous tunneling of catheters has also been described for use in external ventricular drains; however, not all studies support this practice. More research is needed to make definitive recommendations.

## Suspected Pulmonary Infection

Suspected pulmonary infections can be categorized into four main types: (1) community-acquired pneumonia (CAP), (2) hospital-acquired pneumonia (HAP), (3) health care–associated pneumonia (HCAP), and (4) ventilator-associated pneumonia (VAP).[4,5] **Table 19.5** defines the various types of pneumonia. Common pathogens and treatment regimens differ according to the specific type of pneumonia that is diagnosed, so that it is necessary to obtain a careful history and investigate the precise time line of the patient's clinical course. Aspiration pneumonitis frequently masquerades as a pulmonary infection[31] and may require either no antibiotic therapy or therapy that is limited to 72 hours because of a low bacterial burden.

### Assessment

Patients in the neurologic ICU with suspected nosocomial pulmonary infections should be assessed clinically and assigned a clinical pulmonary infection score (CPIS) to guide their diagnostic and therapeutic management.[4] **Table 19.6** describes the CPIS and the clinical assessment criteria used to guide diagnosis. If the CPIS is higher than 6 or an infiltrate exists and more than one clinical assessment criteria exist, then a high degree of suspicion for infection is indicated. If the CPIS is between 2 and 6 or an infiltrate exists along with one clinical assessment criterion, then a low degree of suspicion is warranted.

In the case of a high level of suspicion for a pulmonary infection, a tracheal aspirate Gram strain can yield anywhere from no organisms to numerous predominant organisms. In the case of no or few organisms, a quantitative bronchoscopic bronchoalveolar lavage (BAL) or respiratory therapy "blind" mini-BAL may be an important confirmatory evaluation. If a moderate or large organism burden is demonstrated on the aspirate Gram stain, a BAL can be considered but may not be necessary. Semiquantitative Gram stain results are highly variable between microbiology laboratories, so that a minimally invasive procedure may still be considered necessary. In either case, empiric treatment should be initiated.[4]

In the case of a low level of suspicion for a pulmonary infection, a tracheotomy aspirate Gram stain with no or few organisms has a high negative predictive value, arguing against infection. A worsening clinical status in this scenario or a tracheotomy aspirate Gram stain with moderate to numerous organisms indicates that a quantitative bronchoscopic BAL or mini-BAL is a reasonable diagnostic test to perform.[4] Contraindications to performing a mini-BAL are listed in **Table 19.7**; if any of these are present, a sputum Gram stain or culture is the only suitable alternative diagnostic test. Empiric treatment is warranted if any of these tests demonstrates a significant infectious burden.[4]

**Table 19.5** Types of pneumonia

| Community-acquired pneumonia (CAP) | Pneumonia in persons not satisfying the diagnostic criteria for HAP, HCAP, or VAP |
|---|---|
| Hospital-acquired pneumonia (HAP) | Pneumonia that occurs 48 hours or more after admission and was not present on admission |
| Health care–associated pneumonia (HCAP) | Pneumonia that occurs in a nonhospitalized patient with health care contact or interaction, specifically with at least one of the following:<br>• Intravenous therapy, wound care, or intravenous chemotherapy within the past 30 days<br>• Hospitalization in an acute care hospital for ≥ 2 days within the past 90 days<br>• Residence in a nursing home or long-term care facility<br>• Attendance at a hospital or hemodialysis clinic within the past 30 days |
| Ventilator-associated pneumonia (VAP) | A subtype of HAP that develops > 48 hours after endotracheal intubation |

**Table 19.6** Clinical pulmonary infection score

| Category | Assessment | Score |
|---|---|---|
| Temperature (°C) | > 36.5 and < 38.4 | 0 |
| | > 38.5 and < 38.9 | 1 |
| | > 39.0 or < 36.0 | 2 |
| WBC count (cells per milliliter) | > 4,000 and < 11,000 | 0 |
| | < 4,000 or > 11,000 | 1 |
| Tracheal secretions | Few | 0 |
| | Moderate | 1 |
| | Large | 2 |
| | Purulent | +1 |
| $Pao_2/Fio_2$ | > 240 or + ARDS | 0 |
| | < 240 and – ARDS | 2 |
| Chest X-ray | No infiltrate | 0 |
| | Patchy or diffuse infiltrate | 1 |
| | Localized infiltrate | 2 |

Clinical assessment criteria

- Presence of new or progressive radiographic infiltrate
- Fever > 38°C
- Leukocytosis or leukopenia
- Purulent pulmonary secretions

*Abbreviations*: ARDS, acute respiratory distress syndrome; $Fio_2$, fraction of inspired oxygen; $Pao_2$, partial pressure of arterial oxygen; WBC, white blood cell

**Table 19.7** Contraindications to mini-BAL

| |
|---|
| Coagulopathy or bleeding disorder (INR > 1.5 or platelet count ≤ 50,000/mm³) |
| Refractory hypoxemia ($Sao_2$ < 90%) |
| Myocardial infarction in last 6 weeks |
| New onset of a significant cardiac arrhythmia |
| ICP > 20 cm $H_2O$ |
| PEEP ≥ 15 cm $H_2O$ |
| Endotracheal tube < 7.0 mm or tracheostomy < 7.5 mm |

*Abbreviations*: BAL, bronchoalveolar lavage; ICP, intracranial pressure; INR, International Normalized Ratio; PEEP, positive end-expiratory pressure; $Sao_2$, arterial oxygen saturation

**Table 19.8** Empiric treatment of pulmonary infection if length of stay longer than 5 days or risk for multidrug resistance

| |
|---|
| 1. Antipseudomonal penicillin, cephalosporin, or carbapenems |
| AND |
| 2. Aminoglycoside or fluoroquinolone (renal impairment) |
| AND |
| 3. Vancomycin or linezolid (if methicillin-resistant *Staphylococcus aureus* suspected) |

Risk factors for multidrug resistance:

- Antimicrobial pharmacotherapy within last 90 days
- Current hospitalization > 4 days
- Community or hospital unit antimicrobial resistance
- Immunosuppression (disease-related or therapeutic)

Risks for health care–associated pneumonia

- Hospitalization for > 1 day in the last 90 days
- Resident of nursing home or extended-care facility
- Home infusion therapy
- Home wound care
- Close contact with multidrug-resistant pathogen
- Chronic dialysis in last 30 days

## Treatment

The standard empiric treatment of CAP consists of ceftriaxone with ampicillin, sulbactam, and azithromycin, or moxifloxacin in the case of a penicillin allergy. HAP developing less than 5 days after hospitalization is still considered to be caused by the same bacteria that cause CAP. If the length of stay is longer than 5 days or the risk for multidrug resistance is present, treatment as outlined in **Table 19.8** is indicated.[4]

After empiric treatment has been initiated, the patient should be monitored closely for clinical improvement. If after 48 to 72 hours there is evidence of clinical improvement and culture results are negative or quantitative cultures are below the usual threshold for clinical significance (usually $10^4$ to $10^5$ bacteria per milliliter), antibiotic discontinuation may be considered. If the culture results are positive, antibiotics are adjusted to target the causative agent, with continued treatment for 7 to 8 days, and the patient is reassessed after completing the course of antibiotics. Note that all patients with endotracheal tubes in place will be colonized with bacteria, but not necessarily infected. In the case of *P. aeruginosa* or *Acinetobacter* species, continuing antibiotics for more than 8 days may be reasonable. If clinical deterioration or lack of improvement is observed and the cultures are positive, antibiotics are adjusted according to the causative agent, and consideration is given to repeating the respiratory microbiological assessment while one continues to search for other pathogens, diseases, or potential complications. If the culture results are negative in the setting of clinical deterioration or lack of clinical improvement, one should consider stopping the pneumonia-targeted antibiotics if clinically appropriate.[4]

## Suspected Urinary Tract Infection

Urinary tract infection (UTI) commonly precipitates further infectious sequelae and clinical deterioration in the neurologic ICU. Typical signs and symptoms of a UTI are listed in **Table 19.9**. However, the diagnosis

**Table 19.9** Signs and symptoms of urinary tract infection

| New onset or worsening of fever, and at least one of the following: |
| --- |
| • Rigors |
| • Altered consciousness |
| • Malaise |
| • Lethargy of unknown etiology |
| • Flank pain |
| • Costovertebral angle tenderness |
| • Acute hematuria |
| • Pelvic discomfort |
| • Dysuria |
| • Urgent or frequent urination |
| • Suprapubic pain or tenderness |

of UTI in the neurologically impaired patient and the distinction from asymptomatic bacteriuria in the colonized patient with an indwelling catheter can be challenging.

Clinicians should be particularly suspicious of a possible UTI in patients with spinal cord injury, spasticity, upper motor neuron disease, autonomic dysreflexia, or malaise and in elderly patients with delirium.

### Assessment

Because the clinical diagnosis of UTI in neurologically impaired patients is difficult, laboratory investigation is usually indicated, but it may still be difficult to differentiate UTI from catheter-acquired asymptomatic bacteriuria. Some risk factors for UTI include kidney transplant, recent genitourinary surgery, urinary obstruction, urologic dysfunction, and bladder catheterization. Routine urine screening for catheter-acquired asymptomatic bacteriuria should not be performed except in specific populations, such as pregnant women and patients undergoing urologic procedures in which visible mucosal bleeding is anticipated. Specifically, in patients with indwelling urethral catheters as well as in patients with neurogenic bladder managed with intermittent catheterization, the screening and treatment of catheter-acquired asymptomatic bacteriuria are not recommended in the absence of clinical signs or symptoms suggestive of infection.

The laboratory assessment for UTI includes obtaining a urine sample for microscopic examination (chemistries, blood, pyuria) and culture. In patients with symptoms of sepsis, a Gram stain of the urine may be indicated. In particular, a urine sample is necessary before antimicrobial pharmacotherapy is initiated to distinguish among the diversity of potential causative pathogens and the potential presence of antimicrobial resistance. For patients with an indwelling catheter, samples should be acquired from the port itself, not the drainage bag. Urine samples should be processed promptly because bacterial multiplication may cause the laboratory to overestimate the true pathogenic burden. Rapid urine dipsticks are not appropriate for the investigation of a possible catheter-acquired UTI.

Pyuria in the catheterized patient is not diagnostic of bacteriuria or UTI. Along with odor and cloudiness, the presence or absence of pyuria is not necessarily a reliable differentiator of catheter-acquired asymptomatic bacteriuria from catheter-associated UTI. The absence of pyuria in a symptomatic patient, however, is evidence arguing against a diagnosis of catheter-acquired UTI. Yeast and enterococci tend to cause less pyuria, whereas gram-negative bacteria tend to produce more pyuria.[32,33]

Regardless of whether it is symptomatic, true bacteriuria or candiduria in a catheterized patient will present with a colony count of $10^3$ CFU/mL or higher in culture. However, because the risk for the acquisition of bacteriuria in a catheterized patient is cumulative, at 7% per day, many patients with extended ICU stays will have bacteriuria. Similarly, low colony counts of 1,000 CFU/mL will increase to 100,000 CFU/mL-within 48 hours.[33,34] Neither a high pathogen count nor pyuria is evidence that UTI is the source of fever, and UTI accounts for the minority of fevers identified in the ICU.

In a patient with an indwelling urethral or suprapubic catheter or in a patient undergoing intermittent catheterization, a catheter-acquired UTI can be diagnosed if[1] signs or symptoms of UTI exist with no other identifiable source and if two colony counts of a bacterial species of $10^3$ CFU/mL are present in a single catheter urine sample or in a midstream voided urine sample if the patient has been decatheterized in the last 48 hours. If no clinical signs or symptoms of UTI exist but colony counts of a single bacterial species of more than $10^5$ CFU/mL are found on urine culture in such a patient, a diagnosis of catheter-acquired asymptomatic bacteriuria is appropriate.

## Catheter Management

The overarching goal of catheter management is to reduce the frequency of catheterization. Indwelling catheters should be placed only when they are absolutely indicated. Catheters are not indicated for urinary incontinence except when all other approaches have been ineffective and the patient requests catheter placement. If an indwelling catheter has been in place when UTI symptoms develop and the catheter is still indicated, replacing the catheter may hasten recovery from the infection and reduce the risk for future catheter-acquired bacteriuria or catheter-acquired UTI.

Intermittent catheterization can always be considered as a potential alternative to short- or long-term indwelling catheterization. Silver alloy or antimicrobial-coated urinary catheters may be considered because they delay the onset of bacteriuria, but the data are insufficient to recommend such devices for routine use.

Systemic antimicrobial pharmacotherapy should not be administered routinely for prophylaxis in patients with indwelling catheters, even those undergoing surgical procedures. The risk of selecting for pathogens with antimicrobial resistance is substantial.

Hospitals, long-term care facilities, and associated institutions play an important role in promoting the judicious and responsible use of urinary catheters. Specifically, institutions should provide a list of indications for indwelling catheters and educate their staff on those indications. Regular assessment of staff adherence to evidence-based policies on catheterization is important. Portable bladder scanners can be very useful in determining if catheterization is necessary for postoperative patients. Urinary catheters should be removed as soon as they are no longer indicated, and nurse- or physician-based electronic reminder systems or automatic stop orders may be effective in reducing inappropriate prolonged catheterization.

The use and management of bladder catheterization are complicated, ever changing, and plagued by uncertainty; interested readers are encouraged to refer to Hooton et al[1] for more details on this topic.

## Treatment

The treatment of UTI is guided by a recent, fresh urine sample from a newly placed urinary catheter or a straight catheterization. Patients whose catheter has been recently discontinued may have a urinalysis and culture of a voided midstream urine sample to determine if they are infected antimicrobial pharmacotherapy is determined and initiated. Pyuria, foul odor, and cloudy urine are not indications for antimicrobial treatment in those who are asymptomatic[1] (see **Table 19.9**). However, in neurologically impaired patients, this distinction may be difficult to determine.

In patients with established catheter-acquired UTI who exhibit prompt resolution of symptoms after initiation of antimicrobial pharmacotherapy, 7 days of treatment is recommended.[1] In those patients with a delayed therapeutic response, 10 to 14 days of treatment is recommended.[1] These recommendations stand irrespective of whether the patient remains catheterized. Pharmacotherapy should be selected based on the laboratory findings to limit the antimicrobial spectrum for treatment. If empiric treatment is required, the pharmacotherapy should be selected based on Gram stain results, previous culture results (if available), and the local epidemiology.

Older patients who develop a catheter-acquired UTI without pyelonephritis after an indwelling catheter has been removed may be treated with a 3-day course of antibiotics.[1] In addition, women with catheter-acquired asymptomatic bacteriuria that persists for more than 48 hours after the removal of a short-term indwelling catheter may be considered candidates for antimicrobial pharmacotherapy to reduce the risk for developing a future catheter-acquired UTI.

## Suspected Gastrointestinal Infection

Any patient with fever or leukocytosis and diarrhea who received antibacterial treatment or chemotherapy within the 60 days preceding the onset of symptoms should undergo an assessment for gastrointestinal infection, especially gastrointestinal infection due to *Clostridium difficile*.[2,3,35] Diarrhea is defined as stool that fits the shape of its container, but patients should have two or more unformed stools per day before being considered for testing for *C. difficile* infec-

tion. There are many noninfectious causes of hospital-based diarrhea, such as tube feedings. The antibiotics most frequently associated with *C. difficile* diarrhea are clindamycin, cephalosporins, and fluoroquinolones; however, any antibacterial agent may be the instigating factor for illness.

## Assessment

In the setting of a suspected gastrointestinal infection, a stool sample should be collected for laboratory assessment. These samples should be diarrheal or an unformed stool, except in the case of suspected ileus secondary to *C. difficile*. Assays available include enzyme-linked immunosorbent assay (ELISA) screening for toxin A and B, tissue culture, and polymerase chain reaction (PCR)–based technology.[2] Tissue culture assay is the most sensitive and considered the clinical gold standard test but is not performed at most medical centers. If the ELISA screen is negative, a repeat ELISA should be automatically conducted if the level of clinical suspicion of disease is high. Studies suggest that PCR testing is faster, more sensitive, and more specific than other current methods.[2]

If severe illness is present and results of tests to confirm *C. difficile* infection are negative, inconclusive, or not available, a flexible sigmoidoscopy study is a reasonable next diagnostic alternative. Empiric treatment with oral vancomycin can be considered while diagnostic results are awaited and should be initiated as soon as the diagnosis is suspected or if the infection is severe or complicated. Warning signs of severe infection include a serum lactate level at or above 5 mmol/L and leukocytosis with a cell count above 50,000/ μL.[2] These signs should prompt careful consideration for subtotal colectomy with preservation of the rectum. Early suspicion and early testing should avoid the need for surgical intervention.

Patients who did not present to the hospital with diarrhea and who are immunocompetent rarely require stool cultures for other enteric pathogens (e.g., ova and parasites). Cultures for other pathogens should be ordered only if clinically indicated and epidemiologically appropriate, such as in the case of an immunocompromised host.

Testing for cure of *C. difficile* infection is not recommended, nor is testing in asymptomatic patients. In general, repeat laboratory testing of stool samples should be avoided.

## Treatment

Oral metronidazole is the first line of treatment for mild disease. Patients with moderate to severe disease or a complicated clinical status should receive oral vancomycin. Oral fidaxomicin has recently become available for the treatment of *C. difficile* infection but has not been shown to be superior to vancomycin for acute treatment, and the tablets cannot be crushed and placed in gastrostomy tubes for administration.[36] In general, empiric treatment is not recommended unless moderate to severe disease is present. Treatment will not affect ELISA or PCR laboratory testing. Pharmacotherapy for a laboratory-confirmed, clinically severe, or complicated infection is described in **Table 19.10**.[2] The first recurrence after treatment should be treated with the same regimen as the initial episode but stratified according to disease severity as indicated in **Table 19.10**. Second or third recurrences of infection should be treated with a tapered or pulse regimen of vancomycin. Of note, it is important to avoid the use of metronidazole beyond the first recurrence because the cumulative dose may increase the risk for neurotoxicity. Antiperistaltic agents are not indicated and may actually mask other symptoms or even trigger toxic megacolon.[2]

Minimizing the frequency, duration, and intensity of concomitant antimicrobial pharmacotherapy, in addition to reducing the number of agents used, is important in decreasing the risk for *C. difficile* infections and recurrences. In patients requiring continued antimicrobial therapy for an independent infection, no strong evidence-based recommendations currently exist for the prevention of recurrent *C. difficile* infection. However, expert opinion suggests that metronidazole or vancomycin may be continued for 7 days after the duration of

**Table 19.10** Pharmacotherapy of *Clostridium difficile* infection[2]

| Discontinue inciting/nonessential antimicrobial agents. |
| --- |
| Antiperistaltic agents are not indicated. |
| Initial episode mild to moderate: |
| • Metronidazole, 500 mg orally 3 times per day for 10–14 days |
| Initial episode moderate to severe: |
| • Vancomycin, 125 mg orally 4 times per day for 10–14 days |
| Severe, complicated: |
| • Vancomycin, 500 mg orally 4 times per day |
| • Vancomycin, 500 mg in 100 mL of normal saline per rectum every 6 hours |
| • Metronidazole, 500-mg intravenous bolus every 8 hours |

administration.[16] No evidence exists suggesting that the use of probiotics reduces risk in hospitalized patients, and they may actually increase the risk for bloodstream infections in immunocompromised hosts.

## Special Conditions

*C. difficile* infection is a serious epidemiologic problem in the neurologic ICU, and enhanced contact and isolation precautions should be implemented. Health care workers and neurologic ICU visitors must use gloves and gowns upon entry into the room of a patient with *C. difficile* infection, and soap and water should be used for hand washing because alcohol-based hand gels do not effectively kill spores. Judicious antimicrobial selection is of key importance. Antimicrobials should be chosen that target the pathogens identified, and their selection should be based on the local epidemiology. Cephalosporin, clindamycin, and fluoroquinolone use in particular should be limited where possible.

## Suspected Sinusitis

The assessment of suspected sinusitis in the neurologic ICU does not differ substantially from that performed outside the neurologic ICU. Nevertheless, it is important for clinicians to be aware of the risk for sinusitis in patients with a fever of unknown origin, particularly those patients with nasotracheal or orotracheal intubation.[37,38] The use of nasogastric tubes for extended time periods should be avoided to reduce the risk for nosocomial sinusitis. If the clinical evaluation demonstrates that a fever is present and sinusitis is suspected as the cause, computed tomography (CT) of the facial sinuses is recommended.[3] Minor CT abnormalities of the sinuses are not uncommon, and these abnormalities should be carefully scrutinized before the diagnosis of sinusitis is made. Empiric treatment for sinusitis can be initiated based on the relative time course of the patient's admission to the hospital and whether the patient has received any prior antibiotic therapy. If the patient does not respond to antibiotic treatment, puncture and aspiration of the involved sinuses under aseptic conditions should be considered. Gram stain and culture of the aspirate can be performed to determine both the causative agent and the antimicrobial susceptibility of that agent. Sphenoid sinusitis usually requires more aggressive medical and sometimes surgical treatment.

## Induced Normothermia

The best evidence available suggests that induced normothermia in the setting of neurologic injury is beneficial.[8,9] When compared with normothermia, hyperthermia has been associated with worse neurologic outcomes in both stroke and brain injury patients, and induced hypothermia is associated with numerous morbidities despite its effectiveness in neuroprotection in several experimental models.

Pharmacologic means to avoid pyrexia include acetaminophen, aspirin, and other nonsteroidal antiinflammatory drugs. Corticosteroids, although effective in fever reduction, are not clinically recommended because of their potential adverse effects. All of these antipyretic agents require intact thermoregulatory mechanisms. Antipyretics are more likely to be ineffective if neurologic injury has resulted in impaired thermoregulation, as is often the case in the neurologic ICU. In stroke patients, oral antipyretics have been shown to be only marginally effective, and nonpharmacologic measures are actually more effective.[39]

Pyrexia refractory to pharmacologic measures requires cooling, either externally or internally. Effective external cooling should take advantage of the four modes of heat loss: evaporation (e.g., sponge baths), conduction (e.g., ice packs), convection (e.g., cooling blanket), and radiation (e.g., skin exposure). Internal cooling can be effected with a cold saline infusion centrally. Nonpharmacologic cooling will reduce body temperature below the physiologic set point, which may induce thermogenesis in the form of shivering. Medications such as meperidine, dantrolene, propofol, dexmedetomidine, and paralytics may be useful adjuncts to help control shivering.

Infection can be difficult to detect when fever, a cardinal clinical sign, is suppressed. Unfortunately, no standards have been established for infection surveillance. Monitoring the patient with daily white blood cell counts or chest radiographs, an occasional urinalysis, and blood cultures for an abruptly or steadily increasing white cell count seems reasonable, but there are no evidence-based data to support these practices at this time.

## ■ Conclusion

Guidelines have been established for the diagnosis and management of certain infectious diseases, and these guidelines may prove useful in the neurosurgical critical care unit. However, there are also limitations described in the literature and occasional controversy. This chapter provides a review of the current literature and highlights key tenets of infection diagnosis and treatment strategies. It is imperative that the clinician consider the circumstances surrounding the patient's illness and the pathway needed to optimize care, using the current evidence where applicable.

## References

1. Hooton TM, Bradley SF, Cardenas DD, et al; Infectious Diseases Society of America. Diagnosis, prevention, and treatment of catheter-associated urinary tract infection in adults: 2009 International Clinical Practice Guidelines from the Infectious Diseases Society of America. Clin Infect Dis 2010;50(5):625–663

2. Cohen SH, Gerding DN, Johnson S, et al; Society for Healthcare Epidemiology of America; Infectious Diseases Society of America. Clinical practice guidelines for *Clostridium difficile* infection in adults: 2010 update by the Society for Healthcare Epidemiology of America (SHEA) and the Infectious Diseases Society of America (IDSA). Infect Control Hosp Epidemiol 2010;31(5):431–455

3. O'Grady NP, Barie PS, Bartlett JG, et al; American College of Critical Care Medicine; Infectious Diseases Society of America. Guidelines for evaluation of new fever in critically ill adult patients: 2008 update from the American College of Critical Care Medicine and the Infectious Diseases Society of America. Crit Care Med 2008;36(4): 1330–1349

4. Niederman MS, Craven DE, Bonten MJ, et al; American Thoracic Society; Infectious Diseases Society of America. Guidelines for the management of adults with hospital-acquired, ventilator-associated, and healthcare-associated pneumonia. Am J Respir Crit Care Med 2005; 171(4):388–416

5. Mandell LA, Wunderink RG, Anzueto A, et al; Infectious Diseases Society of America; American Thoracic Society. Infectious Diseases Society of America/American Thoracic Society consensus guidelines on the management of community-acquired pneumonia in adults. Clin Infect Dis 2007;44(Suppl 2):S27–S72

6. Mermel LA, Allon M, Bouza E, et al. Clinical practice guidelines for the diagnosis and management of intravascular catheter-related infection: 2009 update by the Infectious Diseases Society of America. Clin Infect Dis 2009;49(1):1–45

7. Tunkel AR, Hartman BJ, Kaplan SL, et al. Practice guidelines for the management of bacterial meningitis. Clin Infect Dis 2004;39(9):1267–1284

8. Linares G, Mayer SA. Hypothermia for the treatment of ischemic and hemorrhagic stroke. Crit Care Med 2009;37(7, Suppl):S243–S249

9. Badjatia N. Hyperthermia and fever control in brain injury. Crit Care Med 2009;37(7, Suppl): S250–S257

10. Krieger DW, De Georgia MA, Abou-Chebl A, et al. Cooling for acute ischemic brain damage (cool aid): an open pilot study of induced hypothermia in acute ischemic stroke. Stroke 2001;32(8): 1847–1854

11. Dimopoulos G, Falagas ME. Approach to the febrile patient in the ICU. Infect Dis Clin North Am 2009;23(3):471–484

12. Riedel S, Carroll KC. Blood cultures: key elements for best practices and future directions. J Infect Chemother 2010;16(5):301–316

13. Safdar N, Maki DG. Inflammation at the insertion site is not predictive of catheter-related bloodstream infection with short-term, non-cuffed central venous catheters. Crit Care Med 2002;30(12):2632–2635

14. Sakushima K, Hayashino Y, Kawaguchi T, Jackson JL, Fukuhara S. Diagnostic accuracy of cerebrospinal fluid lactate for differentiating bacterial meningitis from aseptic meningitis: a meta-analysis. J Infect 2011;62(4):255–262

15. Srinivas D, Veena Kumari HB, Somanna S, Bhagavatula I, Anandappa CB. The incidence of postoperative meningitis in neurosurgery: an institutional experience. Neurol India 2011;59(2): 195–198

16. Lietard C, Thébaud V, Besson G, Lejeune B. Risk factors for neurosurgical site infections: an 18-month prospective survey. J Neurosurg 2008; 109(4):729–734

17. Dashti SR, Baharvahdat H, Spetzler RF, et al. Operative intracranial infection following craniotomy. Neurosurg Focus 2008;24(6):E10

18. McClelland S III, Hall WA. Postoperative central nervous system infection: incidence and associated factors in 2111 neurosurgical procedures. Clin Infect Dis 2007;45(1):55–59

19. Barker FG II. Efficacy of prophylactic antibiotics against meningitis after craniotomy: a meta-analysis. Neurosurgery 2007;60(5):887–894, discussion 887–894

20. Zarrouk V, Vassor I, Bert F, et al. Evaluation of the management of postoperative aseptic meningitis. Clin Infect Dis 2007;44(12):1555–1559

21. Leib SL, Boscacci R, Gratzl O, Zimmerli W. Predictive value of cerebrospinal fluid (CSF) lactate level versus CSF/blood glucose ratio for the diagnosis of bacterial meningitis following neurosurgery. Clin Infect Dis 1999;29(1):69–74

22. Honda H, Jones JC, Craighead MC, Diringer MN, Dacey RG, Warren DK. Reducing the incidence of intraventricular catheter-related ventriculitis in the neurology-neurosurgical intensive care unit at a tertiary care center in St Louis, Missouri: an 8-year follow-up study. Infect Control Hosp Epidemiol 2010;31(10):1078–1081

23. Wong GK, Ip M, Poon WS, Mak CW, Ng RY. Antibiotics-impregnated ventricular catheter versus systemic antibiotics for prevention of nosocomial CSF and non-CSF infections: a prospective randomised clinical trial. J Neurol Neurosurg Psychiatry 2010;81(10):1064–1067

24. Lozier AP, Sciacca RR, Romagnoli MF, Connolly ES Jr. Ventriculostomy-related infections: a critical review of the literature. Neurosurgery 2008;62(Suppl 2):688–700

25. Friedman WA, Vries JK. Percutaneous tunnel ventriculostomy. Summary of 100 procedures. J Neurosurg 1980;53(5):662–665

26. Wong GK, Poon WS, Wai S, Yu LM, Lyon D, Lam JM. Failure of regular external ventricular drain

exchange to reduce cerebrospinal fluid infection: result of a randomised controlled trial. J Neurol Neurosurg Psychiatry 2002;73(6):759–761

27. Scheithauer S, Bürgel U, Bickenbach J, et al. External ventricular and lumbar drainage-associated meningoventriculitis: prospective analysis of time-dependent infection rates and risk factor analysis. Infection 2010;38(3):205–209

28. Lo CH, Spelman D, Bailey M, Cooper DJ, Rosenfeld JV, Brecknell JE. External ventricular drain infections are independent of drain duration: an argument against elective revision. J Neurosurg 2007;106(3):378–383

29. Beer R, Pfausler B, Schmutzhard E. Management of nosocomial external ventricular drain-related ventriculomeningitis. Neurocrit Care 2009;10(3):363–367

30. Leung GK, Ng KB, Taw BB, Fan YW. Extended subcutaneous tunnelling technique for external ventricular drainage. Br J Neurosurg 2007; 21(4):359–364

31. Raghavendran K, Nemzek J, Napolitano LM, Knight PR. Aspiration-induced lung injury. Crit Care Med 2011;39(4):818–826

32. Tambyah PA, Maki DG. The relationship between pyuria and infection in patients with indwelling urinary catheters: a prospective study of 761 patients. Arch Intern Med 2000;160(5):673–677

33. Stark RP, Maki DG. Bacteriuria in the catheterized patient. What quantitative level of bacteriuria is relevant? N Engl J Med 1984;311(9):560–564

34. Maki DG, Tambyah PA. Engineering out the risk for infection with urinary catheters. Emerg Infect Dis 2001;7(2):342–347

35. Fekety R. Guidelines for the diagnosis and management of *Clostridium difficile*-associated diarrhea and colitis. American College of Gastroenterology, Practice Parameters Committee. Am J Gastroenterol 1997;92(5):739–750

36. Louie TJ, Miller MA, Mullane KM, et al; OPT-80-003 Clinical Study Group. Fidaxomicin versus vancomycin for *Clostridium difficile* infection. N Engl J Med 2011;364(5):422–431

37. Holzapfel L, Chevret S, Madinier G, et al. Influence of long-term oro- or nasotracheal intubation on nosocomial maxillary sinusitis and pneumonia: results of a prospective, randomized, clinical trial. Crit Care Med 1993;21(8):1132–1138

38. van Zanten AR, Dixon JM, Nipshagen MD, de Bree R, Girbes AR, Polderman KH. Hospital-acquired sinusitis is a common cause of fever of unknown origin in orotracheally intubated critically ill patients. Crit Care 2005;9(5):R583–R590

39. Wrotek SE, Kozak WE, Hess DC, Fagan SC. Treatment of fever after stroke: conflicting evidence. Pharmacotherapy 2011;31(11):1085–1091

# Index

*Note:* Page numbers followed by *f* and *t* indicate figures and tables, respectively.

prevention of, 62*t*, 63
treatment of, 62*t*
encephalitis, seasonal distribution of, 51
Arterial thrombosis, in cysticercosis, 82
Arteriovenous malformation, pulmonary,
hereditary hemorrhagic
telangiectasia and, 96, 97*f*
Aspergillosis, 24–25. *See also Aspergillus*
spp.; *Aspergillus flavus; Aspergillus*
*fumigatus*
CNS involvement in, 70–71
diagnostic tests for, 152
disseminated, 70–71
histology of, 77
in HIV-infected (AIDS) patients, 249–250
in HSCT recipients, 264
imaging of, 42, 45*f*, 75–76, 76*f*
in immunocompromised patients, 249–250
intralesional hemorrhage in, 42, 45*f*
laboratory investigation of, 75
prognosis for, 79
risk factors for, 71
spinal epidural abscess in, 173
treatment of, 78, 250
surgical, 77
vertebral column infection, antibiotic
treatment of, 158
vertebral osteomyelitis in, 149
*Aspergillus* spp. *See also* Aspergillosis
blood vessel wall invasion, 71, 71*f*
brain abscess, 26*t*, 68, 74
hyphae of, 68, 68*f*, 71*f*, 77
laboratory identification of, 75
meningitis, 68
in organ transplant recipients, 264–265
*Aspergillus flavus,* 71
*Aspergillus fumigatus,* 71, 71*f*. *See also*
Aspergillosis
in infectious intracranial aneurysms, 138,
138*f*
sinusitis, 137*f*
Asplenia, and meningitis, 113
Astrocytoma(s), T cells in, 7
Ataxia, in schistosomiasis, 88
ATM. *See* Acute transverse myelitis
Autoimmune disease(s), of central nervous
system, 3
Azithromycin, 32*t*

**B**
Back pain
chronic, with vertebral column infection, 159
in schistosomiasis, 88
with spinal epidural abscess, 166

with spinal subdural abscess, 176–177
with vertebral column infection, 150
Bacterial infection(s). *See* Abscess(es), brain,
bacterial; Meningitis, bacterial;
*specific bacteria*
*Bacteroides* spp.
brain abscess, 26*t*, 95, 96*f*
cranial epidural abscess, 128*t*
subdural empyema, 127*t*
Bactiseal, 33
*Balamuthia* spp., 89, 91
diagnostic tests for, 24
*Balamuthia mandrillaris,* 89–90
*Bartonella henselae,* diagnostic tests for, 152
Basilar leptomeningitis
in coccidioidomycosis, 70
in histoplasmosis, 70
treatment of, 77
Batson plexus, 149
BBB. *See* Blood–brain barrier
Behavioral change, with infectious
intracranial aneurysms, 139, 139*t*
Bilharziasis. *See also* Schistosomiasis
spinal epidural abscess in, 174
Biofilm, and shunt infection, 210
Biopsy. *See also* Brain biopsy
in amebiasis, 90
with brain abscess, 77
CT-guided
of spinal epidural abscess, 168
in vertebral column infection, 152
in cysticercosis, 82
open
of spinal epidural abscess, 168
in vertebral column infection, 152
percutaneous, of spinal epidural abscess,
168
rectal, in schistosomiasis, 88
*Bipolaris hawaiiensis,* 73
*Bipolaris spicifera,* 73
*Blastomyces dermatitidis. See also*
Blastomycosis
geographic distribution of, 69, 147
Blastomycosis. *See also Blastomyces*
*dermatitidis;* Chromoblastomycosis
brain abscess in, 74
diagnosis of, 73, 74
geographic distribution of, 69, 147
imaging of, 75
in immunocompromised patients, 252
meningitis in, 74
diagnostic tests for, 23*t*
risk factors for, 23*t*
spinal epidural abscess in, 173–174

Index

Index

Index

**313**

Index